Review Questions & Answers For Veterinary Boards

Small Animal Medicine & Surgery

Edited by

Paul W. Pratt, VMD

Production Manager:
Elisabeth S. Stein

American Veterinary Publications, Inc.
5782 Thornwood Drive
Goleta, CA 93117

This book is for review purposes only. The publisher and authors make no warrant as to results for readers using this book in preparing for scholastic, licensure or certification examinations. While every effort has been made to ensure the accuracy of the information contained herein, the publisher and authors are not legally responsible for errors or omissions. Drug selection, drug dosages, diagnostic methods and treatment methods mentioned in this book are in accord with those in use at the time of publication. However, readers should consult drug package inserts and current veterinary texts and journals for current diagnostic and therapeutic recommendations.

Library of Congress Card Number: 93-70149

ISBN 0-939674-41-6

Printed in the United States of America

Authors

Introduction

Dean C. Frey, DVM
Animal Clinic, 1823 16th Avenue SW, Cedar Rapids, IA 52404

Anesthesiology

Hui-Chu Lin, DVM, MS
Assistant Professor, Large Animal Surgery and Medicine, College of
Veterinary Medicine, Auburn University, Auburn, AL 36849

John C. Thurmon, DVM, MS, Dipl ACVA
Professor, Chief of Anesthesiology, Department of Veterinary Clinical
Medicine, College of Veterinary Medicine, University Illinois,
Urbana, IL 61801

Cardiology

N. Sydney Moise, DVM, MS, Dipl ACVIM
9748 Arden Road, Trumansburg, NY 14886

**Clinical
Pathology**

Barry T. Mitzner, DVM
President, Southeast Vetlab, 18131 SW 98th Court, Miami, FL 33157

Dentistry

Robert B. Wiggs, DVM, Dipl AVDC
Director, Dallas Dental Service Animal Clinic, 12600 Coit Road,
Dallas, TX 75251

Dermatology

Karen A. Moriello, DVM, Dipl ACVD
Associate Professor, Department of Medical Sciences, College of
Veterinary Medicine, University of Wisconsin, Madison, WI 53706

Hematology

Susan M. Cotter, DVM, Dipl ACVIM
Professor, Department of Medicine, School of Veterinary Medicine,
Tufts University, North Grafton, MA 01536

W. Jean Dodds, DVM
President, HEMOPET, 938 Stanford Street, Santa Monica, CA 90403

Medical Diseases

Sharon K. Fooshee, DVM, MS
Animal Health Center of Franklin, 400 Eddy Lane,
Franklin, TN 37064

Dennis W. Macy, DVM, MS, Dipl ACVIM
Professor, Department of Biomedical Sciences, College of Veterinary
Medicine, Colorado State University, Fort Collins, CO 80523

Fred W. Scott, DVM, PhD, Dipl ACVM
Professor, Director of Cornell Feline Health Center, Department of
Microbiology, Immunology and Parasitology, College of Veterinary
Medicine, Cornell University, Ithaca, NY 14853

Robert G. Sherding, DVM, Dipl ACVIM
Professor, Head of Small Animal Medicine, Department of Veterinary
Clinical Sciences, College of Veterinary Medicine,
Ohio State University, Columbus, OH 43210

Continued

Carrie B. Waters, DVM
Resident, Department of Veterinary Clinical Sciences, School of
Veterinary Medicine, Purdue University, West Lafayette, IN 47907

Michael D. Willard, DVM, MS, Dipl ACVIM
Professor, Department of Small Animal Medicine and Surgery, College of
Veterinary Medicine, Texas A&M University, College Station, TX 77845

Neurology   Joe N. Kornegay, DVM, PhD, Dipl ACVIM
Professor, Department of Companion Animal and Special Species Medicine,
College of Veterinary Medicine, North Carolina State University,
Raleigh, NC 27606

Oncology   Susan M. Cotter, DVM, Dipl ACVIM
Professor, Department of Medicine, School of Veterinary Medicine,
Tufts University, North Grafton, MA 01536

Evan T. Keller, DVM, MPVM
Resident, Department of Medical Sciences, School of Veterinary Medicine,
University of Wisconsin, Madison, WI 53706

Ophthalmology   Dennis E. Brooks, DVM, PhD, Dipl ACVO
Associate Professor, Ophthalmology Service Chief, Department of Small
Animal Clinical Sciences, College of Veterinary Medicine,
University of Florida, Gainesville, FL 32610

Pharmacology   Sue Hudson Duran, RPh, MS
Assistant Professor, Director of Pharmacy, Department of Large Animal
Surgery and Medicine, Auburn University, Auburn, AL 36849

Preventive Medicine   Paul C. Bartlett, DVM, PhD, MPH, Dipl ACVPM
Associate Professor, Department of Large Animal Clinical Sciences,
College of Veterinary Medicine, Michigan State University,
East Lansing, MI 48823

Craig Nash Carter, DVM, MS, PhD, Dipl ACVPM
Adjunct Professor, Head of Epidemiology and Informatics, Department of
Veterinary Public Health, College of Veterinary Medicine,
Texas A&M University, POD 3040, College Station, TX 77841

Johnny D. Hoskins, DVM, PhD, Dipl ACVIM
Professor, Department of Veterinary Clinical Sciences, School of
Veterinary Medicine, Louisiana State University, Baton Rouge, LA 70803

**Principles of
Surgery**   Thomas P. Colville, DVM, MS
Director of Veterinary Technology Program, Department of Veterinary and
Microbiological Sciences, North Dakota State University, Fargo, ND 58105

Surgical Diseases   Ronald M. Bright, DVM, MS, Dipl ACVS
Professor, Director of Surgical Services, Department of Urban Practice,
College of Veterinary Medicine, POB 1071, University of Tennessee,
Knoxville, TN 37901

Philip A. Bushby, DVM, MS, Dipl ACVS
Professor, Academic Program Director, College of Veterinary Medicine,
Mississippi State University, Mississippi State, MS 39762

Continued

Joseph Harari, DVM, MS, Dipl ACVS
Assistant Professor, Department of Veterinary Clinical Medicine and
Surgery, College of Veterinary Medicine, Washington State University,
Pullman, WA 99164

James K. Roush, DVM, MS, Dipl ACVS
Assistant Professor, Department of Clinical Sciences, College of
Veterinary Medicine, Kansas State University, Manhattan, KS 66506

Theriogenology   Steven D. Van Camp, DVM, Dipl ACT
Associate Professor, Department of Food Animal and Equine Medicine,
College of Veterinary Medicine, North Carolina State University,
Raleigh, NC 27606

Carrie B. Waters, DVM
Resident, Department of Veterinary Clinical Sciences, School of
Veterinary Medicine, Purdue University, West Lafayette, IN 47907

Urology/Nephrology   Kenneth C. Bovée, DVM, MS
Bower Professor, Department of Medicine, School of Veterinary Medicine,
University of Pennsylvania, Philadelphia, PA 19104

Preface

This series of review books was developed to help candidates prepare for scholastic, licensure and certification examinations. While the books are not definitive texts, they can help candidates organize their preparations, and detect areas in which more study is required.

Time and again while editing the thousands of questions, I found myself saying, "I wish I had these books when I was in veterinary school, and studying for Boards."

I am indebted to our group of 112 contributors, who have taken the time from their busy professional and personal lives to carefully craft questions on their respective subject areas. Their enthusiasm and ingenuity in developing challenging questions are evident throughout the 5 volumes. While I had considered myself fairly well read in our field, I was humbled by the depth and breadth of knowledge illustrated in their questions.

This series contains over 9,400 questions, with accompanying answers. We have gone to great effort to root out all errors and ambiguous statements. Despite these precautions, however, a number of flaws undoubtedly have escaped notice.

We would be grateful if readers would notify us of any errors, ambiguities or questionable statements in these books. We also encourage readers to send their comments/criticism on any aspect of the books. In this way we can improve the quality of future editions. For your convenience, a postage-paid Comments form is included at the back of each book.

Paul W. Pratt, VMD
Editor and Publisher

Contents

Continued

Introduction

D.C. Frey

State and national board examinations have long been surrounded with an air of mystery, misunderstanding and anxiety. *Review Questions & Answers For Veterinary Boards*, a series of 5 volumes, was written to alleviate much of this confusion.

These volumes are not textbooks, nor are they meant to supplant textbooks. Rather, they are guides designed to help readers review, in convenient form, current information on the various subject areas within the scope of a veterinarian's duties.

Who Should Use These Books?

Veterinary Students: Veterinary students can use *Review Questions & Answers For Veterinary Boards* as a review in preparing for final examinations, as each course is concluded.

New Graduates: Graduates can use these books at the conclusion of their veterinary education in preparing for the National Board Examination, and in preparing for licensure examinations required by many states and provinces (see the following section on Licensing of Veterinarians).

Practicing Veterinarians: Veterinarians now working in practice will find these books useful in continuing education. Graduates re-entering the profession will find them helpful in updating their knowledge on various topics. Licensed veterinarians moving to a new locale can use the books to prepare for the licensing examination in their new state or province. The books are also useful in preparing for the American Board of Veterinary Practitioners examination.

Foreign Graduates: Graduates of non-accredited foreign veterinary colleges can use these books in preparing for Education Commission for Foreign Veterinary Graduates (ECFVG) certification.

What Is Covered In These Books?

Review Questions & Answers For Veterinary Boards is a series of 5 volumes covering nearly every aspect of veterinary medicine. The series includes volumes on *Basic Sciences, Clinical Sciences, Small Animal Medicine and Surgery, Large Animal Medicine and Surgery,* and *Ancillary Topics.*

These 5 books contain more than 9,400 questions, divided into the following subject areas:

Anesthesiology: This section covers equipment, techniques and agents used to anesthetize animals. Included are questions on sedation, tranquilization, and general, local and spinal anesthesia.

Behavior: Questions on normal and abnormal behavior of domestic species are included in this section.

Biochemistry: This section contains questions relating to biochemical reactions involved in metabolic processes in animals.

Cage/Aviary Bird Medicine: These questions relate to diseases and husbandry of cage/aviary birds.

Cardiology: These questions concern diagnosis and management of heart disorders.

Clinical Pathology: This section covers all aspects of laboratory diagnosis.

Cytology: This section includes questions on cytologic evaluation of various types of specimens.

Dentistry: This section includes questions on dental anatomy, terminology, periodontal disease, prophylaxis, floating, extraction, endodontics, orthodontics and other dental procedures.

Dermatology: These questions concern skin disease.

Diagnostic Imaging and Recordings: Questions in this section relate to equipment and techniques used in radiography, ultrasonography, endoscopy, electrocardiography, electroencephalography and electromyography.

Diseases of Aquarium Fish: These questions relate to care of freshwater and saltwater aquarium fish.

Embryology: These questions relate to embryonic development of mammals and birds.

Epidemiology: These questions relate to the dynamics of disease in animal populations.

Ethics, Jurisprudence and Animal Welfare: Ethical, legal and animal welfare issues in veterinary medicine are explored in this section.

Gross Anatomy: These questions relate to gross anatomy of all body tissues. Species covered include small animals (dogs, cats), monogastric ungulates (horses, pigs), ruminants (cattle, sheep, goats), and avian/exotics (birds, reptiles).

Hematology: This section includes questions on hematopoiesis, blood and bone marrow cell morphology and coagulation.

Immunology: This section includes questions on immune system structure, function and disorders.

Laboratory Animal Medicine: These questions relate to diseases and husbandry of common laboratory species.

Medical Diseases: These sections contain questions on diagnosis and nonsurgical management of infectious and noninfectious diseases in small and large animals. Disciplines include cardiology, dermatology, neurology, oncology, ophthalmology and urology. Questions cover history taking, physical examination, diagnostic techniques, medical care, followup care and emergency care.

Microbiology: These questions relate to morphology, physiology, culture and identification of bacteria, fungi and viruses of veterinary importance.

Microscopic Anatomy: These questions relate to microscopic anatomy of all body tissues, including blood cells, bone marrow cells and spermatozoa.

Necropsy: Included are questions on techniques used in necropsy of domestic animals.

Neuroanatomy: This section contains questions on gross and microscopic anatomy of the central and peripheral nervous systems.

Neurology: These questions relate to disorders of the central and peripheral nervous systems.

Nutrition: Nutritional requirements and feeding domestic animals are the focus of this section.

Oncology: These questions relate to types and treatment of neoplasia.

Ophthalmology: These questions concern diseases of the eye.

Parasitology: These questions relate to the life cycle, pathologic effects and identification of arthropods, protozoans and helminths of veterinary importance.

Pathology: These questions relate to pathologic processes in various body systems.

Pharmacology: These questions concern the actions of various classes of drugs, calculation of dosages and dilutions, and procedures used in the pharmacy.

Physiology: This section covers the physical and metabolic functions of the various body systems.

Poultry Medicine: These questions relate to diseases and husbandry of domestic fowl and wild waterfowl.

Practice Management: These questions relate to clinic management, practice administration and client relations.

Preventive Medicine: This section focuses on procedures used to prevent disease in domestic species, including use of biologics, anthelmintics, disinfectants and quarantine procedures.

Principles of Surgery: These questions concern wound healing and infection, antimicrobial use, hemostasis, asepsis, sterilization, instruments, suture materials, drains and dressings.

Public Health and Regulatory Medicine: This section covers zoonoses, meat and milk hygiene, and drug residues in animal tissues.

Surgical Diseases: These sections contain questions relating to surgical management of conditions involving the various body systems of small and large animals. Questions cover preoperative preparation, operative technique and postoperative care.

Terminology: This section reviews surgical, medical, anatomic and directional terms, terms used in microbiology and pharmacology, and universally accepted abbreviations.

Theriogenology: This section includes questions on reproductive physiology, function and disease in male and female animals.

Toxicology: These questions relate to toxicants of veterinary importance.

Urology/Nephrology: This section covers diseases of the urinary system.

Zoo, Exotic and Marine Animal Medicine: These questions relate to diseases and care of zoo species, companion exotic species, and marine mammals.

What Types of Questions Are Included In These Books?

The questions in these books were prepared by highly qualified authors, including veterinary educators, content-area specialists and experienced clinicians. The questions have been carefully constructed to test factual knowledge, reasoning skills and clinical judgment. They will also help pinpoint deficiencies in a candidate's studies. The questions are original, and none have been knowingly "recycled" from previous national or state licensure examinations; however, certain overlap is unavoidable and not necessarily a disadvantage.

All of the questions are multiple choice. This format was chosen because it is most commonly used in licensure examinations. Also, it is similar to the format used in the National Board Examination. Questions in these books present 5 answer choices. Each question has only 1 correct answer. There are no "trick" questions.

Multiple-choice questions offer several advantages. Many questions covering a broad range of subjects can be presented in a limited testing period. Also, multiple-choice examinations can be quickly and accurately graded (often by automated optical scanner). Finally, a candidate's answers to multiple-choice questions are not subject to differences of interpretation by the grading examiner, as in essays.

Questions are presented in several styles:

Completion: Together with the question stem, the appended answer forms a complete sentence. For example,

1. The last nucleated stage of maturing mammalian erythrocytes is the:

   a. rubricyte

   b. metarubricyte

   c. reticulocyte

   d. mature erythrocyte

   e. prorubricyte

(The correct answer is b.)

Selection: The question is presented as a complete sentence, and the reader selects the best answer. For example,

2. Which stage of maturing mammalian erythrocytes is the last nucleated stage?

   a. rubricyte

   b. metarubricyte

   c. reticulocyte

   d. mature erythrocyte

   e. prorubricyte

(The correct answer is b.)

Association: Several answer choices are listed, followed by a series of questions relating to these choices. For example,

   a. prorubricyte

   b. metarubricyte

   c. reticulocyte

   d. erythrocyte

   e. rubricyte

3. The final stage of erythrocyte maturation.

4. The last nucleated stage of maturing erythrocytes.

5. The first non-nucleated stage of maturing erythrocytes.

6. The earliest functional stage of maturing erythrocytes.

*7. The stage of maturing erythrocytes **least** commonly seen in peripheral blood.*

(Correct answers: 3. d, 4. b, 5. c, 6. e, 7. a)

Case History: A clinical case is described, and questions pertain to case management. For example,

Questions 8 through 11

A 3-month-old mixed-breed puppy is presented because of diarrhea and coughing. The puppy was recently obtained from an animal shelter, and has been vaccinated (DHLP) but never dewormed. The puppy has a dull haircoat and slight fever, but is well hydrated, alert and playful.

8. The most appropriate initial procedure is to:

   a. make thoracic and abdominal radiographs

   b. perform a physical examination

   c. obtain blood samples for serum chemistry assays

   d. perform an electrocardiographic examination

   e. euthanize the puppy because of probable distemper

9. You examine a fecal sample and find roundworm eggs. The most appropriate drug for deworming this puppy is:

   a. niclosamide

   b. piperazine

   c. sulfadimethoxine

   d. praziquantel

   e. fenbendazole

10. Considering this dog's history and origin, the most likely cause of the coughing is:

   a. infectious tracheobronchitis

   b. lungworm infection

   c. heartworm disease

   d. congenital heart defect

   e. tracheal collapse

11. The most reasonable course of action is to:

   a. hospitalize the puppy for elimination of adult heartworms

   b. hospitalize the puppy for angiocardiographic studies

   c. deworm the puppy and dispense antibacterials

   d. hospitalize the puppy for intravenous antibacterial and fluid therapy

   e. administer dexamethasone and dispense prednisolone

Answers

8. **b** This first step can help guide subsequent diagnostic procedures and treatments.

9. **b** None of the other drugs listed is appropriate for treating roundworm infection.

10. **a** "Kennel cough" is a common problem in commingled dogs obtained from pounds and shelters.

11. **c** This treatment should resolve these relatively minor problems.

How To Use These Books

Review Questions & Answers For Veterinary Boards was meant to be used in reviewing for final examinations or licensure examinations. Before you begin a section, review your texts and course notes pertaining to that subject area. Then, approach each section as you would an actual examination:

- *Carefully read each question.* Look for such key words as "most," "best," "least," "always," "never" and "except." Consider only the facts presented in the question, and don't make assumptions and inferences that may not be true.

- *Carefully evaluate each answer choice.* Each question has only 1 correct answer, with 4 incorrect answers or "distractors." If more than 1 answer choice appears to be correct, closely examine them for clues that would eliminate any as incorrect.

Most of the questions ask you to find a single correct answer among 4 incorrect answers. However, some questions ask you to find an *exception.* For these questions, the answer you are seeking is the single *incorrect* answer among 4 *correct* answers.

- *Select an answer* by circling the letter preceding your answer choice. If you do not wish to mark the book, use the blank answer sheets in the back of the book for practice tests.

- *Compare your answers with the correct answers.* The correct answers are listed separately at the end of each section. Many answers are accompanied by an explanation as to why a specific answer is correct or incorrect.

- *Identify your "weak" areas.* If you cannot correctly answer most of the questions in a particular subject area, it may be wise to spend extra time reviewing that subject before your actual examination. If you do not understand the rationale of why certain answers are correct or incorrect, consult the references in the Recommended Reading list at the beginning of each section.

Preparing for final examinations, licensure examinations and specialty board examinations can be an intimidating task. Faced with stacks of textbooks and lecture notes, you may find it difficult to know where to begin and how to study in an organized, productive fashion. Also, anxiety about examinations can interfere with your preparations.

We hope *Review Questions & Answers For Veterinary Boards* will assist you in preparing for examinations and in updating your knowledge on the many subject areas of veterinary medicine. Good luck in your preparations.

According to Earl Nightingale, "Luck is what happens when preparedness meets opportunity." You have always had the opportunity to succeed. With these books, you can better prepare for success.

Dean C. Frey, DVM
Cedar Rapids, Iowa

This page intentionally left blank.

Licensing of Veterinarians

D.C. Frey

History of Veterinary Licensing

During the early years of the United States, there was no organized system of veterinary education or licensing. Almost anybody could claim to be an "animal doctor" or "healer of animals."

The American Veterinary Medical Association (AVMA) directory lists 42 veterinary teaching institutions in existence during the period of 1852 to 1947. All of these were closed by 1947. The first veterinary school established at a land-grant college was at Iowa State College in 1878. In those early years, there was a great diversity in education and training in what was to become the veterinary profession.

New York was the first state to pass a law, in 1886, requiring prospective veterinary practitioners to pass an examination. In 1888, the U.S. Supreme Court ruled that a state could protect its citizens by imposing licensing conditions upon members of the medical professions.

The National Board Examination

Before 1954, all states and provinces developed their own licensing examinations. In 1954, 3 states first administered the National Board Examination in Veterinary Medicine (NBE) to 210 veterinary candidates.

The AVMA's Consultant Advisory Board and the NBE Committee work with the Professional Examination Service in developing the NBE and Clinical Competency Test. Construction of each examination is a very thorough and exacting process.

Questions are developed at item development workshops held throughout the country each year. Validation workshops and psychometric reviews are conducted until the final printing of the examination by the Professional Examination Service. The NBE is prepared by the Professional Examination Service under contract to the AVMA. It is available for purchase by state and provincial licensing boards.

A companion test, the Clinical Competency Test (CCT), was first administered in 1979. As opposed to the multiple-choice questions of the NBE, the CCT consists of 14 case management problems. Each problem presents an opening clinical scenario, and questions pertain to a sequence of steps in diagnosis and treatment of the animal's problem.

The NBE is a 400-item multiple-choice examination. The content of the NBE is based on a job analysis for entry-level veterinarians. It is administered in 2 parts of 200 questions each. Only 360 questions are used in the final scoring; the 40 questions on which candidates score lowest are deleted in final scoring.

Until December, 1992, the NBE was scored on a "norm-referenced" basis. In this system, candidates scoring 1 or 1.5 standard deviations below the mean of the "criterion population" were failed. The criterion population consisted of candidates taking the examination for the first time in the year in which they were graduating from accredited veterinary colleges.

The philosophy of norm-referenced scoring was that the public interest and the integrity of the profession were protected by failing (not licensing) the lowest-scoring candidates. With this relative-standard system, a given percentage of candidates automatically failed the NBE.

"Criterion-referenced" scoring has since replaced norm-referenced scoring of the NBE. With criterion-referenced scoring, a passing score is based on an absolute standard delineating the qualifications for licensure. All candidates have an opportunity to pass because their scores are compared to a standard, not to the scores of other candidates taking the NBE.

Currently the NBE is required for licensure in nearly every state in the United States, and in 4 Canadian provinces. The CCT is currently required for licensure in 52 states and provinces. Candidates should contact the licensing board of the state or province in which they desire licensure to obtain information on licensing requirements.

In Canada, the Canadian Veterinary Medical Association is responsible for developing examinations. The individual Canadian provinces are responsible for registering qualified veterinarians within the provincial association.

Candidates moving from one state to another can have their NBE and CCT scores reported to their new state by contacting the Interstate Reporting Service, Professional Examination Service, 475 Riverside Drive, New York, NY 10015; telephone (212) 870-3169.

United States

For the convenience of candidates seeking information on licensure, the addresses of state licensing boards follow:

Alabama

Executive Officer
Board of Veterinary Medicine
PO Box 1767
Decatur AL 35602

Alaska

Division of Occupational Licensing
Department of Commerce & Economic
    Development
PO Box D-LIC
Juneau AK 99881

Arizona

Executive Director
Veterinary Medical Examining Board
Room 410
1645 W. Jefferson
Phoenix AZ 85007

Arkansas

Executive Secretary
Arkansas Veterinary Medical Examining
    Board
1 Natural Resources Drive
Little Rock AR 72215

California

Executive Officer
Board of Examiners in Veterinary Medicine
Suite 6
1420 Howe Ave.
Sacramento CA 95825

Colorado

Colorado Veterinary Medical Examining
    Board
Suite 1310
1560 Broadway
Denver CO 80202

Connecticut

Connecticut Board of Veterinary Medicine
150 Washington St.
Hartford CT 06106

Delaware

Board of Veterinary Medicine
PO Box 1401
Dover DE 19903

District of Columbia

District of Columbia Board of Veterinary
    Examiners
Room 923
614 H St. NW
Washington DC 20001

Florida

Executive Director
Florida Board of Veterinary Medicine
1910 N. Monroe St.
Tallahassee FL 32399

Georgia

Executive Director
State Examining Boards
166 Pryor St. SW
Atlanta GA 30303

Hawaii

Executive Secretary
Board of Veterinary Examiners
Box 3469
1010 Richards St.
Honolulu HI 96801

Idaho

Board of Veterinary Medicine
PO Box 7249
Boise ID 83707

Illinois

Veterinary Licensing and Disciplinary Board
Department of Professional Regulation
320 W. Washington
Springfield IL 62786

Indiana

Board Director
Health Professions Bureau
Room 041
402 W. Washington St.
Indianapolis IN 46204

Iowa

Secretary
Iowa Board of Veterinary Medicine
2nd Floor
Wallace Building
Des Moines IA 50319

Kansas

Executive Director
Kansas Board of Veterinary Examiners
North Star Route
Lakin KS 67860

Kentucky

Kentucky Board of Veterinary Examiners
PO Box 456
Frankfort KY 40602

Louisiana

Executive Secretary
Board of Veterinary Medical Examiners
PO Box 15191
Baton Rouge LA 70895

Maine

Division of Licensing and Enforcement
Department of Professional and Financial
    Regulation
State House Station 35
Augusta ME 04333

Maryland

President
State Board of Veterinary Medical
    Examiners
50 Truman Hwy.
Annapolis MD 21401

Massachusetts

Secretary
Board of Registration in Veterinary
    Medicine
Room 1516
100 Cambridge St.
Boston MA 02202

Michigan

Licensing Administrator
Michigan State Board of Veterinary
    Medicine
Department of Commerce
PO Box 30018
Lansing MI 48909

Minnesota

Executive Director
Board of Veterinary Medicine
Room 102
2700 University Ave. West
St. Paul MN 55114

Mississippi

Executive Secretary
Mississippi Board of Veterinary Medicine
209 S. Lafayette St.
Starkville MS 39759

Missouri

Executive Director
Missouri Veterinary Medical Board
PO Box 633
Jefferson City MO 65102

Montana

Board of Veterinary Medicine
Department of Commerce
Lower Level, Arcade Building
111 N. Last Chance Gulch
Helena MT 59620

Nebraska

Director
Bureau of Examining Boards
Department of Health
PO Box 95007
Lincoln NE 68509

Nevada

Nevada State Board of Veterinary Medical
    Examiners
Suite 246
1005 Terminal Way
Reno NV 89502

New Hampshire

Secretary-Treasurer
New Hampshire Board of Veterinary
   Medicine
Caller Box 2042
Concord NH 03302

New Jersey

New Jersey State Board of Veterinary
   Medical Examiners
PO Box 45020
Newark NJ 07101

New Mexico

Executive Director
New Mexico Board of Veterinary Examiners
Suite 400-C
1650 University Blvd. NE
Albuquerque NM 87102

New York

Executive Secretary
New York State Board of Veterinary
   Medical Examiners
Room 3043
Cultural Education Center
Albany NY 12230

North Carolina

Executive Director
North Carolina Veterinary Medical Board
PO Box 12587
Raleigh NC 27605

North Dakota

North Dakota Veterinary Medical
   Examining Board
c/o Board of Animal Health
1st Floor, J Wing
600 East Blvd.
Bismarck ND 58505

Ohio

Executive Secretary
Ohio Veterinary Medical Board
16th Floor
77 S. High St.
Columbus OH 43266

Oklahoma

Executive Secretary
Board of Veterinary Medical Examiners
PO Box 18256
Oklahoma City OK 73154

Oregon

Executive Secretary
Veterinary Medical Examining Board
PO Box 231
Portland OR 97207

Pennsylvania

Chairman
Pennsylvania State Board of Veterinary
   Medicine
PO Box 2649
Harrisburg PA 17104

Rhode Island

Administrator
Division of Professional Regulation
Department of Health
Room 104
3 Capitol Hill
Providence RI 02908

South Carolina

Secretary-Treasurer
State Board of Veterinary Medical
   Examiners
PO Box 11293
Columbia SC 29211

South Dakota

Executive Secretary
State Board of Veterinary Medical
   Examiners
411 S. Fort St.
Pierre SD 57501

Tennessee

Registration Boards Administrator
Board of Veterinary Medical Examiners
283 Plus Park Blvd.
Nashville TN 37217

Texas

Executive Director
Texas State Board of Veterinary Medical
   Examiners
Suite 306
1946 South Interstate Hwy 35
Austin TX 78704

Utah

Division of Occupational and Professional
   Licensing
PO Box 45802
Salt Lake City UT 84145

Vermont
State Veterinary Board
Office of Professional Regulations
109 State St.
Montpelier VT 05609

Virginia
Virginia Board of Veterinary Medicine
1601 Rolling Hills Dr.
Richmond VA 23229

Washington
Program Manager
Veterinary Board of Governors
1300 E. Quince
Olympia WA 98504

West Virgina
Executive Secretary
Board of Veterinary Medicine
712 McCorkle Ave.
South Charleston WV 25303

Wisconsin
Bureau Director
Veterinary Examining Board
PO Box 8935
Madison WI 53708

Wyoming
Secretary-Treasurer
Wyoming Board of Veterinary Medicine
Herschler Bldg.
Cheyenne WY 82002

Canada

Candidates interested in practicing in Canadian provinces should contact those licensing boards at the following addresses:

Alberta
Secretary-Treasurer
Board of Veterinary Medical Examiners
#100
8615 149th St.
Edmonton, Alberta T5R 1B3

British Columbia
Board of Veterinary Medical Examiners
Suite 155
1200 W. 73rd Ave.
Vancouver, British Columbia V6P 6G5

Manitoba
Registrar
Veterinary Medical Board
Agricultural Services Complex
545 University Crescent
Winnipeg, Manitoba R3T 5S6

New Brunswick
Secretary-Treasurer
Board of Veterinary Medical Examiners
PO Box 1065
Moncton, New Brunswick E1C 8P2

Nova Scotia
Board of Veterinary Medical Examiners
Agricultural Centre
Kentville, Nova Scotia B4N 1J5

Ontario
Registrar
College of Veterinarians
Suite 24-25
340 Woodlawn Rd. West
Guelph, Ontario N1H 2X1

Quebec
General Director and Secretary
Board of Veterinary Medical Examiners
Suite 200
795 Avenue du Palais
St. Hyacinthe, Quebec J2S 5C6

Saskatchewan
Secretary-Treasurer
Board of Veterinary Medical Examiners
Suite 11
1025 Boychuk Dr.
Saskatoon, Saskatchewan S7H 5B2

Anesthesiology

H-C. Lin, J.C. Thurmon

Recommended Reading

Hall LW and Clarke KW: *Veterinary Anaesthesia.* 9th ed. Bailliere Tindall, London, 1992.

Haskins SC and Klide AM: Opinions in small animal anesthesia. *Vet Clin No Am* (Small Anim Pract) 22:245-502, 1992.

Lumb WV and Jones EW: *Veterinary Anesthesia.* 2nd ed. Lea & Febiger, Philadelphia, 1984.

Muir WW and Hubbell JA: *Handbook of Veterinary Anesthesia.* Mosby Year Book, St. Louis, 1989.

Short CE: *Principles and Practice of Veterinary Anesthesia.* Williams & Willkins, Baltimore, 1987.

Short CE and Poznak AV: *Animal Pain.* Churchill Livingstone, New York, 1992.

Practice answer sheet is on page 329.

Questions

1. *When using a non-rebreathing system with halothane or isoflurane, the O_2 flow rate should be:*

   a. 2.5-3 times the minute ventilation
   b. 4 times the minute ventilation
   c. 5 times the minute ventilation
   d. 6 times the minute ventilation
   e. equal to the minute ventilation

2. *Concerning the rebreathing bag on an anesthetic machine (circle system), which statement is **least** accurate?:*

   a. It acts as a reservoir bag from which the animal may breath O_2 and anesthetic gas.
   b. It can be used to manually support respiration.
   c. It allows visual assessment of the respiratory rate.
   d. It acts to trap carbon dioxide expired by the animal.
   e. It allows visual assessment of the tidal volume.

Correct answers are on pages 8-9.

3. Concerning the endotracheal tube, which statement is **least** accurate?

   a. It serves as a source of infection if not properly disinfected.
   b. If permitted to protrude excessively out of the mouth, it can extend the dead space.
   c. When inserted too deeply, it can cause bronchial cannulation, collapsing the opposite lung if anesthesia is prolonged.
   d. Inflating the cuff too tightly can restrict blood flow to the mucous membrane where the cuff contacts the trachea, resulting in ulceration.
   e. An endotracheal tube should be placed in all animals receiving injectable anesthetics.

4. Soda lime absorbs 100 ml of CO_2/g. In a 30-lb dog producing 3 ml of CO_2/lb/min, 600 g of soda lime will last about:

   a. 6 hours
   b. 11 hours
   c. 15 hours
   d. 22 hours
   e. 30 hours

5. Concerning use of oxygen in pressurized tanks, which statement is **least** accurate?

   a. The tank must be equipped with a pressure regulator to reduce the pressure so that it can be used safely in an anesthetic machine.
   b. To work effectively, most anesthetic machines must receive a gas supply at a pressure of 100 lb/square inch.
   c. A single-stage regulator permits regulation of the line pressure as gas flows to the anesthetic machine flow meters.
   d. Single-stage regulators are set to work automatically at slightly less than 50 lb/square inch.
   e. The regulator provides the safe operating pressure for the flow meter of the anesthetic machine.

6. Anesthetic vaporizers located within the breathing circuit:

   a. are designed for precision administration of anesthetics

   b. are designed for anesthetics that vaporize poorly or have low potency
   c. can be used safely with halothane
   d. cannot be used safely with methoxyflurane
   e. show the anesthetic concentration by the number located on the top of the Ohio #8 vaporizer (eg, 1=1%, 2=2%, etc)

7. Vaporizers located outside the rebreathing circuit:

   a. are designed to administer anesthetics of either low or high potency
   b. cannot be used safely with methoxyflurane
   c. permit the patient to breath through them
   d. are referred to as nonprecision vaporizers
   e. are more economical to purchase and use than those located within the circuit

8. Mistaken placement of the incorrect gas cylinder on an anesthetic machine is prevented by:

   a. color-coded identification
   b. pin-coded cylinder valve bodies
   c. the diameter-coded cylinder valve outlet
   d. the cylinder label
   e. the cylinder tag

9. What size of O_2 cylinder is attached directly to the anesthetic machine?

   a. E
   b. F
   c. G
   d. H
   e. I

10. An "H" O_2 cylinder with a pressure reading of 2200 lb/square inch is considered full at standard room temperature and pressure, and contains about:

   a. 500 L
   b. 700 L
   c. 5000 L
   d. 7000 L
   e. 70,000 L

11. *Which anesthetic machine part is used to calculate flow of gases to the anesthetic machine and patient?*

    a. flow meter
    b. regulator
    c. pressure gauge
    d. gas cylinder
    e. vaporizer

12. *An example of a precision bubble-through vaporizer located out of the breathing system in which any of the available liquid anesthetics can be used is the:*

    a. Fluotec Mark III
    b. Ohio #8
    c. Vapor
    d. Copper Kettle
    e. Stevens

13. *When using an O_2 flow meter, gas flow should be read at the:*

    a. bottom of the ball or the center of other types of indicators
    b. center of the ball or the top of other indicators
    c. bottom of the ball or the top of other indicators
    d. top of any indicator
    e. center of any indicator

14. *The numbers associated with the control lever on the top of an Ohio #8 vaporizer show:*

    a. the concentration of anesthetic in the vaporizing chamber
    b. the concentration of anesthetic exiting the vaporizer
    c. the relative percentage of anesthetic (oxygen and anesthetic gas) flowing through the vaporizing chamber
    d. the relative percentage of carbon dioxide gas flowing through the vaporizing chamber
    e. a close estimate of the anesthetic concentration being inspired by the patient

15. *Used or depleted soda lime is:*

    a. hard and bluish
    b. soft and white
    c. hard and white
    d. soft and bluish
    e. hard and pink

16. *In comparing the effects of acepromazine and xylazine,:*

    a. acepromazine causes vasoconstriction
    b. xylazine causes alpha-1 blockade
    c. acepromazine initially causes hypertension
    d. acepromazine produces profound analgesia
    e. xylazine produces profound analgesia and deep sedation

17. *In which species are opiates most likely to causes an excitatory response?*

    a. pigs and dogs
    b. horses and pigs
    c. dogs and cattle
    d. cats and horses
    e. cats and dogs

18. *Atropine:*

    a. should be given as a preanesthetic to all patients
    b. is totally effective in controlling bradycardia
    c. is totally effective in controlling salivation in ruminants
    d. can be safely given to horses that have not been fasted
    e. is an anticholinergic acting centrally and peripherally, generally preventing bradycardia caused by vagovagal reflexes

19. *An agent that can be given intravenously for humane euthanasia of dogs is:*

    a. succinylcholine
    b. strychnine
    c. magnesium sulfate
    d. guaifenesin
    e. sodium pentobarbital

Correct answers are on pages 8-9.

20. A 10% solution of thiopental contains the drug at a concentration of:

    a. 0.1 mg/ml
    b. 1 mg/ml
    c. 10 mg/ml
    d. 100 mg/ml
    e. 1000 mg/ml

21. Concerning differences between isoflurane and halothane, which statement is most accurate?

    a. The anesthetic level can be changed more quickly with isoflurane than with halothane.
    b. Isoflurane causes greater sensitization of the heart to catecholamines than does halothane.
    c. Isoflurane is much less volatile than halothane.
    d. Biodegradation occurs to a far lesser degree with halothane than with isoflurane.
    e. Halothane causes greater vasodilation and less myocardial depression than isoflurane.

22. Acepromazine, a phenothiazine tranquilizer, causes hypotension by:

    a. blockade of beta-1 receptors
    b. blockade of beta-2 receptors
    c. blockade of alpha-1 receptors
    d. decreasing cardiac output
    e. agonism of beta-2 receptors

23. Which of the following is the characteristic breathing pattern induced by ketamine administration?

    a. slow, deep breathing
    b. Cheyne-Stokes breathing
    c. tachypnea
    d. apneustic breathing
    e. hyperventilation

24. In what situation is use of ketamine anesthesia **unsuitable**?

    a. muscle trauma
    b. bradycardia
    c. hypotension
    d. castration of a cat
    e. intraocular surgery

25. The agent most likely to produce adequate chemical restraint of vicious dogs is:

    a. xylazine
    b. morphine with acepromazine
    c. morphine
    d. acepromazine
    e. diazepam with tripellenamine

26. Which of the following is the most likely reason for prolonged ketamine anesthesia (delayed recovery) in cats?

    a. hyperthermia
    b. low total plasma protein level
    c. metabolic alkalosis
    d. inadequate urinary clearance
    e. hepatic dysfunction

27. Innovar-Vet is a combination of:

    a. tiletamine and zolazepam
    b. droperidol and fentanyl
    c. meperidine and fentanyl
    d. detomidine and fentanyl
    e. diazepam and ketamine

28. The drug that is a complete narcotic antagonist is:

    a. tolazoline
    b. doxapram
    c. naloxone
    d. yohimbine
    e. nalbuphine

29. Which drug is the most potent analgesic?

    a. fentanyl
    b. meperidine
    c. xylazine
    d. butorphanol
    e. morphine

30. *Which drug combination is used to produce neuroleptanalgesia?*

   a. tranquilizers and barbiturates
   b. tranquilizers and narcotics
   c. sedatives and hypnotics
   d. tranquilizers and muscle relaxants
   e. narcotics and muscle relaxants

31. *About how long does it take for halothane to reach equilibrium between the pulmonary alveoli and vessel-rich organs in an animal that is breathing normally?*

   a. 15 minutes
   b. 30 minutes
   c. 45 minutes
   d. 1 hour
   e. 2 hours

32. *Using an inhalant anesthetic with a minimum alveolar concentration (MAC) of 1.0, the percentage of patients that do **not** move when subjected to a painful stimulus is:*

   a. 10%
   b. 25%
   c. 50%
   d. 75%
   e. 100%

33. *Accidental massive overdose of xylazine can be effectively treated with intravenous fluids and:*

   a. naloxone
   b. detomidine
   c. tolazoline
   d. doxapram
   e. epinephrine

34. *Concerning use of atropine and glycopyrrolate as anticholinergic preanesthetics, which statement is most accurate?*

   a. Atropine does not cross the blood-brain barrier.

   b. Atropine crosses the blood-brain barrier more slowly than glycopyrrolate and has only peripheral effects.
   c. Atropine is longer acting than glycopyrrolate.
   d. Glycopyrrolate crosses the blood-brain barrier in larger amounts than atropine and has primarily central effects.
   e. Glycopyrrolate crosses the blood-brain barrier more slowly than atropine and has primarily peripheral effects.

35. *The inhalant anesthetic that induces the **least** cardiovascular depression during general anesthesia is:*

   a. halothane
   b. methoxyflurane
   c. enflurane
   d. isoflurane
   e. desflurane

36. *The inhalant anesthetic that **does not** require a vaporizer for administration is:*

   a. halothane
   b. methoxyflurane
   c. nitrous oxide
   d. enflurane
   e. isoflurane

37. *In cats, the sedative effect of xylazine can be effectively reversed with the alpha antagonist:*

   a. doxapram
   b. naloxone
   c. butorphanol
   d. buprenorphine
   e. tolazoline

38. *Postoperative pain may result in any of the following **except**:*

   a. hypoventilation
   b. hypoxia
   c. alkalosis
   d. acidosis
   e. hyperventilation

Correct answers are on pages 8-9.

39. A high $PaCO_2$ in a patient during anesthesia suggests:

    a. hyperventilation
    b. metabolic alkalosis
    c. hypoventilation
    d. metabolic acidosis
    e. respiratory alkalosis

40. Continuous positive-pressure ventilation is **contraindicated** in patients with:

    a. acute pulmonary edema
    b. diffuse emphysema
    c. neonatal respiratory distress syndrome
    d. peripheral circulatory failure
    e. asthma

41. Balanced anesthesia is characterized by:

    a. sedation, analgesia and muscle relaxation
    b. narcosis, analgesia and muscle relaxation
    c. neuroleptanalgesia
    d. hypnosis and muscle relaxation
    e. tranquilization, analgesia and muscle relaxation

42. In rabbits, injectable anesthetics are best injected into the:

    a. femoral vein
    b. jugular vein
    c. auricular vein
    d. cephalic vein
    e. right ventricle

43. In rabbits,:

    a. atropine effectively controls salivation
    b. the safety margin between the anesthetic and lethal dose of pentobarbital is very narrow
    c. pentobarbital is a potent analgesic
    d. the trachea is easily intubated under light pentobarbital anesthesia
    e. intravenous fluid infusion is not recommended during anesthesia

44. Concerning ketamine anesthesia in birds, which statement is **least** accurate?

    a. A dosage of 30-40 mg/kg IM is required for such diagnostic procedures as radiography and laparoscopy.
    b. Ketamine may be given IV to large birds.
    c. Induction is smooth and muscle relaxation is enhanced when ketamine is combined with diazepam.
    d. There are considerable species variations in the response to ketamine, and owls appear to be especially sensitive.
    e. Injectable anesthesia is the method of choice for lengthy or involved surgical procedures in birds.

45. Concerning anesthesia in birds, which statement is **least** accurate?

    a. Inhalant anesthetics are best delivered with a non-rebreathing system, such as a Bain apparatus.
    b. The trachea of birds is easily intubated.
    c. Birds do not have a larynx.
    d. As compared with mammals, birds have a higher lung surface-to-volume ratio and a thinner blood-air barrier, making it more efficient for gas exchange.
    e. Birds require more time to recover from inhalation anesthesia than do mammals.

46. The most common change in acid-base status in an anesthetized patient is:

    a. metabolic acidosis
    b. metabolic alkalosis
    c. respiratory alkalosis
    d. respiratory acidosis
    e. mixed acid-base disturbance

47. The most reliable indication of the depth of anesthesia and well-being of birds is:

    a. respiratory rate and character and ventilatory response to stimulation
    b. electrocardiographic pattern
    c. blood gas and acid-base status

d. palpebral reflex present in deep anesthesia
e. pedal reflex present in deep anesthesia

48. **Which inhalant anesthetic is considered most desirable for birds?**

a. ether
b. nitrous oxide
c. isoflurane
d. methoxyflurane
e. halothane

49. **When using injectable agents for restraint and analgesia in small animals, xylazine combined with an opioid is useful because this combination:**

a. produces no detrimental cardiovascular effect
b. does not depress respiration
c. is completely compatible with ketamine
d. does not alter the dosage requirement of other drugs that might be used
e. has specific antagonists that can nearly completely reverse the depressant effects, if necessary

50. **Primates are most easily intubated if positioned in:**

a. dorsal recumbency
b. left lateral recumbency
c. right lateral recumbency
d. sternal recumbency
e. the prone position

51. **The larynx of primates is considered:**

a. very sensitive to stimulation, making it difficult to intubate
b. about as sensitive to stimulation as that of a dog
c. weakly sensitive to stimulation, making intubation rather simple
d. the primary cause of difficult intubation because of its proximity to the uvula
e. easy to intubate because of its shape and location

52. **The agent of choice for anesthesia of reptiles is:**

a. xylazine
b. thiopental
c. pentobarbital
d. ketamine
e. acepromazine

53. **Abolition of the awareness of pain is referred to as:**

a. hypnosis
b. sedation
c. narcosis
d. analgesia
e. tranquilization

54. **Deep anesthesia with isoflurane generally depresses ventilation and causes CO_2 retention. Clinical management of this problem should include:**

a. IV infusion of sodium bicarbonate
b. assisted or controlled ventilation
c. IV fluid administration
d. acepromazine as a preanesthetic drug
e. a lighter plane of anesthesia and assisted or controlled ventilation

55. **If a patient inhaled 50% N_2O at the standard temperature and pressure, the partial pressure of N_2O in the alveolus should be approximately:**

a. 180 mm of Hg
b. 355 mm of Hg
c. 450 mm of Hg
d. 460 mm of Hg
e. 760 mm of Hg

56. **Shock is initially treated with:**

a. rapid infusion of fluids
b. epinephrine
c. dobutamine
d. alpha-2 antagonists
e. corticosteroids

Correct answers are on pages 8-9.

57. *All anesthetic machines should be equipped*
     with:

    a. a static electricity arrestor

    b. an electrocardiograph

    c. a waste gas scavenging system

    d. a blood pressure monitor

    e. a nitrous oxide flow meter and flush valve

58. *The normal resting heart rate and respiratory*
     rate of cats are:

    a. 40-60 beats/minute, 10-15 breaths/minute

    b. 60-90 beats/minute, 40-60 breaths/minute

    c. 60-80 beats/minute, 10-20 breaths/minute

    d. 110-150 beats/minute, 20-40 breaths/minute

    e. 150-200 beats/minute, 40-60 breaths/minute

59. *When inducing anesthesia in a Greyhound*
     dog, the barbiturate of choice is:

    a. thiamylal

    b. thiopental

    c. pentobarbital

    d. methohexital

    e. phenobarbital

Answers

1. **a**	24. **e**
2. **d**	25. **b**
3. **e**	26. **d**
4. **b**	27. **b**
5. **b**	28. **c**
6. **b**	29. **a**
7. **a**	30. **b**
8. **b**	31. **a**
9. **a**	32. **c**
10. **d**	33. **c**
11. **a**	34. **e**
12. **d**	35. **e**
13. **b**	36. **c**
14. **c**	37. **e**
15. **a**	38. **c**
16. **e**	39. **c**
17. **d**	40. **d**
18. **e**	41. **b**
19. **e**	42. **c**
20. **d**	43. **b**
21. **a**	44. **e**
22. **c**	45. **e**
23. **d**	46. **d**

47. **a**
48. **c**
49. **e**
50. **a**
51. **a**
52. **d**
53. **d**

54. **e**
55. **b**
56. **a**
57. **c**
58. **d**
59. **d**

Notes

Notes

Section

2

Cardiology

N.S. Moise

Recommended Reading

Fox PR *et al: Canine and Feline Cardiology*. Churchill Livingstone, New York, 1988.
Kirk RW *et al: Current Veterinary Therapy XI*. Saunders, Philadelphia, 1992.
Tilley LP and Owens JM: *Manual of Small Animal Cardiology*. Churchill Livingstone, New York, 1985.

> *Practice answer sheet is on page 331.*

Questions

1. Which of the following is an angiotensin-converting enzyme inhibitor?

   a. hydralazine
   b. prazosin
   c. enalapril
   d. nitroglycerin
   e. propranolol

2. Which combination of drugs may elevate serum potassium levels?

   a. furosemide and hydrochlorothiazide
   b. enalapril and spironolactone
   c. hydralazine and furosemide
   d. digoxin and furosemide
   e. enalapril and digoxin

3. Digoxin toxicity is most likely to be induced by treatment of animals with:

   a. hypokalemia and renal disease
   b. hyperkalemia and hyperthyroidism
   c. hyperkalemia and liver disease
   d. hyponatremia and hyperkalemia
   e. hypercalcemia and hypoadrenocorticism

4. Which of the following is most likely to be found in dogs with chronic heart failure?

   a. increased serum dobutamine level
   b. decreased serum insulin level
   c. decreased serum angiotensin II level
   d. decreased serum renin level
   e. increased serum aldosterone level

Correct answers are on pages 14-15.

5. Which of the following is **not** an action of digoxin?

   a. increases the rate of sinus node discharge
   b. decreases serum renin and aldosterone levels
   c. positive inotropy
   d. increases parasympathetic tone
   e. increases atrioventricular conduction time (slows conduction velocity)

6. Which condition is associated with a diastolic murmur?

   a. mitral insufficiency
   b. pulmonic stenosis
   c. patent ductus arteriosus
   d. aortic insufficiency
   e. ventricular septic defect

7. Which condition is associated with bounding pulses and a wide pulse pressure?

   a. subaortic stenosis
   b. patent ductus arteriosus
   c. valvular pulmonic stenosis
   d. tricuspid insufficiency
   e. atrial septal defect

8. Which association between electrocardiographic findings and cardiac changes is most accurate?

   a. deep S wave in Lead I with left ventricular enlargement
   b. wide QRS complex in Lead II with a deep S wave in left ventricular enlargement
   c. tall R wave in Lead II with left ventricular enlargement
   d. tall P waves in Lead II with left ventricular enlargement
   e. wide P waves in Lead II with right ventricular enlargement

9. Differential cyanosis (cyanosis in one part of the body but not another) is associated with:

   a. subaortic stenosis
   b. right-to-left shunting with patent ductus arteriosus
   c. left-to-right shunting with ventricular septal defect
   d. right-to-left shunting with atrial septal defect
   e. tricuspid dysplasia

10. A 10-year-old male Labrador Retriever has a 2-month history of episodes of dyspnea that worsens with exercise. The owners observe that during these episodes the dog makes a loud, harsh sound. On physical examination, the dog has obvious stridor but no sign of pulmonary edema. The most likely cause of these signs is:

    a. congestive heart failure
    b. pneumonia
    c. infectious tracheobronchitis
    d. tracheal collapse
    e. laryngeal paralysis

11. A 4-year-old male cat is admitted with hind limb paralysis. The owners returned home from work and found the cat crying as if in pain. The femoral pulses are absent and the nail beds of the hind limb digits are purple. Of the following courses of action, which is **least** appropriate?

    a. perform emergency surgery to relieve acute caudal aortic thromboembolism
    b. make thoracic radiographs
    c. perform an echocardiographic examination
    d. treat the cat with aspirin
    e. treat the cat with heparin

12. A 3-year-old Pomeranian has a honking cough that worsens with excitement. A grade-II systolic murmur is heard loudest at the fifth intercostal space on the left. The most likely cause of the cough is:

    a. pulmonary edema
    b. tracheal collapse
    c. pneumonia
    d. laryngeal paralysis
    e. pleural effusion

13. Golden Retrievers, Newfoundlands, German Shepherds and Boxers are predisposed to:

   a. tricuspid dysplasia
   b. subaortic stenosis
   c. patent ductus arteriosus
   d. valvular pulmonic stenosis
   e. mitral insufficiency

14. In dogs with mitral insufficiency and dilative cardiomyopathy, treatment with which drug improves clinical signs and prolongs life?

   a. furosemide
   b. enalapril
   c. hydralazine
   d. digoxin
   e. nitroglycerin

15. A 5-month-old cat has a grade-III systolic murmur heard at the fourth intercostal space on the right hemithorax. The electrocardiogram is normal but thoracic radiographs show generalized cardiomegaly, with enlargement of the pulmonary artery and veins and slight pulmonary edema. The most likely cause of these signs is:

   a. heartworm disease
   b. mitral insufficiency
   c. ventricular septal defect
   d. subaortic stenosis
   e. patent ductus arteriosus

16. An English Bulldog has a grade-IV systolic murmur with a point of maximum intensity over the cranial left third intercostal space. The dog's femoral pulses are adequate. The electrocardiogram shows a deep S wave in Leads I, II, III and aVF, and a mean electrical axis of 160 degrees. The most likely cause of these findings is:

   a. subaortic stenosis
   b. pulmonic stenosis
   c. ventricular septal defect
   d. patent ductus arteriosus
   e. atrial septal defect

17. Which drug is usually indicated in treatment of dangerous ventricular tachycardia?

   a. digoxin
   b. lidocaine
   c. atropine
   d. propranolol
   e. diltiazem

18. Which drug is a calcium channel blocker used in treatment of hypertrophic cardiomyopathy in cats?

   a. atenolol
   b. diltiazem
   c. digoxin
   d. propranolol
   e. procainamide

19. Concerning adjustment of digoxin doses, which statement is most accurate?

   a. The dose should be decreased with renal disease and increased in aged animals.
   b. The dose should be increased in aged animals and based on the animal's estimated lean body weight.
   c. The dose should be decreased with renal disease and based on the animal's estimated lean body weight.
   d. The dose should be increased with renal disease and decreased in aged animals.
   e. The dose should be decreased with renal disease and based on the animal's actual body weight.

20. Which of the following most accurately describes the side effects of propranolol?

   a. vomiting, diarrhea, seizures
   b. listlessness, anorexia, bradycardia
   c. seizures
   d. seizures, tachycardia, nervousness
   e. vomiting, diarrhea, depression

Correct answers are on pages 14-15.

21. An owner telephones regarding her dog with dilative cardiomyopathy. For the past 10 days the dog has been treated with digoxin, furosemide and enalapril. The owner complains that the dog is vomiting, and has diarrhea, and will not get up. The dog is drinking water and appears hydrated. What is the most likely cause of these signs?

a. excessive diuresis with furosemide
b. toxicity from the digoxin
c. progression of the disease process, with ischemia or thromboembolism
d. unrelated gastrointestinal disease
e. toxicity from concurrent use of enalapril with furosemide

22. Dilative cardiomyopathy in cats is most commonly associated with a dietary deficiency of:

a. taurine
b. carnitine
c. guanine
d. selenium
e. cobalt

23. Which of the following is **not** associated with heartworm infection?

a. pulmonary hypertension
b. no clinical signs
c. dilatation of the pulmonary arteries
d. right ventricular hypertrophy
e. systemic hypertension

24. A 12-year-old German Shepherd has a sudden onset of weakness, dyspnea and exercise intolerance. The femoral pulses are weak and the heart rate is regular at 190 beats/minute. The heart sounds are muffled. You observe jugular vein distention and suspect ascites. The mucous membranes are pale pink. The most likely cause of these signs is:

a. auricular hemangiosarcoma
b. splenic lymphoma
c. dilative cardiomyopathy
d. hypertrophic cardiography
e. benign (idiopathic) pericardial effusion

25. Of the following cardiac anomalies, which is **not** part of the complex known as tetralogy of Fallot?

a. ventricular septal defect
b. cor triatriatum
c. pulmonary stenosis
d. dextroposition of the aorta
e. right ventricular hypertrophy

Answers

1. c

2. b Enalapril is an angiotensin-converting enzyme inhibitor that decreases levels of aldosterone and causes potassium retention. Spironolactone is a potassium-sparing diuretic.

3. a Hypokalemia increases binding of digoxin to myocytes and, therefore, increases toxicity. Because digoxin is cleared by the kidneys, renal disease increases digoxin levels and toxicity.

4. e Serum aldosterone concentrations are elevated because of stimulation of the renin-angiotensin-aldosterone system.

5. a Digoxin can decrease the sinus rate.

6. d

7. b Animals with patent ductus arteriosus have a large difference between systolic and diastolic blood pressures.

8. c

9. b The ductus arteriosus leaves the aorta after the brachiocephalic trunk and subclavian

artery; therefore, the head is oxygenated and cranial tissues are pink, while the caudal body is cyanotic.

10. **e** Laryngeal paralysis is common in older Labrador Retrievers. Affected dogs characteristically show upper airway obstruction that causes noise known as stridor.

11. **a** Surgery to resolve thromboembolism has a high mortality.

12. **b** Collapsing trachea characteristically occurs in this breed. Affected animals have a honking cough.

13. **b**

14. **b**

15. **c** Ventricular septal defect is relatively common in cats. The location of this murmur is consistent with a ventricular septal defect. The radiographs confirm the volume overload state.

16. **b** The point of maximum intensity is over the pulmonic valve and the ECG shows marked right heart enlargement. Also, English Bulldogs are predisposed to pulmonic stenosis.

17. **b**

18. **b**

19. **c**

20. **b**

21. **b**

22. **a**

23. **e**

24. **a** Hemangiosarcoma of the right auricle is a common cause of pericardial effusion in German Shepherds.

25. **b** Cor triatriatum is not part of the tetralogy of Fallot anomaly. In cor triatriatum, the pulmonary veins enter an accessory left atrium. The true left atrium and the accessory left atrium connect through a narrow opening, obstructing pulmonary venous return.

Notes

Notes

3

Clinical Pathology

B.T. Mitzner

Recommended Reading

Cowell RL and Tyler RD: *Diagnostic Cytology of the Dog and Cat.* American Veterinary Publications, Goleta, CA, 1989.

Goldston RT *et al: Practitioner's Laboratory.* Veterinary Medicine Publishing, Lenexa, KS, 1983.

Henry JB *et al: Clinical Diagnosis and Management by Laboratory Methods.* 17th ed. Saunders, Philadelphia, 1984.

Mitzner BT: In-house Laboratory. Column published regularly in *DVM Newsmagazine.*

Osborne CA and Stevens JB: *Handbook of Canine and Feline Urinalysis.* Ralston Purina, St. Louis, 1981.

Schalm OW: *Manual of Feline and Canine Hematology.* Veterinary Practice Publishing, Santa Barbara, CA, 1980.

Practice answer sheet is on page 333.

Questions

1. *Specimens for hematologic analysis should be collected in vacuum tubes with a stopper of what color?*

   a. lavender
   b. blue
   c. red
   d. green
   e. gray

2. *Before staining, blood smears should be fixed in:*

   a. acetone
   b. xylene
   c. isopropyl alcohol
   d. ethanol
   e. methanol

3. *When scanning a blood smear, a finding of 4-6 white blood cells per high-power field indicates an estimated white blood cell count of:*

   a. 7000-10,000/μl
   b. 2000-4000/μl
   c. 13,000-15,000/μl
   d. 16,000-18,000/μl
   e. >20,000/μl

Correct answers are on pages 28-30.

4. The blood smear of a normal patient should have how many platelets per oil-immersion field?

   a. <3
   b. 3-5
   c. 6-10
   d. 11-15
   e. >16

5. Methods for obtaining the total white blood cell count include all of the following **except**:

   a. estimation from blood smear
   b. dilution pipet
   c. volumetric impedence analyzer
   d. filtration
   e. Unopette method

6. Why are blood cell counts done with automated hematology analyzers likely to be more accurate than those done manually?

   a. automated counts are free from human influence
   b. automated analyzers count a greater number of cells
   c. automated analyzers use light to count cells
   d. cells become distorted during preparation for microscopic viewing
   e. specimens for manual counts require further dilution to be as accurate as specimens counted with an automated system

7. Automated blood cell counts require manual or electronic coincidence correction. Concerning automated blood cell counts, which statement is most accurate?

   a. As the count gets higher, accuracy increases.
   b. The procedure corrects for any clots that might have formed in the sample.
   c. Coincidence correction is only necessary for specimens that have been held overnight.
   d. As the count gets higher, the probability of 2 or more cells simultaneously passing through the aperture becomes greater.
   e. As the count gets higher, certain cells in the diluent tend to sediment out of solution.

8. The most important periodic maintenance procedure required by impedence-type hematology analyzers is:

   a. oiling the vacuum pump
   b. changing the vacuum tubing
   c. deproteinizing the counting aperture
   d. cleaning the dilutor probe
   e. adjusting the vacuum pressure

9. When using an impedence-type hematology analyzer, the background count is performed on:

   a. a normal blood sample
   b. a diluted control sample
   c. deionized water
   d. an aliquot of isotonic diluent
   e. an aliquot of cleaning solution

10. Hematology quality-control tests are used to assess the:

    a. performance of the operator
    b. accuracy of the counting method
    c. accuracy of the sample dilutions
    d. integrity of the reagents
    e. performance of the entire system

11. Most errors that occur with automated hematology analyzers can be traced back to:

    a. improper specimen collection
    b. inadequate premixing of the specimen
    c. improper dilution of the specimen
    d. lack of familiarity with the analyzer
    e. improper transposition of results

12. Most practices use a refractometer to perform a quick "total solids" measurement. When the specimen is taken from a spun hematocrit tube, the measurement includes **only**:

    a. total protein
    b. total protein and fibrinogen
    c. plasma protein
    d. albumin
    e. albumin and globulin

13. *When using a refractometer to measure total solids, a lipemic sample:*

    a. decreases the result
    b. increases the result
    c. has no effect on the result
    d. makes the result impossible to read
    e. gives accurate results in fasted patients only

14. *Which cell type is **not** found in an avian blood smear?*

    a. erythrocyte
    b. thrombocyte
    c. heterophil
    d. neutrophil
    e. eosinophil

15. *Which cell type is **not** in the red cell series?*

    a. prorubricyte
    b. metamyelocyte
    c. rubricyte
    d. reticulocyte
    e. erythrocyte

16. *Which of the following is a platelet precursor?*

    a. megakaryocyte
    b. metamyelocyte
    c. metarubricyte
    d. thrombocyte
    e. myeloblast

17. *What artificial change in the complete blood count is most likely to occur if the blood sample is collected from an excited or agitated patient?*

    a. leukocytosis
    b. decreased hematocrit
    c. platelet aggregation
    d. left shift
    e. leukopenia

18. *A Barr body is a small, spherical extension of the nucleus of some peripheral granulocytes. Barr bodies indicate that the patient:*

    a. is anemic
    b. is stressed
    c. is female
    d. is in critical condition
    e. has vitamin B_{12} deficiency

19. *Rouleaux formation (stacking or linear clumping of erythrocytes) is a common finding in:*

    a. dogs
    b. cats
    c. cattle
    d. horses
    e. pigs

20. *In which species are nucleated erythrocytes a normal finding?*

    a. cats
    b. pigs
    c. rabbits
    d. chickens
    e. horses

21. *Which cell type is **least** likely to be found on a peripheral blood smear from a dog with autoimmune hemolytic anemia?*

    a. reticulocyte
    b. spherocyte
    c. target cell
    d. erythrocyte
    e. metamyelocyte

22. *The formula* $\dfrac{PCV(\%) \times 10}{RBC\ count}$ *is used to calculate:*

    a. the maturation index
    b. the reticulocyte count
    c. the mean corpuscular volume
    d. corrected nucleated red blood cell count
    e. the mean corpuscular hemoglobin

Correct answers are on pages 28-30.

23. *Microcytic anemia is characterized by:*

   a. nucleated red blood cells
   b. abnormally small red blood cells
   c. abnormally large red blood cells
   d. pale red blood cells
   e. schistocytes

24. *Variation in the size of erythrocytes is known as:*

   a. macrocytosis
   b. poikilocytosis
   c. polychromasia
   d. erythrocytosis
   e. anisocytosis

25. *Abnormally shaped erythrocytes are collectively referred to as:*

   a. stomatocytes
   b. poikilocytes
   c. macrocytes
   d. heterocytes
   e. polychromatocytes

26. *In a complete blood count, a left shift refers to:*

   a. movement of the microscope slide to the left
   b. decreased numbers of platelets
   c. an abundance of immature white blood cell forms
   d. increased numbers of nucleated red blood cells
   e. a trend toward macrocytosis

27. *An abundance of eosinophils on a peripheral blood smear is most commonly associated with:*

   a. neoplastic disease
   b. infection
   c. trauma
   d. allergic conditions
   e. stress

28. *How long should microhematocrit tubes be centrifuged?*

   a. 1 minute
   b. 5 minutes
   c. 10 minutes
   d. 3 minutes
   e. depends on centrifuge calibraton

29. *If the sealant clay fails to stay in the microhematocrit tube during centrifugation, the most likely cause is:*

   a. worn tube cushions or gasket
   b. old clay sealant
   c. tube of incorrect diameter
   d. centrifuge not properly balanced
   e. not enough clay sealant used

30. *Punctate reticulocytes are most frequently found in:*

   a. dogs
   b. cats
   c. horses
   d. pigs
   e. cattle

31. *Which stain is **not** appropriate for routine staining of blood smears?*

   a. Wright's
   b. Wright's-Giemsa
   c. Diff-Quik
   d. trichrome
   e. Giemsa

32. *As a minimum standard, blood collection tubes containing EDTA should be filled:*

   a. to the top
   b. one-fourth of the way to the top
   c. half way to the top
   d. three-quarters of the way to the top
   e. to any desired level, as the amount is not critical

33. *The most common bleeding disorders seen in companion animals are related to:*

   a. decreased clotting factor activity

b. thrombocytopenia

c. platelet dysfunction

d. hemophilia A and B

e. hypocalcemia

34. *The activated clotting time (ACT) is prolonged in animals with:*

a. platelet dysfunction

b. anemia

c. platelet deficiency

d. clotting factor deficiency

e. reticulocytosis

35. *Bleeding time is the best test to detect:*

a. platelet dysfunction

b. anemia

c. platelet deficiency

d. clotting factor deficiency

e. reticulocytosis

36. *Specimens for coagulation testing should be collected in tubes containing:*

a. EDTA

b. ammonium heparin

c. sodium citrate

d. potassium oxalate

e. no anticoagulant

37. *Which of the following is **not** a test of hemostasis?*

a. activated clotting time

b. prothrombin time

c. partial thromboplastin time

d. bleeding time

e. erythrocyte sedimentation rate

38. *While a serum specimen is preferred for chemistry analysis, a plasma specimen may be used for most chemistry assays, provided that the specimen is:*

a. collected from a fasted patient

b. collected in a tube containing lithium heparin

c. collected in a tube containing EDTA

d. collected only from the jugular vein

e. analyzed within 15 minutes after collection

39. *Which abnormality is **least** likely to be found in a non-separated blood sample collected for serum chemistry analysis?*

a. increased potassium level

b. increased aspartate aminotransferase activity

c. increased phosphorus level

d. decreased glucose level

e. decreased cholesterol level

40. *Which method **cannot** be used to avoid or clear most lipemic blood specimens?*

a. allow the specimen to stand upright in the refrigerator for several hours or overnight

b. treat the specimen with chemical "clearing agents"

c. use an ultracentrifuge to separate the specimen

d. obtain the specimen from a fasted patient

e. collect the specimen in a heparinized tube

41. *Which technique is most likely to prevent hemolysis during blood collection?*

a. use a large-gauge (<19-ga) needle

b. use a small-gauge (>21-ga) needle

c. soak the skin well with alcohol before venipuncture

d. shake the specimen vigorously after collection

e. use a large (>10 ml) collection tube

42. *Which clinicopathologic abnormality is **least** likely to be found in a patient with advanced renal disease?*

a. increased blood urea nitrogen level

b. increased serum creatinine level

c. decreased serum calcium level

d. decreased hematocrit

e. increased serum phosphorus level

Correct answers are on pages 28-30.

43. Which of the following does **not** reflect liver function?

    a. serum albumin level
    b. serum alanine aminotransferase activity
    c. serum alkaline phosphatase activity
    d. serum creatinine level
    e. serum aspartate aminotransferase activity

44. Serum amylase activity generally is **not** increased in animals with:

    a. pancreatitis
    b. renal disease
    c. dehydration
    d. pancreatic abcess
    e. colitis

45. Icteric patients usually exhibit an increased:

    a. serum bilirubin level
    b. serum albumin level
    c. serum creatinine level
    d. serum lipase activity
    e. serum creatine phosphokinase activity

46. Total serum bilirubin reflects serum levels of:

    a. direct bilirubin
    b. direct bilirubin and conjugated bilirubin
    c. conjugated bilirubin and unconjugated bilirubin
    d. indirect bilirubin and unconjugated bilirubin
    e. indirect bilirubin

47. Total plasma protein values in excess of 10 g/dl are usually asociated with:

    a. increased serum albumin levels
    b. increased serum creatinine levels
    c. increased red blood cell hemoglobin content
    d. increased serum globulin levels
    e. dehydration

48. Increased serum amylase and lipase activities usually suggest:

    a. liver disease
    b. kidney disease
    c. intestinal disease
    d. pancreatic disease
    e. pulmonary disease

49. Elevated serum creatine phosphokinase activity is usually associated with:

    a. renal disease
    b. liver disease
    c. intestinal disease
    d. muscular disease
    e. pancreatic disease

50. Decreased serum cholinesterase activity often accompanies:

    a. renal disease
    b. trauma
    c. organophosphate insecticide toxicity
    d. diabetes mellitus
    e. pancreatitis

51. The d-xylose test is used as a screening test to detect:

    a. malabsorption syndrome
    b. diabetes mellitus
    c. adrenal disease
    d. liver tumors
    e. renal disease

52. In an endpoint analysis,:

    a. several light-absorbence readings are taken at intervals
    b. a standard is not necessary
    c. a conversion coefficient is required
    d. a stable, colored product is formed at the conclusion
    e. light absorbence is not proportional to solute concentration

53. Which of the following is **not** used to calculate anion gap?

    a. serum sodium level
    b. serum calcium level
    c. serum CO_2 level

d. serum potassium level

e. serum chloride level

54. *The constituents in most serum chemistry control samples are stable for approximately 7 days after reconstitution. Which control sample is stable for the shortest time after reconstitution?*

a. glucose

b. albumin

c. creatinine

d. carbon dioxide

e. urea nitrogen

55. *A microscope should be professionally cleaned:*

a. yearly or more often, as needed

b. every 5 years

c. when more than 30 samples a week are examined for 6 consecutive months

d. when the focal field is obscured

e. when the focusing mechanism breaks

56. *The proper immersion oil for normal light microscopy is:*

a. type A

b. type B

c. mineral oil

d. linseed oil

e. SAE 30 automotive oil

57. *Which of the following is **not** an acceptable fecal flotation solution?*

a. sodium nitrate

b. Sheather's (sugar)

c. zinc sulfate

d. potassium chromate

e. glycerin

58. *In an infected animal, life cycle stages of which parasite are **least** likely to be found on a fecal flotation preparation?*

a. *Giardia cati*

b. *Toxocara canis*

c. *Trichuris vulpis*

d. *Ancylostoma caninum*

e. *Isospora*

59. *Ova of* Capillaria plica *are most likely to be found in:*

a. feces

b. urine

c. saliva

d. blood

e. nasal discharge

60. *Ova of which parasite are usually seen in the larvated form?*

a. *Ancylostoma* (hookworm)

b. *Isospora* (coccidia)

c. *Dipylidium* (tapeworm)

d. *Strongyloides* (threadworm)

e. *Toxocara* (roundworm)

61. *The parasite that appears as a punctate small rod-like or ring-like structure on the periphery of red blood cells in peripheral blood smears is:*

a. *Ehrlichia canis*

b. *Babesia bigemina*

c. *Anaplasma marginale*

d. *Hemobartonella felis*

e. *Tritrichomonas fetus*

62. *Which method is most reliable for detection of* Ehrlichia canis *infection?*

a. blood smear examination

b. buffy coat examination

c. indirect fluorescent antibody test on serum

d. wet preparation of peripheral blood stained with new methylene blue

e. serum titer

63. *The parasite* Hemoproteus *is most likely to infect the erythrocytes of:*

a. horses

b. cattle

c. dogs

d. birds

e. cats

Correct answers are on pages 28-30.

64. Microfilariae of Dirofilaria immitis (canine heartworm) are most often confused with those of:

    a. *Dipetalonema*
    b. *Trypanosoma*
    c. *Babesia*
    d. *Hemobartonella*
    e. *Ehrlichia*

65. Which method is **not** used for detection of heartworm microfilariae?

    a. direct blood smear
    b. buffy coat examination
    c. modified Knott's technique
    d. filtration/concentration method
    e. enzyme-linked immunosorbent assay

66. The test of choice for routine surveillance of dogs treated monthly with heartworm preventives is:

    a. Knott's technique
    b. filtration/concentration
    c. enzyme-linked immunosorbent assay of high sensitivity
    d. enzyme-linked immunosorbent assay of high specificity
    e. filtration/concentration plus enzyme-linked immunosorbent assay

67. Cigar-shaped mites in a skin scraping from a dog are most likely of the genus:

    a. *Sarcoptes*
    b. *Notoedres*
    c. *Otodectes*
    d. *Demodex*
    e. *Psoroptes*

68. Which method is **least** appropriate for urine collection?

    a. mid-stream free catch
    b. manual expression of the bladder
    c. aspiration of urine from a cage floor or litterbox

    d. bladder catheterization
    e. cystocentesis

69. In which type of patient should cystocentesis **not** be performed?

    a. 3-month-old puppy
    b. obese Beagle
    c. female dog in heat
    d. adult male cat with disease of the bladder wall
    e. old dog with a fever

70. A normal-colored but slightly opaque urine sample is most likely to contain:

    a. many white blood cells and/or phosphates crystals
    b. much fat
    c. many uric acid crystals
    d. much bilirubin
    e. many yeast organisms

71. A urine specimen with a "fruity" odor is most likely to contain:

    a. metabolized fruit juice
    b. bacteria
    c. hemolyzed blood
    d. acetone
    e. myoglobin

72. A specific gravity reading consistent with isosthenuria is:

    a. <1.001
    b. 1.001-1.008
    c. 1.008-1.012
    d. 1.012-1.025
    e. >1.025

73. What is the most common cause of erroneous results from urine testing with dipsticks?

    a. light damage to the strip
    b. moisture damage to the strip
    c. failure to time the reaction correctly

d. insufficient quantity of urine applied

e. cross reactions of various urine constituents

d. ascorbic acid

e. creatinine

74. What is the normal pH of canine and feline urine?

a. 7 or greater
b. 7 or less
c. 8-10
d. 10 or greater
e. highly variable pH, from 4 to 9

75. Highly alkaline urine samples may result in false-positive results when testing for:

a. protein
b. blood
c. glucose
d. ketones
e. urobilinogen

76. Myoglobin, a breakdown product of muscle, is eliminated in the urine and produces a positive reaction on which pad of a urine dipstick?

a. blood
b. bilirubin
c. ketone
d. glucose
e. urobilinogen

77. When present in the urine, bilirubin can be broken down by:

a. heating of the specimen
b. exposure of the specimen to light
c. blood in the specimen
d. drugs in the specimen
e. chemicals used to preserve the specimen

78. When present in urine, which substance can **mask** a positive glucose reaction on urine dipsticks?

a. ketones
b. blood
c. penicillin

79. The urine nitrite test is based on the ability of bacteria to convert nitrate to nitrite and is a crude indicator of urinary tract infection in people. Why is it of limited use in dogs and cats?

a. Dogs and cats are rarely affected by bacterial infections of the urinary tract.
b. The acidic pH of dog and cat urine prevents this reaction.
c. The bacteria tend to react with other proteins in the urine of dogs and cats.
d. The diets of most dogs and cats do not contain sufficient nitrate to cause a positive reaction.
e. Enzymes in the urine of dogs and cats break down nitrate.

80. For best results, urine specimens for microscopic analysis should be centrifuged for:

a. 5 minutes at 10,000 RPM
b. 5 minutes at 6000 RPM
c. 1 minute at 3000 RPM
d. 400 RCF for 5 minutes
e. time and speed are of no significance

81. Squamous epithelial cells found in a urine sample usually originate from the:

a. kidney
b. renal pelvis
c. ureter
d. bladder
e. genital tract

82. Transitional epithelial cells found in urine may originate from all of the following sites **except** the:

a. renal pelvis
b. ureter
c. renal tubules
d. bladder
e. proximal urethra

Correct answers are on pages 28-30.

83. *White blood cell casts in a urine sample suggest:*

    a. lymphoid neoplasia of the bladder
    b. disease of the ureter
    c. disease of the kidney
    d. calculi
    e. bacterial cystitis

84. *Cystine crystals are most likely to be found in the urine of:*

    a. female Collies
    b. female Doberman Pinschers
    c. female Cocker Spaniels
    d. male Dachshunds
    e. male Labrador Retrievers

85. *Calcium oxalate crystals in urine sediment are most often associated with:*

    a. ethylene glycol (antifreeze) toxicity
    b. gout
    c. bacterial cystitis
    d. end-stage renal disease
    e. organophosphate insecticide poisoning

86. *The sensitivity of enzyme-linked immunosorbent assay is related to the:*

    a. stability of the reagents
    b. ease with which an assay can be performed
    c. number of components in the assay
    d. overall accuracy of the assay in detecting true-positive samples
    e. ability of the assay to detect minimal concentrations of the antigen in question

87. *The higher the specificity of a test kit, the* **less** *likely that:*

    a. false-negative results will occur
    b. it will be easy to use
    c. it will be accurate
    d. false-positive results will occur
    e. results will be reliable

88. *All commercially available feline leukemia virus (FeLV) test kits are designed to detect:*

    a. FeLV antibodies
    b. FeLV-infected red blood cells
    c. FeLV antigens
    d. FOCMA antibodies
    e. FeLV-infected lymphoid cells

89. *A positive enzyme-linked immunosorbent assay for feline leukemia virus (FeLV) may indicate any of the following* **except**:

    a. the cat may be transiently infected
    b. the cat may be chronically infected
    c. the cat will definitely die from FeLV infection
    d. the cat may become a latent carrier
    e. the cat may be contagious for other cats

90. *You test a cat's serum for feline leukemia virus using a microwell-type enzyme-linked immunosorbent assay kit. Color develops in the negative control and patient sample wells, as well as in the positive well. What is the most likely cause of these results?*

    a. failure to properly time the test
    b. inadequate washing of wells after addition of the enzyme conjugate
    c. prolonged storage of the kit at room temperature
    d. nonspecific cross-reactive antibodies in the cat's serum
    e. failure to add the enzyme conjugate

91. *The commercially available enzyme-linked immunosorbent assay kits for heartworm infection in dogs are designed to detect:*

    a. antibodies to microfilariae
    b. antibodies to adult heartworms
    c. antibodies to migrating microfilariae
    d. microfilarial antigens
    e. adult heartworm antigens

92. *A 7-year-old outdoor male cat has a history and clinical signs strongly suggestive of heartworm infection. However, filter tests for*

heartworm microfilariae and enzyme-linked immunosorbent assay are both negative. What is the most likely explanation?

a. the cat likely does not have heartworm infection
b. the cat may have small numbers of adult heartworms
c. the test procedures were performed incorrectly
d. the tests are designed for use only in dogs
e. the cat is probably infected with feline leukemia virus

93. You test a 2-year-old clinically normal cat from a single-cat household for feline leukemia virus infection with an enzyme-linked immunosorbent assay kit designed for in-office use. The test is positive. What is the most appropriate advice for the cat's owner?

a. isolate the cat and repeat the test in 1-2 months
b. euthanize the cat before it develops full-blown infection
c. the result was probably inaccurate
d. isolate the cat but do not bother to retest, as the second test will likely be positive
e. do not breed this cat

94. Concerning cats whose saliva tests are positive for feline leukemia virus, which statement is most accurate?

a. They will soon die.
b. They are only transiently infected.
c. They have a latent infection.
d. They can transmit the virus to other cats.
e. They are probably not contagious.

95. A commonly used antimicrobial susceptibility testing method is:

a. chromatographic separation
b. agar dilution
c. Kirby-Bauer
d. McFarland's standard technique
e. anaerobic subculture

96. The medium of choice for antimicrobial susceptibility testing is:

a. triple sugar-iron agar with 5% sheep blood
b. Mueller-Hinton agar
c. MacConkey agar
d. Sabouraud's dextrose agar
e. Hektoen agar

97. When interpreting the results of an antimicrobial susceptibility test, a drug that is appropriate for treatment is indicated by a disk:

a. with a large zone of inhibition
b. with a small zone of inhibition
c. with a zone diameter designated as inhibitory, according to standard charts for antimicrobial susceptibility
d. with a zone of inhibition indicating poor ability to diffuse through the agar
e. that inhibits growth of the greatest number of organisms

98. Precise antimicrobial susceptibility testing requires that the agar plate containing the antimicrobial disks be inoculated:

a. and incubated immediately after the differential media plates have been inoculated
b. with a standard suspension of a single organism selected from the preincubated blood agar plate
c. with a mixed culture of all the organisms present on the preincubated blood agar plate
d. after preincubation of triple sugar-iron agar slants and broth subcultures
e. after preincubation of Sabouraud's dextrose slants and Hektoen broth subcultures

99. For long-term storage, antimicrobial sensitivity disks should be held at:

a. room temperature
b. 2-25 C
c. <2 C
d. >25 C
e. any convenient temperature

Correct answers are on pages 28-30.

100. *In cytologic specimens stained with Romanowsky-type stains (Diff-Quik, DipStat, Wright's), which practice is most likely to result in excessive pink staining?*

    a.   inadequate washing of stained slide

    b.   delayed fixation
    c.   exposure to formalin vapors
    d.   smear is too thick
    e.   stain or diluent is too acidic

Answers

1. **a** Lavender-top tubes contain EDTA anticoagulant.

2. **e**

3. **a**

4. **b**

5. **d**

6. **b**

7. **d**

8. **c** Protein accumulation in the aperture can result in erroneous hematocrit readings and an increased frequency of obstructions.

9. **d** Contamination of the diluent with bacteria or other particles results in counting errors. As the count increases, errors increase exponentially.

10. **e** The entire system includes the reagent, instrument and operator.

11. **b** While all of the other choices can cause errors, inadequate mixing is the most common error. An automatic specimen rotator improves mixing.

12. **b**

13. **b**

14. **d** The avian heterophil is analogous to the mammalian neutrophil.

15. **b** The metamyelocyte is a granulocyte precursor. The others are erythrocyte precursors.

16. **a**

17. **a** Physiologic leukocytosis occurs when marginated granulocytes enter the general circulation as a result of excitement or stress.

18. **c**

19. **d**

20. **d** All avian erythrocytes are nucleated.

21. **e** The metamyelocyte is a granulocyte precursor. The other cells are all of the erythrocyte series.

22. **c**

23. **b**

24. **e**

25. **b**

26. **c** Immature forms include band and stab cells.

27. **d** Eosinophilia occurs commonly in response to antigen antibody reactions, as well as with inflammation of certain organs, such as the lungs, which tend to be allergy "targets."

28. **e** Calibration should be performed every 1-3 months to account for changes in the centrifuge that occur as a result of "wear and tear."

29. **a**

30. **b**

31. **d** Trichrome stain is typically used for visualization of parasites in feces.

32. **c** Filling a tube less than half way results in a dilution error that could, among other things, artificially lower the hematocrit value.

33. **b** Thrombocytopenia refers to a reduction in platelet numbers.

34. **d**

35. **a** Bleeding time is also prolonged with platelet deficiency, but a direct count of platelets is a better method to assess thrombocytopenia.

36. **c**

37. **e** Erythrocyte sedimentation rate is not a test of hemostasis.

38. **b**

39. **e** Serum values of potassium, aspartate aminotransferase and phosphorus increase as a result of red blood cell leakage and hemolysis. Glucose levels decrease up to 5% per hour as a result of anaerobic glycolysis by red blood cells.

40. **e**

41. **b** Large-bore needles result in "spiraling" of the cells as they enter the needle. Alcohol and rough handling can result in cell lysis. A 10-ml tube would likely create too much negative pressure when collecting blood from a small animal.

42. **c** Some renal diseases are related to increased serum calcium levels.

43. **d** The serum creatinine level is a better assessment of renal function.

44. **e** Because amylase is eliminated through the kidneys, any disorder that reduces renal blood flow or impairs kidney function can result in elevated serum amylase activity.

45. **a**

46. **c**

47. **d**

48. **d**

49. **d**

50. **c** Organophosphate insecticides can be cholinesterase inhibitors.

51. **a**

52. **d**

53. **b** Anion gap = (Na + K) – (Cl + total CO_2).

54. **d** Ammonia (NH_3) is also unstable. Such enzymes as alanine aminotransferase and aspartate aminotransferase usually show some loss of activity after a few days unless the reconstituted control is frozen.

55. **a**

56. **b** Type B is a high-viscosity oil and is the best choice for light microscopy.

57. **d**

58. **a** *Giardia* is more likely to be found in direct saline smears.

59. **b**

60. **d**

61. **d**

62. **c** *Ehrlichia* morulae can occasionally be found in peripheral blood smears, but they are rare.

63. **d**

64. **a**

65. **e** Enzyme-linked immunosorbent assays detect adult heartworm antigens.

66. **d** In a low-incidence population, a test with a high positive predictive value is the best choice. Tests of high specificity have a high positive predictive value.

67. **d**

68. **c** Urine specimens collected from the floor or litterbox are likely to be contaminated.

69. **d** Needle puncture of the wall of a diseased bladder may predispose to bladder rupture.

70. **a**

71. **d** The urine of diabetic patients with ketoacidosis may have a fruity odor.

72. **c**

73. **b**

74. **b** The diet of carnivores usually produces acidic urine.

75. **a**

76. **a**

77. **b**

78. **d** Dogs and cats can synthesize ascorbic acid; therefore, an ascorbic acid-resistant urine dipstick is best for veterinary use.

79. **d** Nitrate occurs naturally in plants. Dogs and cats are primarily carnivores.

80. **d** RCF refers to relative centrifugal force. An RCF of 400 can be attained with a 6-inch-radius arm rotated at 1500 RPM.

81. **e**

82. **c**

83. **c**

84. **d** Cystinuria occurs almost exclusively in male dogs. Dachshunds, Basset Hounds, Chihuahuas, Yorkshire Terriers and Irish Terriers have been affected.

85. **a** Calcium oxalate crystals may also be found in small numbers in normal urine.

86. **e**

87. **d**

88. **c** All of these kits test for the p27 FeLV antigen.

89. **c** Some infected cats will die from FeLV infection; however, many more will recover and become immune.

90. **b** Unbound enzyme conjugate was probably left behind in all 3 wells. The unbound conjugate reacted with the added substrate to produce color.

91. **e**

92. **b** The test kits currently on the market lack the sensitivity to repeatedly detect only 1-2 adult worms.

93. **a** Many of these animals are transiently infected and seroconvert in time.

94. **d** FeLV is transmitted primarily through the saliva of infected cats.

95. **c**

96. **b**

97. **c** The extent to which an antimicrobial diffuses through agar is a property of the individual drug. Drugs that diffuse more slowly yield smaller zones of inhibition; however, they may still be effective choices for treatment.

98. **b** Direct sensitivity tests (those performed with mixed cultures) may only yield equivocal results.

99. **c** Unopened disk cartridges are best stored in the freezer. Once opened, however, it may be more convenient to store them with the dispenser in the refrigerator.

100. **e** All of the other choices listed would tend to cause excessive blue staining.

Notes

Section

4

Dentistry

R.B. Wiggs

Recommended Reading

Bojrab MJ and Tholen M: *Small Animal Oral Medicine and Surgery*. Lea & Febiger, Philadelphia, 1990.

Emily P and Penman S: *Handbook of Small Animal Dentistry*. Pergammon Press, Oxford, 1990.

Harvey CE: Feline dentistry. *Vet Clin No Am* (Small Anim Pract) 22:1265-1495, 1992.

Harvey CE: *Veterinary Dentistry*. Saunders, Philadelphia, 1985.

Holmstrom SE *et al: Veterinary Dental Techniques*. Saunders, Philadelphia, 1992.

Marretta-Manfra S: Dentistry. *Problems in Veterinary Medicine*. 2:1-278, 1990.

Wiggs RB: Canine oral anatomy and physiology. *Comp Cont Ed Pract Vet* 11:1475-1482, 1989.

Practice answer sheet is on page 335.

Questions

For Questions 1 through 5, select the correct answer from the 5 choices below.

a. dolichocephalic breeds
b. brachygnathic breeds
c. mesaticephalic breeds
d. prognathic breeds
e. brachycephalic breeds

1. Borzoi, Greyhound and Saluki.

2. Labrador Retriever and German Shepherd.

3. Boxer, Pekingese, Pug and Bulldog.

4. Have an overbite (maxilla too long in relation to the mandible).

5. Have an underbite (mandible too long in relation to the maxilla).

For Questions 6 through 10, select the correct answer from the 5 choices below.

a. posterior crossbite
b. base-narrow mandibular canines
c. wry mouth
d. anterior crossbite
e. open bite

Correct answers are on pages 38-40.

6. *Malocclusion in which one side of the mandible or maxilla is disproportionate to its other side, and the incisor midline of the mandible does not match the incisor midline of the maxilla.*

7. *When the mouth is closed as fully as possible, a gap or space remains between the upper and lower incisors.*

8. *Malocclusion of the permanent incisors resulting from retained deciduous teeth displacing their normal eruption position, with no indications of disproportionate jaw length.*

9. *Malocclusion in which the upper fourth premolars lie medial to the lower first molars.*

10. *Malocclusion of the permanent lower canine teeth resulting from retained deciduous teeth displacing their normal eruption position and causing trauma to the hard palate.*

For Questions 11 through 15, select the correct answer from the 5 choices below.

    a. $2 \times (I\ 3/3;\ C\ 1/1;\ P\ 3/2) = 26$
    b. $2 \times (I\ 3/3;\ C\ 1/1;\ P\ 4/4;\ M\ 2/3) = 42$
    c. $2 \times (I\ 3/3;\ C\ 1/1;\ P\ 3/2;\ M\ 1/1) = 30$
    d. $2 \times (I\ 3/3;\ C\ 1/1;\ P\ 3/3) = 28$
    e. $2 \times (I\ 3/3;\ C\ 1/1;\ P\ 4/4;\ M\ 3/3) = 44$

11. *Dental formula for deciduous or temporary teeth of dogs.*

12. *Dental formula for permanent teeth of dogs.*

13. *Dental formula for deciduous or temporary teeth of cats.*

14. *Dental formula for permanent teeth of cats.*

15. *Dental formula for permanent teeth of swine.*

For Questions 16 through 20, select the correct answer from the 5 choices below.

    a. premolars
    b. molars
    c. incisors
    d. carnassials
    e. canines or cuspids

16. *Teeth anatomically suited to grooming, nibbling and cutting.*

17. *Teeth anatomically suited to holding, grasping and tearing.*

18. *Teeth anatomically suited to holding, shearing and cutting.*

19. *Teeth anatomically suited to grinding.*

20. *Largest shearing cheek teeth.*

For Questions 21 through 25, select the correct answer from the 5 choices below.

    a. enamel
    b. dentin
    c. cementoenamel junction
    d. enamodentinal junction
    e. cementum

21. *The outside coating of the normally exposed portion of a cat's tooth.*

22. *The hard portion of the tooth that constitutes the majority of the tooth's hard structure.*

23. *The modified bone-like structure on the outer surface of the root of a dog's tooth.*

24. *Juncture on the outside of the tooth where crown and root meet.*

25. *Juncture of the enamel and the hard tissue immediately deep to it.*

For Questions 26 through 30, select the correct answer from the 5 choices below.

    a. apex
    b. crown
    c. root
    d. neck
    e. pulp cavity

26. *Normally exposed portion of the tooth.*

27. *Juncture of the crown and root.*

28. *Portion of the tooth normally embedded in the periodontium.*

29. *Deep tip of the root.*

30. *Open area within the tooth, occupied by soft tissues.*

31. *In regard to periodontal disease, all of the following are considered part of the peridontium **except**:*

    a. alveolar bone
    b. pulp
    c. cementum
    d. peridontal ligament
    e. gingiva

For Questions 32 through 36, select the correct answer from the 5 choices below.

    a. root canal
    b. pulp
    c. apical foramen
    d. pulp chamber
    e. apical delta

32. *Interior soft tissue of the tooth.*

33. *Normal part of the cavity within the tooth root.*

34. *Normal portion of the cavity within the tooth crown.*

35. *A single opening in the apex of a tooth root that provides passage for vascular, neural and connective tissues.*

36. *A multiple opening at the apex of the tooth.*

For Questions 37 through 41, select the correct answer from the 5 choices below.

    a. gingival margin
    b. free gingival margin
    c. epithelial attachment
    d. sulcus
    e. mucogingival junction

37. *Normally occurring crevice between the tooth and gingiva.*

38. *Line demarcating attached and free gingiva.*

39. *Connection of the gingiva at the bottom of the tooth sulcus.*

40. *Line demarcating attached gingiva and alveolar mucosa.*

41. *Thin, knife-like edge of the free gingiva.*

42. *Teeth are suspended in surrounding hard tissues by the:*

    a. cementum
    b. gingiva
    c. alveolar bone
    d. peridontal ligament
    e. pulp

Correct answers are on pages 38-40.

43. *The fluid found in the sulcus surrounding teeth is produced by the:*

   a. crevicular epithelium
   b. parotid salivary gland
   c. lingual epithelium
   d. sublingual salivary gland
   e. zygomatic salivary gland

44. *Oral parakeratinized tissue is much tougher than nonkeratinized tissue. Which of the following is **not** keratinized?*

   a. free gingiva
   b. gingival margin
   c. alveolar mucosa
   d. attached gingiva
   e. gingival papilla

For Questions 45 through 49, select the correct answer from the 5 choices below.

   a. dental elevator
   b. probe
   c. curette
   d. explorer
   e. sickle scaler

45. *Used to scale below the gum line (subgingival).*

46. *Used to scale above the gum line (supragingival).*

47. *Aids in removal of a tooth.*

48. *Used to check teeth for decay, canal exposures and cavities.*

49. *Used to check the depth of the gingival sulcus.*

50. *How often should curettes and hand-scaling instruments be sharpened?*

   a. with each use
   b. once daily
   c. once weekly
   d. once monthly
   e. when chipped or broken

For Questions 51 through 55, select the correct answer from the 5 choices below.

   a. rotosonic
   b. sonic
   c. piezoelectric
   d. magnetostrictive
   e. sickle scaler

51. *Claw-like scaler held by a modified "pen grasp."*

52. *Scaler vibrating at 20-40 kHz, producing an elliptic oscillating pattern through a ferromagnetic rod.*

53. *Scaler vibrating at 20-40 kHz, producing a linear oscillating pattern through changes in shape of a crystal by electric charge.*

54. *Scaler with a tip that vibrates at less than 20 kHz.*

55. *Six-sided soft steel bur, used on a high-speed handpiece.*

For Questions 56 through 58, select the correct answer from the 5 choices below.

   a. bisecting-angle technique
   b. lateral oblique technique
   c. perpendicular technique
   d. intersecting-angle technique
   e. parallel technique

56. *The intraoral film and tooth are perpendicular to the primary x-ray beam.*

57. *The x-ray beam is perpendicular to the intersecting angle equidistant between the intraoral film and tooth.*

58. The x-ray beam is perpendicular to the extraoral film, with the animal's head tilted at a 45-degree angle to avoid superimposition of the opposite quadrant, resulting in some foreshortening of the image.

59. As an animal ages, several classic changes occur in the normal tooth and its supporting system. Which of the following most accurately describes these changes?

    a. enlargement of the pulp cavity, thickening of the dentin, loss of definition of the lamina dura
    b. narrowing of the pulp cavity, thickening of the dentin, loss of definition of the lamina dura
    c. narrowing of the pulp cavity, thinning of the dentin, loss of definition of the lamina dura
    d. enlargement of the pulp cavity, thickening of the dentin, thickening of the lamina dura
    e. narrowing of the pulp cavity, thinning of the dentin, thickening of the lamina dura

60. Periodontal disease is a disease of the structures that support the tooth. Approximately what percentage of dogs and cats over 3 years of age have periodontal disease of a degree that would benefit from treatment?

    a. 5%
    b. 10%
    c. 15%
    d. 25%
    e. 85%

61. The major underlying cause of periodontal disease in dogs is:

    a. endocrine
    b. viral
    c. traumatic
    d. bacterial
    e. immune mediated

62. The factor primarily contributing to periodontal disease is:

    a. tartar
    b. plaque
    c. calculus
    d. salivary polysaccharides
    e. salivary minerals

63. All of the following predispose to periodontal disease **except**:

    a. overcrowded and rotated teeth
    b. retained deciduous teeth
    c. hard, crunchy diet
    d. malocclusions
    e. some endocrine and systemic diseases

For Questions 64 through 66, select the correct answer from the 5 choices below.

    a. polishing
    b. sulcal lavage
    c. subgingival curettage
    d. scaling
    e. root planing

64. Curettage of rough and disease cementum.

65. Curettage of the sulcal epithelium.

66. Flushing of the sulcus with a solution.

For Questions 67 through 71, select the correct answer from the 5 choices below.

    a. splinting
    b. closed curettage
    c. gingivoplasty
    d. open curettage
    e. odontoplasty

67. Removal of hyperplastic gingival tissue.

68. Root planing in association with a releasing flap.

69. Root planing without a gingival flap.

70. Removal of a portion of the tooth structure.

71. Bonding of loose teeth together to stabilize them during a healing process.

Correct answers are on pages 38-40.

Questions 72 through 77

In extracting teeth, it is important to know how many roots each type of tooth has.

72. How many roots do the incisor teeth of dogs have?

   a. 1
   b. 2
   c. 3
   d. usually 1, but sometimes 2
   e. usually 3, but sometimes 2

73. How many roots do the cuspid or canine teeth of dogs have?

   a. 1
   b. 2
   c. 3
   d. usually 1, but sometimes 2
   e. usually 3, but sometimes 2

74. How many roots do the upper fourth premolar teeth of dogs have?

   a. 1
   b. 2
   c. 3
   d. usually 1, but sometimes 2
   e. usually 3, but sometimes 2

75. How many roots do the lower fourth premolar teeth of dogs have?

   a. 1
   b. 2
   c. 3
   d. usually 1, but sometimes 2
   e. usually 3, but sometimes 2

76. How many roots do the upper first molar teeth of dogs have?

   a. 1
   b. 2
   c. 3
   d. usually 1, but sometimes 2
   e. usually 3, but sometimes 2

77. How many roots do the lower first molar teeth of dogs have?

   a. 1
   b. 2
   c. 3
   d. usually 1, but sometimes 2
   e. usually 3, but sometimes 2

78. Periodontal disease or injury resulting in communication between the oral cavity and a cavity dorsal to the upper corner incisor of a dog is most likely to lead to formation of:

   a. an oronasal fistula
   b. an oroantral fistula
   c. a periodontal fistula
   d. an endodontic fistula
   e. a gingivobuccal fistula

79. Periodontal disease or injury resulting in communication between the oral cavity and a cavity dorsal to the upper canine tooth of a dog is most likely to lead to formation of:

   a. an oronasal fistula
   b. an oroantral fistula
   c. a periodontal fisutla
   d. an endodontic fistula
   e. a gingivobuccal fistula

80. Periodontal disease or injury resulting in communication between the oral cavity and a cavity dorsal to the upper fourth premolar tooth of a dog is most likely to lead to formation of:

   a. an oronasal fistula
   b. an oroantral fistula
   c. a periodontal fistula
   d. an endodontic fistula
   e. a gingivobuccal fistula

81. In which species are incisors an open-rooted type of tooth that continually erupts throughout the animal's life?

   a. cats
   b. dogs
   c. rabbits
   d. horses
   e. cattle

For Questions 82 through 84, select the correct answer from the 5 choices below.

   a. composite
   b. acrylic
   c. porcelain
   d. glass ionomer
   e. amalgam

82. Has a silver and mercury base.

83. Most commonly used to treat cervical line lesions in cats.

84. A tooth-colored material commonly used to treat lesions or close access sites in dogs' teeth.

85. Which substance should **not** be used for routine brushing of the teeth of a 14-year-old dog with congestive heart failure?

   a. enzymatic tooth paste
   b. baking soda
   c. 0.12% chlorhexidine gluconate solution
   d. 0.4% stannous fluoride gel
   e. zinc ascorbate solution

86. Enamel hypoplasia of the permanent teeth of dogs may be associated with any of the following **except**:

   a. viral infection
   b. high fever
   c. vitamin C supplementation
   d. trauma
   e. fluorosis

87. An adult dog is presented to you for treatment of a tooth with a broken crown and exposed pulp. The injury occurred several weeks before presentation. What is the most appropriate type of treatment?

   a. composite filling
   b. application of a crown
   c. extraction or root canal therapy
   d. amalgam filling
   e. glass ionomer filling

88. The articulation between the mandible and the skull is termed the:

   a. maxillomandibular joint
   b. temporomandibular joint
   c. premaxillary mandibular joint
   d. incisomaxillary joint
   e. incisomandibular joint

89. All of the following are salivary glands of dogs **except** the:

   a. sublingual salivary gland
   b. mandibular salivary gland
   c. parotid salivary gland
   d. maxillary salivary gland
   e. zygomatic salivary gland

90. The most common malignant oral tumor of dogs is the:

   a. adenosarcoma
   b. squamous-cell carcinoma
   c. fibrosarcoma
   d. mast-cell tumor
   e. melanoma

91. The most common malignant oral tumor of cats is the:

   a. adenocarcinoma
   b. squamous-cell carcinoma
   c. fibrosarcoma
   d. mast-cell tumor
   e. melanoma

Correct answers are on pages 38-40.

92. The most common benign oral tumor of dogs is the:

    a. osseous epulis
    b. papilloma
    c. fibrous epulis
    d. acanthomatous epulis
    e. melanoma

93. All of the following are indications for tooth extraction **except**:

    a. advanced periodontal disease
    b. retained deciduous teeth
    c. abscessed tooth
    d. chipped tooth without pulpal exposure or pulpitis
    e. root fractured near the periodontal sulcus

94. All of the following are considered tumors of dental origin **except** the:

    a. ranula
    b. odontoma
    c. dentigerous cyst
    d. odontogenic cyst
    e. ameloblastoma

95. The cause of cervical line lesions, neck lesions or erosions in the teeth of cats is:

    a. raw meat diet
    b. reflux of gastric acid into the mouth during vomiting of hairballs
    c. high-fiber diet
    d. high-protein diet
    e. unknown

96. The most common oral fracture in cats is fracture of the:

    a. temporomandibular joint
    b. maxillary bone
    c. mandibular symphysis
    d. body of the mandible
    e. ramus of the mandible

Answers

1. **a** These breeds have a long, narrow muzzle.
2. **c** These breeds have a muzzle of medium length and width.
3. **e**
4. **b** These breeds have a short, wide muzzle.
5. **d**
6. **c**
7. **e**
8. **d** Some upper incisors are caudal to the lower incisors.
9. **a**
10. **b**
11. **d**
12. **b**
13. **a**
14. **c**
15. **e** A phenotypically correct dentition consists of a formula of I3, C1, P4, M3 in each of the 4 jaw quadrants. Swine are the most common animals in this classification.
16. **c**
17. **e**
18. **a**
19. **b**
20. **d**
21. **a** Enamel covers the crown of the tooth.
22. **b** Dentin constitutes the bulk of the tooth under the enamel and cementum.
23. **e**
24. **c** This is the neck of the tooth.
25. **e**

26. **b**

27. **d**

28. **c**

29. **a**

30. **e** This inner cavity consists of the root canal (root) and the pulp chamber (crown).

31. **b** The periodontium comprises the supporting structures of the tooth.

32. **b**

33. **a**

34. **d**

35. **c**

36. **e**

37. **d**

38. **b**

39. **c**

40. **e**

41. **a**

42. **d** The periodontal ligament connects the root's cementum to alveolar bone.

43. **a** Epithelium lines the sulcus, producing fluid rich in immunoglobulins.

44. **c** The parakeratinized attached gingiva helps protect the nonkeratinized alveolar mucosa.

45. **c** A curette with a rounded toe is safer to use subgingivally.

46. **e** A sickle scaler with a sharp tip and edges should be used supragingivally.

47. **a** An elevator is used to loosen the periodontal ligament for tooth extraction.

48. **d** An explorer has a sharp, hooked end.

49. **b** A probe is marked in millimeters to measure pockets.

50. **a** Instruments must be sharp to remain effective.

51. **e** This is a hand instrument.

52. **d** This is an ultrasonic scaler.

53. **c**

54. **b**

55. **a**

56. **e**

57. **a**

58. **b** The image does not have the same height as the tooth.

59. **b** Increased dentin narrows the pulp cavity. Older animals have loss of definition of the lamina dura.

60. **e** Over 85% have stage-I or more severe periodontal disease.

61. **d** Bacteria in plaque cause the initial infection.

62. **b** Plaque is associated with bacterial infection.

63. **c** Crowding facilitates retention of plaque and inflammation. Hard, crunchy foods help reduce plaque and calculus accumulation.

64. **e** Root planing involves use of a curette in several different directions to scale the root.

65. **c** Subgingival curettage involves use of a curette to gently remove diseased tissue from the sulcus lining.

66. **b** Sulcular lavage flushes out debris, plaque and prophylaxis paste.

67. **c**

68. **d**

69. **b**

70. **e** Odontoplasty involves restructuring the shape of a tooth.

71. **a**

72. **a**

73. **a**

74. **c**

75. **b**

76. **c**

77. **b**

78. **a** This causes fistulation into the rostral nasal cavity.

79. **a** This causes fistulation into the rostral nasal cavity.

80. **b** This causes fistulation into the maxillary sinus.

81. **c** Lagomorph incisors are continually erupting and open rooted. Horses and cattle have continually erupting cheek teeth.

82. **e**

83. **d** Glass ionomer needs no mechanical undercuts and releases fluoride.

84. **a**

85. **b** Baking soda (sodium bicarbonate) can cause sodium loading.

86. **c** Enamel hypoplasia is caused by insult during tooth development. Vitamin C supplementation should cause no insult.

87. **c** Pulpal tissue exposed for several weeks is infected and necrotic. It should be removed and the cavity filled with inert material or the tooth should be extracted.

88. **b**

89. **d**

90. **e**

91. **b**

92. **c**

93. **d** Without pulpal insult, the tooth should be preserved.

94. **a**

95. **e**

96. **c** Mandibular symphyseal separation is commonly associated with falls in cats.

Notes

Dermatology

K.A. Moriello

Recommended Reading

DeBoer DJ: Advances in clinical dermatology. *Vet Clin No Am* 20:1397-1707, 1990.
Muller GH *et al: Small Animal Dermatology.* 4th ed. Saunders, Philadelphia, 1989.
Willemse T: *Clinical Dermatology of the Dog and Cat.* Lea & Febiger, Philadelphia, 1991.

Practice answer sheet is on page 337.

Questions

1. *Concerning dermatophyte cultures, which statement is **least** accurate?*

   a. Cultures of samples obtained by haircoat brushing with a toothbrush are the most reliable method for cats, especially suspected asymptomatic carriers.

   b. When culturing isolated lesions from dogs, it is best to swab the area with alcohol to minimize the number of contaminant fungi.

   c. A red color change on dermatophyte test medium is diagnostic for a dermatophyte.

   d. Dermatophyte test medium contains Sabouraud's dextrose agar, a pH indicator (phenol red), and antibacterial and antifungal agents.

   e. Fungal pathogens are never heavily pigmented, either macroscopically or microscopically.

2. *Concerning diagnosis of ectoparasitism, which statement is **least** accurate?*

   a. Deep skin scrapings are required to find *Demodex* mites.

   b. Scabies mites may be found on either superficial or deep skin scrapings.

   c. Flea combs are useful for finding fleas, lice and *Cheyletiella* mites.

   d. Ticks are best found using acetate tape (*eg,* Scotch tape) preparations.

   e. Ear mites may be found via direct examination of the ear canal with an otoscope or via microscopic examination of ear debris.

Correct answers are on pages 48-50.

3. Concerning intradermal testing in dogs and cats, which statement is **least** accurate?

   a. Antihistamines and acepromazine may cause a false-negative reaction.
   b. Oral or parenteral glucocorticoids, but not topical glucocorticoids, may cause a false-negative reaction.
   c. Fear, pseudopregnancy or estrus may cause a false-negative reaction.
   d. Inflammation associated with severe superficial pyoderma may cause a false-positive reaction.
   e. Testing with antigen mixtures, outdated allergens or overdilute allergen concentrations may cause a false-negative reaction.

4. Concerning the haircoat of dogs and cats, which statement is **least** accurate?

   a. Shedding occurs in a mosaic pattern in dogs and cats.
   b. The cycle of hair growth and shedding is controlled by photoperiod, ambient temperature, nutrition, hormones, genetics and the general state of health.
   c. Cats and dogs have simple hair follicles.
   d. The growing period of a hair is called anagen.
   e. The resting period of a hair is called telogen.

5. Concerning the structure and function of the skin in dogs and cats, which statement is **least** accurate?

   a. Langhans' cells are part of the skin pigmentary system.
   b. The epidermis of dogs and cats is thinner than that of people.
   c. Melanocytes are fewer in number in feline skin than in canine skin.
   d. Cats and dogs do not have eccrine sweat glands in haired skin.
   e. The tail gland (supracaudal gland, preen gland) in dogs and cats produces an oily substance believed to be important in olfactory recognition.

6. Which organism is the primary pathogen of pyoderma in dogs?

   a. Staphylococcus intermedius
   b. Staphylococcus hyicus
   c. Staphylococcus aureus
   d. Staphylococcus epidermidis
   e. Staphylococcus xylosus

7. "Hot spots" are intensely pruritic areas of self-trauma. Concerning pyotraumatic dermatitis or "hot spots," which statement is **least** accurate?

   a. Flea infestation, ear mite infestation, atopy and anal sac problems are possible underlying causes of pyotraumatic dermatitis.
   b. Dogs with recurrent areas of pyotraumatic dermatitis, especially on the face, may be atopic.
   c. "Hot spots" in dogs with a thick or long haircoat (eg, Golden Retrievers) are treated differently than those in short-haired dogs.
   d. Staphylococcus intermedius is the bacterium most commonly isolated from the lesions.
   e. Glucocorticoids and topical astringents are the treatments of choice for "hot spots."

8. Concerning treatment of bacterial folliculitis, superficial pyoderma or impetigo in dogs, which statement is **least** accurate?

   a. Concurrent use of antibiotics with glucocorticoids is contraindicated.
   b. Superficial pyoderma should be treated for at least 3-4 weeks or at least 1 week after clinical resolution of lesions.
   c. Tetracycline, ampicillin and gentamicin are suitable for treatment of staphylococcal infections.
   d. Topical antibacterial shampoos, such as benzoyl peroxide or chlorhexidine, are useful adjuvant antibacterial therapies.
   e. Recurrent bacterial infections indicate an underlying cause of the pyoderma, such as atopy or hypothyroidism.

9. The most common underlying cause of deep pyoderma in dogs is:

   a. demodicosis
   b. dermatophytosis

c. inadequately treated superficial pyoderma

d. *Proteus* infection

e. hypothyroidism

10. Which of the following is the **least** likely cause of a nonhealing wound on the thorax of a cat?

a. sporotrichosis

b. atypical mycobacterial infection

c. *Actinomyces* infection

d. nocardiosis

e. demodicosis

11. Of the following sets of diseases and causative microorganisms, which set is **incorrect**?

a. cat bite abscess, *Pasteurella multocida*

b. feline dermatophytosis, *Microsporum canis*

c. bubonic plague, *Yersinia pestis*

d. Lyme disease, *Ixodes dammini*

e. bacterial granulomas (botryomycosis), coagulase-positive staphylococci

12. Concerning viral, rickettsial and protozoal skin diseases of small animals, which statement is **least** accurate?

a. Cutaneous manifestations of feline immunodeficiency virus infection include pustular dermatitis, gingivitis and stomatitis.

b. Lesions of feline poxvirus infection most commonly involve the face, limbs and paws, and consist of crusted papules, plaques and nodules.

c. Rocky Mountain spotted fever (*Rickettsia rickettsii* infection) should be included in the differential diagnoses for dogs with diffuse erythema, petechiation, and necrosis and ulceration of the mucous membranes.

d. A clinical sign of toxoplasmosis in cats is cutaneous nodules on the legs.

e. Leishmaniasis is an exfoliative dermatitis of the face, feet and pinnae of dogs. It is characterized by silver-white, asbestos-like scales in areas of alopecia, depigmentation of the nose, long brittle nails and cutaneous nodules, and has not been observed in the United States.

13. Which of the following is **not** a superficial mycosis of cats or dogs?

a. *Microsporum canis* or *Microsporum gypseum* infection

b. candidiasis

c. otic *Malassezia* infection

d. cutaneous *Malassezia* infection

e. sporotrichosis

14. Dermatophytosis is common in cats but uncommon in dogs. Many cases of so-called dermatophytosis in dogs are actually:

a. superficial staphylococcal pyoderma

b. seborrhea

c. flea-allergy dermatitis

d. zinc deficiency

e. pemphigus foliaceus

15. A trauma-induced chronic subcutaneous nodule-mass with a fistulous tract that contains granules is known as:

a. a kerion

b. a mycetoma

c. a foreign body

d. phaeohyphomycosis

e. a histiocytoma

16. Of the following sets of diseases and forms of therapy, which set is **incorrect**?

a. sporotrichosis, sodium or potassium iodide

b. blastomycosis, ketoconazole and/or amphotericin B

c. feline dermatophytosis, lime sulfur or chlorhexidine dips

d. pythiosis, ketoconazole

e. cutaneous *Malassezia* infection, selenium disulfide shampoo and/or ketoconazole

17. A dog has extreme pruritus of the feet, with some footpads crusted and some not crusted. The **least** likely cause of these signs is:

a. hookworm dermatitis

b. *Pelodera* dermatitis

c. irritant contact reaction

d. contact allergy

e. biotin deficiency

Correct answers are on pages 48-50.

18. Of the following sets of common names and scientific names, which set is **incorrect**?

    a. spinous ear tick, *Otobius megnini*
    b. brown dog tick, *Rhipicephalus sanguineus*
    c. American dog tick, *Dermacentor variabilis*
    d. Rocky Mountain wood tick, *Dermacentor andersoni*
    e. deer tick, *Ixodes scapularis*

19. Concerning mite infestations in cats and dogs, which statement is **least** accurate?

    a. Cheyletiellosis is characterized by scaling, with or without pruritus.
    b. Scabies in dogs is an intensely pruritic skin disease with a predilection for thinly haired areas of the body.
    c. *Otodectes* infestations in cats and dogs require treatment of the ears and the body for eradication.
    d. Demodicosis is a contagious mite infestation.
    e. Notoedric mange in cats has a predilection for the head, and mites are easily found on skin scrapings.

20. Concerning demodicosis in dogs and cats, which statement is **least** accurate?

    a. Most cases of localized demodicosis in dogs resolve without treatment.
    b. Amitraz is the drug of choice for treatment of generalized demodicosis in dogs.
    c. Dogs with generalized demodicosis should not be bred because the tendency to develop generalized demodicosis is heritable.
    d. Most cases of adult-onset demodicosis in cats are associated with underlying disease, such as diabetes mellitus.
    e. Adult-onset demodicosis in dogs usually stems from an untreated or unrecognized case of juvenile demodicosis.

21. Which of the following has **not** been implicated in the pathogenesis of flea-allergy dermatitis?

    a. Type-1 hypersensitivity
    b. Type-4 hypersensitivity
    c. late-phase immediate hypersensitivity reactions
    d. cutaneous basophil hypersensitivity
    e. Type-3 reactions

22. Concerning use of direct immunofluorescence testing for diagnosis of autoimmune skin diseases in dogs and cats, which statement is **least** accurate?

    a. It is the test of choice for diagnosis of autoimmune skin diseases.
    b. Tissues for direct immunofluorescence testing can be preserved in Michel's fixative or liquid nitrogen.
    c. Specimens preserved in Michel's fixative or liquid nitrogen cannot be used for routine histopathologic examination.
    d. Samples from primary lesions are required for diagnosis.
    e. False-positive reactions may ocur in some inflammatory or neoplastic skin diseases.

23. Concerning atopy in dogs or cats, which statement is **least** accurate?

    a. Atopy is a familial disease with definite breed predispositions in dogs, such as terriers.
    b. Atopic animals typically show facial, pedal, axillary and inguinal pruritus, but some dogs may show only pruritus of the ears.
    c. Clinical signs may be seasonal or nonseasonal.
    d. The primary skin lesions in atopy are hair loss, superficial pyoderma, miliary dermatitis and seborrhea.

24. Concerning food allergy in dogs and cats, which statement is **least** accurate?

    a. Food allergies are immunologically mediated.
    b. Food allergies appear to be more common in cats than in dogs.
    c. Food allergies may involve cutaneous, respiratory and/or gastrointestinal signs.
    d. Food allergies are diagnosed reliably by radioallergosorbent testing or enzyme-linked immunosorbent assay of serum.
    e. The pruritus of food allergy responds poorly to glucocorticoids.

25. A 6-year-old Persian cat is depressed, slightly anorectic and lame. Findings of physical examination are unremarkable except for the skin. You find marked crusting of the inner aspect of the pinnae, intact pustules, periocular and nasal crusting, and exudative paronychia. The haircoat is matted, with marked exfoliation. Results of a complete blood count, serum chemistry panel and urinalysis are within normal limits. An antinuclear antibody test is negative. Cytologic examination of the contents of an intact pustule reveals full fields of neutrophils, no bacteria, and rafts of acantholytic cells. Histopathologic examination reveals subcorneal and intragranular pustular dermatitis, with acantholysis but no evidence of bacteria. Direct immunofluorescence testing reveals deposition of immunoglobulins intercellularly. The most likely cause of these findings is:

   a. systemic lupus erythematosus
   b. pemphigus foliaceus
   c. discoid lupus erythematosus
   d. pemphigus vulgaris
   e. drug eruption

26. Which disease is **not** usually associated with generalized mucocutaneous ulceration?

   a. discoid lupus erythematosus
   b. mucocutaneous candidiasis
   c. bullous pemphigoid
   d. systemic lupus erythematosus
   e. graft vs host disease

27. Concerning eosinophilic granuloma complex in cats, which statement is **least** accurate?

   a. The treatment of choice is levamisole.
   b. Linear granuloma is the only form of this complex that is a true granulomatous skin disease.
   c. Recurrent eosinophilic plaques are often a manifestation of atopy and/or flea-allergy dermatitis.
   d. Squamous-cell carcinomas may develop at the margin of indolent ulcers.
   e. Peripheral eosinophilia does not always accompany lesion development.

28. Which hormone initiates anagen in hair follicles?

   a. estrogen
   b. thyroxine
   c. testosterone
   d. cortisol
   e. insulin

29. The most definitive test for thyroid disease in dogs is:

   a. total baseline thyroid hormone concentrations
   b. free serum thyroxine (T_4) and triiodothyronine (T_3) concentrations
   c. thyroid-stimulating hormone response test
   d. thyroid biopsy
   e. thyrotropin-releasing hormone response test

30. An 8-year-old male Golden Retriever is presented for evaluation of recurrent superficial pyoderma. The dog is only pruritic when the pyoderma is present, and the pyoderma always responds to antibiotics. A review of the case history indicates that the appropriate drug, dosage and treatment length have been used. The pyoderma recurs within 2-3 months of discontinuation of the antibiotic regimen. The dog is slightly obese and the haircoat is normal. Which test is **not** indicated in the initial diagnostic evaluation of this patient?

   a. complete blood count
   b. serum chemistry profile
   c. intradermal test
   d. thyroid function evaluation
   e. skin biopsy

31. Which of the following is **not** a cutaneous sign of hyperadrenocorticism in cats or dogs?

   a. calcinosis cutis
   b. thin, fragile skin
   c. symmetric alopecia
   d. hypertrichosis
   e. comedones

Correct answers are on pages 48-50.

32. *Growth hormone-responsive alopecia is diagnosed by:*

    a. xylazine response test
    b. dexamethasone response test
    c. baseline serum growth hormone concentrations
    d. ACTH response test
    e. high-dosage dexamethasone response test

33. *Concerning dermatoses related to sex hormones in dogs, which statement is **least** accurate?*

    a. Hyperestrogenism is used to describe a syndrome of vulvar enlargement, gynecomastia, bilaterally symmetric alopecia and abnormal estrous cycles; the treatment of choice is ovariohysterectomy.
    b. Estrogen-responsive dermatosis is used to describe bilaterally symmetric alopecia in the genital and perineal regions of spayed bitches. This alopecia may become generalized. The vulva and nipples are infantile.
    c. Male feminization occurs in male dogs with certain types of Sertoli-cell tumors and is characterized by bilaterally symmetric alopecia, gynecomastia, a pendulous prepuce and attraction of other male dogs.
    d. Testosterone-responsive dermatosis is usually seen in older castrated dogs. Bilaterally symmetric alopecia in the perineal and genital regions may progress to involve the trunk and legs.
    e. The test of choice for sex hormone-related dermatoses is measurement of serum or plasma concentrations of androgens, estrogens and progesterone.

34. *The drug of choice for thyroid hormone replacement in dogs and cats is:*

    a. thyroxine and triiodothyronine
    b. thyroxine
    c. desiccated thyroid
    d. triiodothyronine
    e. dietary supplementation of iodine

35. *Cutaneous asthenia is characterized by:*

    a. alopecia
    b. abnormal skin elasticity and fragility
    c. exfoliation
    d. abnormal haircoat shedding and hair replacement
    e. hyperesthesia and self-trauma

36. *Concerning dermatomyositis in dogs, which statement is **least** accurate?*

    a. The disease has a hereditary component.
    b. It has been documented in Collies and Shetland Sheepdogs.
    c. It resolves with large doses of glucocorticoids.
    d. Skin lesions consist of hair loss, crusting, papules and pigmentary changes on the face, ear tips, tail, sides of the paws, and stifle. Lesions may be transient or permanent.
    e. Muscle signs may or may not be clinically evident. Temporal muscle atrophy, difficulty in eating, megaesophagus and stunted growth may be seen.

37. *Concerning color-dilution alopecia, which statement is **least** accurate?*

    a. The disease is hereditary.
    b. It has been documented in blue, red and fawn Doberman Pinschers, blue Dachshunds, Chow Chows, Standard Poodles, blue Great Danes, Italian Greyhounds and Whippets.
    c. The defect in melanization and critical structure of the hair results in abnormal hair color.
    d. Clinical signs include papules, cystic hair follicles, alopecia, seborrhea and recurrent pyoderma.
    e. Clinical signs are evident within the first year of life.

38. *Concerning pigmentary diseases of dogs and cats, which statement is **least** accurate?*

    a. Albinism is a hereditary lack of pigment that is transmitted as a recessive trait.

b. Siamese, Himalayan, Balinese and Burmese cats exhibit acromelanism.

c. Lentigo in orange cats is a benign condition characterized by asymptomatic macular melanosis.

d. Hyperpigmentation in the skin may be caused by inflammation, trauma or endocrine diseases.

e. Vogt-Koyanagi-Harada syndrome is a hereditary syndrome in Persian cats with yellow eyes and blue smoke color. Affected cats have a bleeding disorder and are predisposed to infections.

39. *Concerning primary seborrhea and secondary seborrhea in dogs, which statement is most accurate?*

a. Primary seborrhea is pruritic, while secondary seborrhea is not pruritic.

b. Primary seborrhea is a disorder of keratinization inherent to the epidermal cells.

c. Primary seborrhea is generally greasy, while secondary seborrhea is exfoliative.

d. Secondary seborrhea is an inherited exfoliative condition that occurs primarily in Arctic breeds of dogs.

e. Secondary seborrhea is usually treated with dietary zinc supplementation and lime sulfur dips.

40. *Which topical agent acts to "poison" the basal epidermal cells and thereby helps to reestablish normal keratinization?*

a. tar
b. sulfur
c. salicylic acid
d. benzoyl peroxide
e. selenium disulfide

41. *Concerning acne on the skin of cats, which statement is **least** accurate?*

a. It is characterized by comedones on the chin and lip margins.

b. Unlike the syndrome in dogs and people, this condition tends to occur most commonly in adult cats.

c. Severely affected cats may develop suppurative folliculitis and furunculosis requiring antibiotic therapy.

d. Lesions should be scraped for *Demodex* mites, a fungal culture should be performed to rule out dermatophytosis, and cytologic examination of follicular debris should be performed to rule out bacterial or yeast infections.

e. It must be treated to prevent complications.

42. *The cause of endocrine alopecia in cats is:*

a. thyroid hormone insufficiency
b. cortisol excess
c. estrogen insufficiency
d. progesterone excess
e. unrelated to hormonal imbalance

43. *Which of the following has **not** been associated with zinc-responsive dermatoses in dogs?*

a. oversupplementation of young growing dogs with vitamins and minerals

b. diets with high calcium levels or a high proportion of cereal grains

c. prolonged enteritis or diarrhea

d. generic dog food with a high phytate content or poor nutritional composition

e. hereditary predisposition in Dachshunds and Collies

44. *Which of the following is **least** likely to cause bilateral chronic otitis externa in dogs?*

a. atopy
b. food allergy
c. foreign body
d. seborrheic dermatitis
e. pemphigus foliaceus

Correct answers are on pages 48-50.

45. A 12-week-old Labrador Retriever puppy is extremely depressed and anorectic. It has a rectal temperature of 104.5 F and the skin is painful to the touch. The ears, face and muzzle are swollen, and intact vesicles and pustules are present. There is periocular swelling and ulceration. Marked generalized lymphade-nopathy is present and numerous lymph nodes have abscessed. Nodular draining lesions are present on the trunk. According to the owner, lesions developed 4 days after vaccination. A complete blood count reveals leukocytosis and neutrophilia. Lymph node aspiration reveals suppurative inflammation. Cytologic examination of material from a pustule shows degenerative neutrophils but no bacteria. A skin scraping is negative for Demodex mites. The most likely cause of these findings is:

   a. occult juvenile demodicosis
   b. juvenile cellulitis
   c. septicemia
   d. systemic lupus erythematosus
   e. drug reaction

46. What is the treatment of choice for viral papillomatosis in dogs?

   a. benign neglect (no treatment)
   b. excision
   c. crushing or traumatizing several lesions in an attempt to cause regression of other lesions
   d. intralesional glucocorticoids
   e. autogenous wart vaccine

47. A 10-year-old white cat is presented to you for examination. The cat's ear margins are red, crusty, ulcerative and bleeding. Closer examination reveals small ulcers and proliferative masses on the cat's nose. The most likely cause of these lesions is:

   a. basal-cell tumor
   b. squamous-cell carcinoma
   c. mast-cell tumor
   d. seborrheic dermatitis
   e. sunburn

48. Which of the following is **not** a common skin tumor of cats?

   a. basal-cell carcinoma
   b. squamous-cell carcinoma
   c. fibrosarcoma
   d. mast-cell tumor
   e. lipoma

49. What is the most common skin tumor of dogs?

   a. lipoma
   b. mast-cell tumor
   c. squamous-cell tumor
   d. sebaceous-gland adenoma with hyperplasia
   e. papilloma

50. Which skin tumor is most likely to resolve without treatment?

   a. histiocytoma in a 6-month-old dog
   b. sebaceous adenoma in a 12-year-old Poodle
   c. mast-cell tumor in a 14-year-old cat
   d. intracutaneous cornifying epithelioma in a Norwegian Elkhound
   e. trichoepithelioma in a cat

Answers

1. **c** The red color indicator in dermatophyte test medium is not diagnostic for a pathogen. It only indicates that the organism is using the protein in the agar. Definitive diagnosis of a dermatophyte infection requires microscopic examination of the specimen.

2. **d** Ticks are best found by direct visualization of the parasite. Many ticks are found by palpation of the skin.

3. **b** Topical (ocular, otic, cutaneous) glucocorticoid preparations can cause false-negative skin test reactions.

4. **c** Cats and dogs have compound hair follicles, consisting of a large guard hair surrounded by secondary hairs. Horses and cattle have simple hair follicles.

5. **a** Langhans' cells are important immune cells in the skin.

6. **a** *Staphylococcus intermedius* was once classified as *Staphylococcus aureus*. New techniques in bacterial identification have determined that dogs have a special species of staphylococcal organisms different from *Staphylococcus aureus*.

7. **e** "Hot spots" are areas of bacterial infection and require antibiotic therapy, especially in long-haired dogs. These lesions are best treated with at least 3 weeks of antibiotic therapy. In some instances, a short (1- to 3-day) course of glucocorticoid therapy may be needed while the cause of pruritus is treated, *eg*, fleas. Astringents are best avoided in treatment of these lesions, as they impede wound healing and epithelialization of the lesion. The area should be kept clean with an antibacterial scrub and kept moist with an antibacterial cream.

8. **c** These drugs are unsuitable for treatment of bacterial infections. Tetracycline and ampicillin are rarely effective. Gentamicin cannot be administered for long enough periods without adverse effects.

9. **a** Demodicosis is the most common cause.

10. **e** Demodicosis in cats does not cause deep pyoderma or nonhealing wounds.

11. **d** *Ixodes dammini* is a tick that acts as the vector for the causative agent of Lyme disease, *Borrelia burgdorferi*.

12. **e** Leishmaniasis is enzootic in certain areas of Texas and Oklahoma. This disease is of extreme zoonotic importance.

13. **e** Sporotrichosis is an intermediate mycosis. Animals are infected by traumatic inoculation of the organism into the skin.

14. **a** Bacterial pyoderma in dogs commonly appears as circular areas of hair loss and scaling. These lesions are commonly misdiagnosed as dermatophytosis.

15. **b** Mycetomas are characterized by cold, subcutaneous swellings with draining fistulous tracts containing granules. They can resemble bacterial granulomas or botryomycosis.

16. **d** Pythiosis is not susceptible to commonly used antifungal agents. Currently, amputation or euthanasia is recommended.

17. **e** Zinc deficiency is the most common nutritional cause of crusted footpad lesions. The pruritus in zinc deficiency is due to secondary bacterial skin infection. Biotin deficiencies have only been reported experimentally.

18. **e** *Ixodes dammini* is the deer tick.

19. **d** Demodicosis in dogs is not considered a contagious mite infestation. Mites are transmitted during the first few days of life.

20. **e** Adult-onset demodicosis refers to development of clinical demodicosis in an adult dog with no prior history of demodicosis. Usually some underlying systemic disease debilitates the dog and allows development of demodicosis.

21. **e** Type-3 reactions are antigen-antibody reactions and are not involved in the pathogenesis of flea-bite hypersensitivity.

22. **a** Direct immunofluorescence testing is supportive but not diagnostic of autoimmune skin disease. Histopathologic examination of skin biopsy specimens is the most useful diagnostic test.

23. **d** Primary skin lesions in atopy are rare. Alopecia, superficial pyoderma and seborrhea are all secondary to the self-trauma associated with the pruritus that accompanies this disease.

24. **d** Food allergies are diagnosed by food elimination trials.

25. **b** The clinical signs, histopathologic findings and results of direct immunofluorescence testing are most consistent with pemphigus foliaceus.

26. **a** Discoid lupus erythematosus is primarily a depigmenting disease of the nose of dogs. Bilateral nasal ulceration may occur, but generalized mucocutaneous ulceration is extremely rare.

27. **a** This disease complex may be caused by any number of allergic diseases. It is best to determine and treat the underlying cause of the pruritus, *eg*, food allergy, atopy, flea allergy. If antiinflammatory drugs are required, glucocorticoids should be given.

28. **b** Thyroxine and its metabolites initiate hair growth (anagen) in hair follicles.

29. **d** Though it is invasive, thyroid biopsy is the best method of evaluating the function and structure of a dog's thyroid gland.

30. **c** Because this patient is only pruritic when the pyoderma is present, the pruritus is due to the secondary superficial pyoderma. At this point, an intradermal test is not indicated because an underlying pruritic cause of the pyoderma is not suspected. The other diagnostic tests will assist in identifying a nonpruritic underlying cause of recurrent pyoderma.

31. **d** Hypertrichosis is the most common clinical sign of hyperadrenocorticism in horses but not in dogs or cats.

32. **a** Intravenous xylazine causes a release of growth hormone in dogs. In deficient dogs, no increase in growth hormone levels is noted.

33. **e** Serum sex hormone concentrations do not correlate with clinical signs and/or the responsiveness of these animals to neutering or hormone replacement. The dysfunction is believed to be at the cell receptor level or due to an abnormal metabolite of the hormone.

34. **b** Thyroxine (T4) is the drug of choice for treatment of hypothyroidism. Though triiodothyronine (T3) is the active form, supplementation with T3 results in peripheral hyperthyroidism and central hypothyroidism due to idiosyncrasies of metabolism.

35. **b** Cutaneous asthenia is an inherited collagen defect that results in abnormally loose and extendable skin. Affected animals are unsuitable as pets because of impaired wound healing.

36. **c** There is no effective treatment for this disease. Affected dogs should not be bred.

37. **e** Clinical signs do not develop until the animal is at least 3 years of age.

38. **e** The syndrome described is Chediak-Higashi syndrome. Vogt-Koyanagi-Harada syndrome is an autoimmune skin disease of dogs that is characterized by uveitis and depigmentation of the lips, gum, nose and eyelid margins.

39. **b**

40. **a** Tar acts as a cellular poison that slows epidermal proliferation, thereby "normalizing" keratinization.

41. **e** Not all affected animals should be treated. If the lesions are not severe, no treatment is necessary. There is no evidence that early or aggressive treatment alters the course of the disease. Cats with severe folliculitis/furunculosis should be treated with topical hot packs and a course of systemic antibiotic therapy.

42. **e** "Feline endocrine alopecia" is a misnomer. There is no documented hormonal excess or deficiency. Many cases of symmetric alopecia are caused by pruritus, while others are a behavioral "overgrooming" disorder.

43. **e** Zinc-responsive dermatosis is hereditary in Siberian Huskies and Alaskan Malamutes, and requires lifelong therapy in these dogs. With the other 4 causes, therapy may be temporary, depending upon whether the underlying cause can be eliminated.

44. **c** The other conditions listed almost always cause bilateral otitis externa. Unilateral otitis externa is more likely to occur with a foreign body.

45. **b** Juvenile cellulitis is an idiopathic skin disease of young dogs. The lesions are almost always sterile and affected dogs do not respond to antibiotic therapy. Corticosteroids are used in treatment.

46. **a** Viral papillomatosis is a self-limiting disease of puppies. Most lesions spontaneously regress and require no medical intervention. If breathing or eating is affected, lesions should be excised. Autogenous vaccines should be avoided because skin tumors often develop at the site of injection.

47. **b** Squamous-cell carcinoma is the most likely cause. The lesions have become ulcera- tive and destructive, suggesting an active neoplasm. Cats with sunburn exhibit erythema without destructive ulcerative lesions.

48. **e** Unlike dogs, cats rarely develop lipomas.

49. **a**

50. **a** Histiocytomas are benign self-limiting tumors that resolve without treatment.

Section 6

Hematology

S.M. Cotter, W.J. Dodds

Recommended Reading

Cotter SM: Clinical transfusion medicine. *Adv Vet Sci Comp Med* 36:188-224, 1991.
Duncan JR and Prasse KW: *Veterinary Laboratory Medicine.* 2nd ed. Iowa State University Press, Ames, 1986.
Ettinger S: *Textbook of Veterinary Internal Medicine.* 3rd ed. Saunders, Philadelphia, 1990.
Jain NC *et al: Schalm's Veterinary Hematology.* 4th ed. Lea & Febiger, Philadelphia, 1986.
Kaneko JJ: *Clinical Biochemistry of Domestic Animals.* 4th ed. Academic Press, New York, 1989.
Young KM *et al*, in Morgan RV: *Handbook of Small Animal Practice.* 2nd ed. Churchill Livingstone, New York, 1992.
Meyers JR *et al: Veterinary Laboratory Medicine.* Saunders, Philadelphia, 1992.

> **Practice answer sheet is on page 339.**

Questions

1. Smears of blood from dogs with autoimmune hemolytic anemia often show:

    a. rouleaux formation
    b. spherocytosis
    c. Heinz bodies
    d. elliptocytosis
    e. hypochromasia

2. The red blood cells of animals with iron-deficiency anemia are classically:

    a. hyperchromic and normocytic
    b. polychromatophilic
    c. hypochromic and macrocytic
    d. hypochromic and microcytic
    e. hypochromic and normocytic

3. The nonregenerative anemia that accompanies chronic renal failure is caused by:

    a. chronic blood loss
    b. erythropoietin deficiency
    c. erythrophagocytosis
    d. elevated blood urea nitrogen
    e. hypoparathyroidism

4. A common cause of chronic blood loss anemia in young animals is:

    a. parasitism (fleas, hookworms)
    b. rodenticide toxicosis (warfarin)
    c. primary bleeding disorder
    d. immune-mediated hemolytic disease
    e. copper deficiency

Correct answers are on pages 57-58.

5. *Basophilic stippling of erythrocytes is characteristic of:*

   a. magnesium poisoning
   b. copper toxicosis
   c. lead poisoning
   d. hemobartonellosis
   e. babesiosis

6. *The cause of feline infectious anemia is:*

   a. feline leukemia virus
   b. coronavirus
   c. parvovirus
   d. *Hemobartonella felis*
   e. feline immunodeficiency virus

7. *Dehydration is characterized by:*

   a. increased packed cell volume and decreased plasma protein level
   b. decreased packed cell volume and decreased plasma protein level
   c. decreased packed cell volume and increased plasma protein level
   d. increased packed cell volume and normal plasma protein level
   e. increased packed cell volume and increased plasma protein level

8. *The "LE cell" is characteristic of:*

   a. acute leukemia
   b. chronic leukemia
   c. Hodgkin's disease
   d. systemic lupus erythematosus
   e. lymphosarcoma

9. *Monocytosis is a characteristic sign of:*

   a. systemic toxicity
   b. severe viral disease
   c. severe parasitic infection
   d. acute lymphoblastic leukemia
   e. systemic inflamatory response

10. *Cyclic hematopoiesis of gray Collie dogs is characterized by:*

   a. cyclic thrombocytosis
   b. cyclic leukocytosis
   c. cyclic neutropenia
   d. intermittent polycythemia
   e. erythrophagocytosis

11. *The congenital, hereditary anemia of Basenji dogs is called:*

   a. glucose-6-phosphate dehydrogenase deficiency
   b. phosphofructokinase deficiency
   c. porphyria
   d. pyruvate kinase deficiency
   e. methemoglobinemia

12. *Tropical pancytopenia is a tick-borne rickettsial infection known as:*

   a. babesiosis
   b. ehrlichiosis
   c. trypanosomiasis
   d. piroplasmosis
   e. anaplasmosis

13. *The most common severe inherited coagulation defect of companion animals is:*

   a. hemophilia A
   b. von Willebrand's disease
   c. factor X deficiency
   d. Christmas disease
   e. factor XII deficiency

14. *The most common inherited bleeding disorder of people and dogs is:*

   a. thrombocytopenic purpura
   b. von Willebrand's disease
   c. hemophilia
   d. factor VII deficiency
   e. factor X deficiency

15. *A common cause of bleeding tendency in aged patients is:*

   a. rodenticide toxicosis (warfarin)
   b. capillary fragility

c. platelet dysfunction secondary to uremia (end-stage kidney disease)

d. hepatosplenomegaly secondary to production of defective red blood cells

e. cardiopulmonary failure

16. *Adverse effects of trimethoprim-sulfa antibacterials include bleeding tendency because they:*

a. inhibit vitamin K-dependent clotting factors

b. enhance fibrinolysis

c. cause thrombocytopenia and platelet dysfunction

d. sterilize the bowel

e. impair production of von Willebrand factor

17. *The recently developed second-generation rodenticides are more toxic because they:*

a. affect platelet function as well as coagulation

b. affect coagulation and fibrinolysis

c. are more potent and slowly metabolized

d. are more potent and rapidly metabolized

e. are hepatotoxic

18. *Patients with hypothyroidism have a bleeding tendency primarily related to:*

a. altered hepatic protein synthesis

b. reduced platelet function and von Willebrand factor activity

c. capillary fragility

d. chronic intravascular coagulation

e. hyperactive fibrinolysis

19. *Parvovirus infection in people and animals can produce:*

a. septic arthritis

b. urticaria

c. abruptio placentae

d. muscle atrophy

e. transient bone marrow failure

20. *Coagulation profiles performed in animals with liver disease typically show:*

a. low von Willebrand factor activity

b. reduced fibrinolysis

c. elevated prothrombin time

d. thrombocytosis

e. hypercoagulability

21. *Inherited platelet function defects have been recognized in:*

a. German Shepherds and Doberman Pinschers

b. Beagles and Basenjis

c. Otterhounds and Basset Hounds

d. Poodles and Cocker Spaniels

e. Lhasa Apsos and Keeshonds

22. *The dog breed most commonly affected with von Willebrand's disease is the:*

a. Scottish Terrier

b. Shetland Sheepdog

c. Standard Poodle

d. Doberman Pinscher

e. Akita

23. *A typical sign of thrombocytopenic bleeding is:*

a. hematoma formation and joint pain

b. epistaxis and exercise intolerance

c. petechiae and ecchymoses

d. melena and retinal hemorrhage

e. hematuria and splenomegaly

24. *Aspirin is used to prevent and treat thrombosis because it:*

a. impairs coagulation

b. impairs platelet function

c. enhances fibrinolysis

d. stimulates thrombopoiesis

e. produces thrombocytopenia

25. *The most common cause of chronic recurrent thrombocytopenia is:*

a. onion poisoning

b. parvoviral infection

c. adverse reaction to modified-live-virus vaccine

d. bone marrow failure

e. immune-mediated disease

Correct answers are on pages 57-58.

26. If a hemophiliac male is bred to an unrelated normal female, the proportion of offspring that would show signs of bleeding is:

a. one-quarter
b. none
c. all of the males
d. all
e. one-half

27. A 1-year-old Collie was found lying on the porch after being outside unattended for 2 hours. The dog is pale and blood is obtained on abdominocentesis. The packed cell volume is 35%, platelet count is 150,000/μl (normal is 200,000-400,000/μl), prothrombin time is 12 seconds (control, 11 seconds), and activated partial thromboplastin time is 17 seconds (control, 18 seconds). Fibrin split products are not detected. The most likely cause for the bleeding is:

a. warfarin toxicity
b. immune-mediated thrombocytopenia
c. von Willebrand's disease
d. bleeding from trauma, with normal coagulation
e. disseminated intravascular coagulation

28. All of the following signs may occur in cats with acetaminophen toxicity except:

a. facial edema
b. Heinz-body formation
c. hepatic necrosis
d. aplastic anemia
e. hemolytic anemia

29. A 5-year-old spayed Poodle has petechiae on the gums and ventral abdomen. Following venipuncture, the dog bleeds for a prolonged period, but once bleeding ceases it does not recur. These findings suggest a defect in which component of the hemostatic mechanism?

a. extrinsic pathway factors
b. plasminogen
c. antithrombin III
d. platelets
e. fibrinogen

30. To evaluate a patient's hemostatic mechanism, which anticoagulant is routinely used?

a. citrate
b. EDTA
c. sodium heparin
d. cumarin
e. lithium heparin

31. Which mechanism best explains interference with platelet function by aspirin?

a. prevention of adherence of platelets to collagen
b. decreased synthesis of thromboxane (TXA_2)
c. immune-mediated platelet lysis
d. increased synthesis of prostacyclin (PGI_2)
e. blocked binding of fibrin to platelet phospholipid

32. Which hematopoietic growth factor has proven beneficial to patients with renal failure?

a. interleukin-3
b. interleukin-2
c. granulocyte, monocyte colony-stimulating factor
d. thrombopoietin
e. erythropoietin

33. The best stain to demonstrate reticulocytes is:

a. Wright's
b. Giemsa
c. new methylene blue
d. hematoxylin
e. any Romanowsky stain

34. When the mean corpuscular volume (MCV) is decreased in an anemic animal, the most likely cause is:

a. immune-mediated hemolytic anemia
b. nonregenerative anemia from any cause
c. iron deficiency
d. myelodysplasia
e. Heinz-body anemia

35. Which of the following is **not** likely to be found in urine described as dark or red?

    a. unconjugated bilirubin
    b. conjugated bilirubin
    c. urobilinogen
    d. hemoglobin
    e. red blood cells

36. A complete blood count in a dog shows packed cell volume 35%, WBC count 1800/μl, 10% neutrophils, 50% lymphocytes, 20% monocytes and 20% eosinophils. The most **significant** abnormality in this hemogram is:

    a. eosinophilia
    b. neutropenia
    c. lymphocytosis
    d. monocytosis
    e. anemia

37. Addison's disease (hypoadrenocorticism) is a condition in which the adrenal cortex is unable to produce sufficient glucocorticoids and mineralocorticoids. Considering the effects of corticosteroids on the hemogram, what would you expect to see in an animal with Addison's disease?

    a. neutrophilia
    b. lymphopenia
    c. eosinophilia
    d. monocytosis
    e. thrombocytopenia

38. The stimulus for movement of granulocytes from the marginal pool to the circulating pool is:

    a. granulocyte colony-stimulating factor
    b. complement
    c. immunoglobulin
    d. corticosteroid
    e. epinephrine

39. A 4-month-old male Dachshund is presented because of lameness and swollen joints. Joint aspiration produces bloody fluid. You order a coagulation screen, the results of which are normal except for prolonged prothrombin time and activated partial thromboplastin time.

Which of the following has **not** been ruled out by these findings?

    a. von Willebrand's disease
    b. hemophilia A
    c. hemophilia B
    d. factor VII deficiency
    e. factor V deficiency

40. Hemoglobinuria in an anemic animal indicates:

    a. IgM on red cells
    b. circulating immune complexes
    c. renal glomerular damage
    d. intravascular hemolysis
    e. decreased hepatic conjugation of bilirubin

41. What is the mechanism of action of corticosteroids in treatment of autoimmune hemolytic anemia?

    a. they suppress erythrophagocytosis and antibody binding
    b. they bind to antibodies to block binding sites
    c. they suppress chemotaxis and neutrophil function
    d. they suppress release of IgG from plasma cells
    e. they bind to macrophages to prevent attachment to antibodies

42. A dog given a blood transfusion 3 weeks ago now needs another transfusion. Concerning a major crossmatch, which statement is most accurate?

    a. Lack of reactivity indicates that the donor and recipient have the same blood type.
    b. Lack of reactivity indicates that the recipient does not have antibodies against donor red blood cell antigens.
    c. Lack of reactivity indicates that the recipient will not form antibodies against donor red blood cells.
    d. Crossmatching involves mixing donor plasma with recipient red blood cells and checking for agglutination.
    e. Crossmatching is not necessary if the donor is negative for DEA-1 (that is, if the donor is A-negative).

Correct answers are on pages 57-58.

43. A 7-year-old male Airedale with weakness, pale mucous membranes and splenomegaly has a packed cell volume of 12% and a reticulocyte count of 3%. The WB count is 3800/μl, with 25% neutrophils, 68% lymphocytes (many atypical) and 7% monocytes. The platelet count is 72,000/μl. The procedure most likely to confirm the diagnosis is:

a. direct antiglobulin test
b. cytologic examination of a bone marrow aspirate
c. serum iron level
d. serum creatinine level
e. antiplatelet antibody test

44. In cats, the best indication of regenerative anemia is:

a. punctate reticulocytes
b. aggregate reticulocytes
c. circulating nucleated red blood cells
d. increased mean corpuscular volume
e. *Hemobartonella*

45. A stray dog is presented to you after it was found in a collapsed state. Before you examine the dog, your technician collects a blood sample and tells you the packed cell volume is 52% and the total plasma protein level is 9.5 g/dl. The most appropriate initial interpretation of these findings is:

a. dehydration
b. hyperglobulinemia
c. hyperalbuminemia
d. polycythemia
e. laboratory error

46. Which of the following is most likely to be present within minutes after acute severe blood loss?

a. decreased packed cell volume
b. decreased red blood cell count
c. increased neutrophil count
d. decreased platelet count
e. decreased lymphocyte count

47. Which of the following is most likely to cause blood to appear chocolate brown?

a. hemoglobinemia from a transfusion reaction
b. increased unconjugated bilirubin from hemolysis
c. increased conjugated bilirubin from cholestasis
d. methemoglobin from nitrate poisoning
e. cyanosis from carbon monoxide poisoning

48. When the mean corpuscular volume (MCV) is increased in a dog, the condition you are most likely to encounter in the animal is:

a. reticulocytosis
b. red cell aplasia
c. pernicious anemia
d. hemolysis
e. spherocytosis

49. After splenectomy, an animal is more likely to have:

a. anemia
b. lymphocytosis
c. spherocytosis
d. reticulocytosis
e. red blood cell parasites

50. A friend says her cat is eating kitty litter. The 2-year-old cat seems otherwise healthy. What is the most appropriate advice?

a. litter ingestion can cause Heinz-body anemia in cats
b. the cat should not be allowed to eat litter, as it often contains lead
c. this is a behavioral problem of no medical consequence
d. this is a sign of iron deficiency; give an iron supplement
e. have a blood count done to check for anemia

Answers

1. **b**

2. **d**

3. **b**

4. **a**

5. **c**

6. **d**

7. **e**

8. **d**

9. **e**

10. **c**

11. **d**

12. **b**

13. **a**

14. **b**

15. **c**

16. **c**

17. **a**

18. **b**

19. **e**

20. **c**

21. **c**

22. **d**

23. **c**

24. **b**

25. **e**

26. **b** All female offspring would be normal carriers; all males would be normal (x-linked inheritance).

27. **d** Bleeding is unlikely with a platelet count over 100,000/μl.

28. **d** The marrow is not affected.

29. **d** Platelet abnormalities are characterized by petechiae, mucosal bleeding, and sometimes bleeding from venipuncture.

30. **a** Citrate loosely binds calcium.

31. **b** Thromboxane is important in platelet agglutination.

32. **e** Erythropoietin is deficient in renal failure, resulting in anemia.

33. **c** The stain shows residual RNA as a web-like reticulum.

34. **c** Iron-deficiency anemia is microcytic hypochromic.

35. **a** Unconjugated bilirubin in not water soluble, so it is not passed into the urine.

36. **b** Absolute neutropenia is present. Numbers of the other white blood cells are only relatively (not absolutely) increased.

37. **c** Corticosteroids cause eosinopenia and lymphopenia, and insufficiency of endogenous corticosteroids is likely to cause the converse.

38. **e** Physiologic neutrophilia can occur with excitement (epinephrine release).

39. **e** Because both PT and APTT are prolonged, the defect must involve the common pathway (fibrinogen, prothrombin, factor V or X) or multiple factors (vitamin K antagonists).

40. **d** Destruction of circulating red blood cells releases hemoglobin.

41. **a** Corticosteroids do not directly suppress antibody production but tend to suppress antibody binding and macrophage function.

42. **b** The major crossmatch (donor cells with recipient plasma) only detects antibodies already present to any of several antigens on red blood cells.

43. **b** Nonregenerative anemia, neutropenia and thrombocytopenia often indicate bone marrow disease. Abnormal lymphocytes could indicate malignancy in the bone marrow.

44. **b** Aggregate reticulocytes indicate active production of red blood cells by the bone marrow.

45. **a** Both the packed cell volume and total plasma protein level increase in dehydration.

46. **c** Epinephrine release causes neutrophilia. Decreased blood cell numbers are not evident for several hours because both plasma and cells are lost proportionately.

47. **d** This color change is characteristic of any oxidant toxin.

48. **a** Reticulocytes are larger than mature red blood cells.

49. **e** The spleen normally aids in removal of red blood cell parasites.

50. **e** Pica is a nonspecific sign of anemia in cats.

Notes

Section

7

Medical Diseases

Recommended Reading

August JR: *Consultations in Feline Medicine*. Saunders, Philadelphia, 1991.

Ettinger SJ: *Textbook of Internal Medicine*. 3rd ed. Saunders, Philadelphia, 1989.

Feldman EC and Nelson RW: *Canine and Feline Endocrinology and Reproduction*. Saunders, Philadelphia, 1987.

Greene CE: *Infectious Diseases of the Dog and Cat*. Saunders, Philadelphia, 1990.

Holzworth J: *Diseases of the Cat*. Saunders, Philadelphia, 1987.

Kirk RW and Bonagura JD: *Current Veterinary XI*. Saunders, Philadelphia, 1992.

O'Brien TR: *Radiography of Abdominal Disorders of the Dog and Cat*. Saunders, Philadelphia, 1978.

Pedersen NC: *Feline Husbandry: Diseases and Management in the Multiple-Cat Environment*. American Veterinary Publications, Goleta, CA, 1991.

Pedersen NC: *Feline Infectious Diseases*. American Veterinary Publications, Goleta, CA, 1988.

Sherding RG: *The Cat: Diseases and Clinical Management*. Churchill-Livingstone, New York, 1989.

Strombeck DR and Guilford WG: *Small Animal Gastroenterology*. 2nd ed. Stonegate Publishing, Davis, CA, 1990.

Practice answer sheets are on pages 341-344.

Dogs

M.D. Willard

Questions

1. *The most common and most severe side effect of amphotericin B therapy is:*

   a. hepatic failure

   b. renal failure

   c. blood dyscrasias

   d. phlebitis due to extravasation of the drug

   e. cardiac failure

Correct answers are on pages 154-179.

Dogs, continued

2. A 57-kg, male mixed-breed dog has acute, severe hypovolemic shock. There is a large amount of blood in the abdomen, but you are uncertain of its origin. The most appropriate course of action is to:

   a. infuse 1 unit of packed red blood cells intravenously and give an injection of vitamin K_3
   b. apply a compression bandage to the abdomen
   c. infuse large volumes of physiologic saline solution intravenously
   d. immediately perform an exploratory laparotomy
   e. perform autotransfusion of blood withdrawn from the abdomen until the patient's condition is stabilized

3. Concerning blastomycosis in dogs, which statement is **least** accurate?

   a. Commonly used serologic tests have poor sensitivity and specificity.
   b. Pulmonary miliary interstitial patterns are commonly found on radiographs of animals with disseminated blastomycosis.
   c. Cytologic examination of cutaneous lesions and material aspirated from enlarged lymph nodes is often diagnostic.
   d. Culture of the yeast is rarely needed for diagnosis.
   e. On radiographs, osseous blastomycosis may closely resemble osseous neoplasia.

4. In a dog with severe hepatic cirrhosis of unknown origin and associated encephalopathy and ascites, treatment should **not** include:

   a. dexamethasone
   b. lactulose
   c. oral neomycin
   d. a low-protein diet
   e. a low-salt diet

5. Concerning barium enemas in dogs with lymphocytic-plasmacytic colitis, which statement is most accurate?

   a. Iodide contrast agents provide better detail and are safer than other contrast agents.
   b. You can expect to see an "apple-core" lesion in many affected dogs.
   c. You can expect to see thickening of the colonic wall in many affected dogs.
   d. This procedure is not sensitive in detecting mucosal disease.
   e. This procedure is best done immediately after colonoscopy and biopsy of the colon (assuming there are no gross lesions), while the dog is still anesthetized.

6. A dog has a large wound on the medial aspect of the right rear leg. The owner noticed the wound 3 days previously, at which time he removed a large wooden splinter from it. Now the wound is discolored blue-black and has obvious crepitus in the surrounding tissues. What is the most appropriate treatment for this animal?

   a. enrofloxacin plus gentamicin
   b. amikacin
   c. metronidazole plus cefazolin
   d. povidone-iodine soaks twice daily
   e. massage of the affected area and warm compresses 3 times daily

7. Which of the following is **not** a likely reason why a dog with exocrine pancreatic insufficiency may fail to respond to therapy with oral pancreatic enzyme supplementation?

   a. failure to preincubate the food with the supplemental pancreatic enzymes
   b. small intestinal bacterial overgrowth
   c. poor-quality supplemental pancreatic enzymes
   d. use of an enteric-coated supplemental pancreatic enzyme preparation
   e. use of a high-fat diet

8. What is the most likely cause of chronic hematemesis in a middle-aged dog?

   a. bacterial peritonitis
   b. coagulopathy
   c. gastric ulceration
   d. hepatic failure

e. bacterial cholangitis

9. A dog has a large wound on its side. The wound shows dark discoloration, a malodorous exudate and crepitus. The pathogens most likely to be isolated from this wound are:

a. *Pseudomonas aeruginosa, Proteus*
b. *Blastomyces dermatitidis, E coli*
c. *Bacteroides, Clostridium*
d. *Actinomyces, Nocardia*
e. *E coli, Staphylococcus*

10. A 9-year-old intact male Bull Mastiff has had dyschezia and tenesmus for 5 months. The problem has not worsened. The feces are normal in consistency and appearance, but it takes the dog 2-5 minutes to defecate. The dog appears normal on physical examination, but you cannot adequately perform an abdominal or rectal examination because of the dog's large size (69 kg). What is the most likely cause of these signs?

a. poor diet
b. perineal hernia
c. perianal fistulae
d. anal sacculitis
e. prostatomegaly

11. A mature castrated dog has had a fever (39.3-40.1 C) of unknown origin for 3 days but otherwise is in good condition. The dog lives in a kennel in the northern midwestern United States. The client requests that you initiate antibiotic therapy for a suspected bacterial infection, rather than perform any diagnostic tests. Which drug is the best choice for this animal?

a. cefazolin
b. amikacin
c. lincomycin
d. tetracycline
e. trimethoprim

12. A dog is clinically normal but then suddenly develops acute, fulminating hepatic failure. A finding that would **not** be expected in this dog after 1 day's illness is:

a. vomiting
b. coagulopathy
c. hepatic encephalopathy
d. hypoglycemia
e. polyuria, polydipsia

13. A 3-year-old hunting dog has a chronic pleural effusion. The fluid grossly resembles blood and contains small clots of exudate; cytologic examination reveals many degenerate neutrophils. The dog has lost some weight and has a persistent fever (39.0-39.4 C). There is no evidence of pulmonary parenchymal involvement. The most likely cause of these signs is:

a. tuberculosis
b. malignancy
c. blastomycosis
d. nocardiosis
e. pythiosis

14. In a 2-year-old dog with abdominal distention, abdominocentesis yields fluid with the following characteristics: specific gravity, 1.009; total protein concentration, <1 g/dl; nucleated cell count, 450/μl. The most likely cause of this effusion is:

a. lymphangiectasia
b. right-sided cardiac failure
c. left-sided cardiac failure
d. abdominal neoplasia
e. ruptured urinary tract

15. A 3-year-old Shih Tzu is continually licking at its anal region, and the owner has seen white "grains" on the hair of the perineal region and on the feces. You find no abnormalities after a thorough physical examination. The most appropriate course of action is to:

a. make plain caudal abdominal radiographs
b. administer fenbendazole
c. perform a heartworm examination
d. perform a direct fecal smear
e. administer praziquantel

Correct answers are on pages 154-179.

Dogs, continued

16. A dog has a voluminous peritoneal effusion with the following characteristics: specific gravity, 1.020; total protein concentration, 2.1 g/dl; nucleated cell count, 2780/μl. Which procedure would be most useful in determining the cause of effusion in this dog?

   a. urine protein:creatinine ratio
   b. plain abdominal radiographs
   c. endoscopic biopsy of the duodenum
   d. culture of the peritoneal fluid
   e. preprandial and postprandial serum bile acid determinations

17. Concerning blastomycosis in dogs, which statement is most accurate?

   a. Ketoconazole should be used if there is substantial hepatic disease.
   b. Amphotericin B is an effective treatment.
   c. Infected dogs pose a substantial human health risk.
   d. Griseofulvin is useful but must be used for 4-6 months to achieve a cure.
   e. Many clinical infections are mild and self-limiting, and need not be treated.

18. A dog that has been depressed, anorectic and vomiting bile for 2 days has a modest amount of peritoneal fluid with the following characteristics: specific gravity, 1.035; total protein concentration, 3.8 g/dl; nucleated cell count, 49,000/μl. Which procedure is **not** indicated in this dog at this time?

   a. abdominal ultrasonographic examination
   b. plain abdominal radiographs
   c. culture of the peritoneal fluid
   d. preprandial and postprandial bile acid determinations
   e. complete blood count and serum chemistry profile

19. Which drug is **least** likely to cause iatrogenic hepatic disease, as detected by clinical signs or significantly altered liver-derived enzyme activity?

   a. chloramphenicol

   b. betamethasone
   c. phenobarbital
   d. primidone
   e. thiacetarsamide

20. A dog has a voluminous peritoneal effusion with the following characteristics: specific gravity, 1.007; total protein concentration, <1 g/dl; nucleated cell count, <100/μl. Which procedure is **least** likely to yield useful information?

   a. urine protein:creatinine ratio
   b. thoracic radiography
   c. endoscopic biopsy of the duodenum
   d. preprandial and postprandial serum bile acid determinations
   e. abdominal ultrasonography

21. The drug most likely to cause gastrointestinal ulceration or erosion in a dog is:

   a. erythromycin
   b. prednisolone
   c. ibuprofen
   d. thiacetarsamide
   e. quinacrine

22. A 9-year-old dog that has been vomiting for 3 days has moderate amounts of straw-colored peritoneal effusion with the following characteristics: specific gravity, 1.033; total protein concentration, 3.8 g/dl; nucleated cell count, 35,000/μl. Most of the cells in the fluid are nondegenerate neutrophils. The dog is otherwise normal. The most appropriate course of action is to:

   a. make positive-contrast radiographs using barium sulfate to search for intestinal leakage
   b. perform simultaneous bilirubin determinations on peritoneal fluid and serum
   c. perform simultaneous creatinine determinations on peritoneal fluid and serum
   d. make positive-contrast radiographs using an iodide agent to search for intestinal leakage

e. perform an exploratory laparotomy as soon as possible

23. *Concerning liver biopsy in dogs with suspected hepatic disease, which statement is **least** accurate?*

   a. Biopsy is often useful to detect metastatic malignancies.
   b. Blood coagulation should be assessed before liver biopsy.
   c. It may be useful to perform another biopsy after treatment so as to assess therapeutic efficacy.
   d. Localized masses in the liver are an indication for biopsy.
   e. There is little or no benefit in biopsying a liver that is clearly smaller than normal.

24. *A middle-aged dog that is kept outside on a large farm is found recumbent. The dog has a distended abdomen, but ballottement does not produce a fluid wave. After several attempts at abdominocentesis, you finally obtain 5 ml of bloody fluid containing 3 small blood clots. This dog most likely:*

   a. has a hepatic rupture, with subsequent bleeding
   b. has a coagulopathy, possibly due to rodenticide poisoning
   c. has a chronically bleeding abdominal neoplasm
   d. has a splenic rupture, with subsequent bleeding
   e. does not have chronic abdominal bleeding

25. *A 3-year-old dog with a dry, unproductive cough began coughing 3 days previously. The animal is otherwise normal. The most appropriate **initial** course of action is to:*

   a. make thoracic radiographs
   b. administer prednisolone to reduce tracheal irritation
   c. perform a complete blood count to seek evidence of tracheal infection
   d. administer tetracycline to treat for *Bordetella bronchiseptica* infection
   e. administer theophylline for bronchodilation

26. *A 4-year-old Labrador Retriever that travels throughout the United States has numerous ticks attached to it. The dog has a fever of 39.5 C and has been depressed for 1 day. Which statement concerning this dog is most accurate?*

   a. A normal platelet count would essentially rule out ehrlichiosis and borreliosis.
   b. The dog could have a negative *Rickettsia rickettsii* titer and still have Rocky Mountain spotted fever.
   c. Aggressive therapy with ampicillin and gentamicin is the most reasonable next step if a complete diagnostic workup is declined by the owner.
   d. Absence of hyperglobulinemia would make ehrlichiosis a much less likely diagnosis.
   e. A positive *Borrelia* titer would be excellent evidence of clinical borreliosis.

27. *A 3-year-old dog that is markedly depressed and anorectic has vomited bile 10 times in the past day. The dog is hypothermic (36 C), has very injected sclerae, and has a peritoneal effusion with the following characteristics: specific gravity, 1.032; total protein concentration, 5.3 g/dl; nucleated cell count, 125,000/μl. The most likely cause of these signs is:*

   a. alimentary tract leakage
   b. severe hepatic cirrhosis
   c. abdominal carcinomatosis
   d. abdominal hemangiosarcoma
   e. severe pancreatitis

28. *Concerning aspergillosis in dogs, which statement is most accurate?*

   a. Cytologic examination of smears of nasal swabs or washes is a preferred method of diagnosis.
   b. It is best distinguished from nasal carcinoma by the fact that aspergillosis typically does not cause destruction of nasal turbinates, evident on radiographs.
   c. A chronic nasal discharge, often containing blood, is the most common sign.
   d. Amphotericin B is the treatment of choice.
   e. Resection of lesions, with administration of thiabendazole, is the treatment of choice.

Correct answers are on pages 154-179.

Dogs, continued

29. *A 2-year-old male German Shepherd that has traveled throughout the United States has had diarrhea for 5 months. The diarrhea occurs 1-3 times daily and is soft and brown without mucus, blood or straining. The dog has lost 6% of its body weight despite a good appetite. The animal is otherwise normal. A complete blood count and serum chemistry profile, including creatinine, blood urea nitrogen, total protein, albumin, glucose, alanine aminotransferase, alkaline phosphatase, calcium and phosphorus determinations, are normal. The **least** likely cause of these signs is:*

  a. giardiasis
  b. lymphocytic-plasmacytic enteritis
  c. lymphosarcoma
  d. exocrine pancreatic insufficiency
  e. colonic adenocarcinoma

30. *A 7-year-old German Wire-Haired Pointer has had diarrhea for 8 months. The diarrhea occurs 2-4 times daily and is soft and brown without mucus, blood or straining. The dog has lost 4% of its body weight despite a reasonable appetite. The animal is otherwise normal. Three fecal flotations have been negative. A complete blood count and serum chemistry profile are normal, except for hypoalbuminemia (1.3 g/dl; normal, 2.4-4.5 g/dl) and hypoproteinemia (3.0 g/dl; normal, 5.0-7.5 g/dl). The **least** likely cause of these signs is:*

  a. exocrine pancreatic insufficiency
  b. lymphocytic-plasmacytic enteritis
  c. lymphangiectasia
  d. lymphosarcoma
  e. eosinophilic enteritis

31. *Concerning babesiosis in dogs in the United States, which statement is most accurate?*

  a. A core bone marrow biopsy is the most practical method of diagnosis.
  b. It can be differentiated from immune-mediated hemolytic anemia in that babesiosis is characterized by a negative Coombs' test and nonregenerative anemia.
  c. Doxycycline is the preferred treatment.

  d. Infected dogs are human health hazards.
  e. Babesiosis may often be diagnosed by examining a peripheral blood smear.

32. *Beginning 2 days previously, a 3-year-old dog suddenly began to regurgitate solid food but not liquids. There are no prodromal signs, and the dog consistently regurgitates within 5 minutes of eating. The animal seems otherwise normal. The most appropriate **initial** course of action is to:*

  a. treat conservatively with a central-acting antiemetic
  b. make plain thoracic radiographs
  c. do a complete blood count and serum chemistry profile
  d. make plain abdominal radiographs
  e. treat with subcutaneous fluids and oral kaolin-pectin (Kaopectate)

33. *A 4-year-old spayed Doberman Pinscher has become anorectic and has started drinking and urinating excessively over the past 6 days. Until that time the dog was normal. In addition, it has begun vomiting bile-stained fluid every 2-3 days. Laboratory findings include hypoalbuminemia (2.2 g/dl; normal, 2.5-4.4 g/dl), hyperbilirubinemia (3.2 mg/dl; normal, <1 mg/dl), decreased blood urea nitrogen level (2 mg/dl; normal, 5-20 mg/dl), increased serum alanine aminotransferase activity (8 times normal), and increased serum alkaline phosphatase activity (8 times normal). The liver is smaller than normal on abdominal radiographs. The most likely cause of these abnormalities is:*

  a. chronic pancreatitis causing obstruction of the bile duct
  b. vacuolar hepatopathy causing cirrhosis
  c. hepatic lipidosis causing cirrhosis
  d. hepatic lymphosarcoma
  e. chronic active hepatic causing cirrhosis

34. *In dogs with blastomycosis, which body system is **least** often affected?*

  a. lymph nodes
  b. eyes
  c. lungs

d. central nervous system

e. skin

35. *A mixed-breed dog has had a relatively severe, dry cough for the past 10 days. The cough began 4-5 days after the animal was housed at a kennel. The most likely cause of this dog's disease is:*

a. herpesvirus

b. *Streptococcus pneumoniae*

c. *Klebsiella pneumoniae*

d. *Pasteurella multocida*

e. *Bordetella bronchiseptica*

36. *A 6-week-old Schnauzer recently began to regurgitate food at almost every meal. There is no bile or blood in the material and there is no obvious retching associated with the act. The dog seems otherwise normal. Which statement concerning this dog is most accurate?*

a. Barium contrast radiographs of the stomach and intestines are indicated.

b. Fluid and electrolyte abnormalities are the most likely reason this dog would die within the next few weeks.

c. Aspiration pneumonia is the most likely reason this dog would die within the next few weeks.

d. This problem is likely to spontaneously resolve within the next 1-4 weeks.

e. Endoscopic examination should be performed as the next step.

37. *The most reasonable treatment for a dog that appears to be rapidly exsanguinating due to gastrointestinal ulceration is to:*

a. apply a tight bandage around the abdomen

b. administer vitamin K_1

c. resect the ulcer

d. reduce the blood pressure with acepromazine

e. autotransfuse blood

38. *Concerning borreliosis in dogs, which statement is most accurate?*

a. Renal failure is a common complication of chronic disease.

b. A positive indirect fluorescent antibody titer is the most reliable method of diagnosis.

c. Thrombocytopenia is a common finding.

d. Recurrent, intermittent nonerosive arthritis is the major clinical sign of chronic disease.

e. Skin lesions at the site of the tick bite are useful in presumptive diagnosis.

39. *The disease in which metronidazole treatment is **not** indicated is:*

a. giardiasis

b. salmon poisoning

c. inflammatory bowel disease

d. clostridial enteritis

e. small intestinal bacterial overgrowth

40. *Concerning botulism in dogs, which statement is most accurate?*

a. Antitoxin is most effective if administered within 3 days of the onset of clinical signs.

b. Diagnosis is best made by culturing the causative bacterium from the feces.

c. Progressive, ascending flaccid paralysis is the most common sign.

d. Affected dogs usually have markedly increased serum alanine aminotransferase and creatine phosphokinase activities.

e. Affected dogs usually have diminished pain perception, in addition to quadriplegia.

41. *A 12-year-old German Shepherd has been severely constipated for 1 week. The dog strains for several minutes without passing any stool. It has been fed only commercial dog food and has been kept indoors, except for a 35-minute leash walk daily. On abdominal palpation, the colon is distended to 2 times its normal size throughout its length. The most appropriate **initial** course of action is to:*

a. perform a digital rectal examination

b. obtain a complete blood count and serum chemistry profile

c. make plain abdominal radiographs

d. administer a warm-water enema and then urecholine parenterally

e. administer mineral oil per os and feed the dog a fiber-enriched diet

Correct answers are on pages 154-179.

Dogs, continued

42. In a 5-month-old dog with a moderately severe congenital portosystemic shunt, which laboratory finding would **not** be expected?

   a. markedly increased postprandial serum bile acid concentration
   b. markedly increased serum alanine aminotransferase activity
   c. moderate hypoalbuminemia
   d. decreased blood urea nitrogen level
   e. moderate hypocholesterolemia

43. Concerning brucellosis in dogs, which statement is most accurate?

   a. Most infections with *Brucella canis* are inapparent.
   b. The rapid slide agglutination test is sensitive and specific in dogs.
   c. Aggressive therapy with tetracycline is relatively reliable for eliminating the infection.
   d. *Brucella canis* infections in people are typically severe.
   e. Infected male dogs typically only shed the organism for 2-3 weeks or less.

44. Four young dogs that are unrelated and owned by different clients have developed severe bloody diarrhea within the past 4 days in your clinic. The dogs are also anorectic and depressed. One of your kennel assistants develops acute gastroenteritis. The most likely cause of diarrheic disease in these dogs, especially if the kennel person contracted the infection from the dogs, is:

   a. *E coli* infection
   b. salmonellosis
   c. *Campylobacter jejuni* infection
   d. *Giardia* infection
   e. *Yersinia* infection

45. An 8-year-old male German Shepherd that is constantly kept indoors has had a distended abdomen for at least 5-8 days. The oral mucosae are very pale and there is a palpable fluid wave in the abdomen. Abdominocentesis yields frank blood. The dog is not in obvious distress but is weak. The clients say the dog has been like this for the past 9 days. The most appropriate **initial** course of action is to:

   a. autotransfuse blood withdrawn from the abdominal cavity
   b. perform abdominal ultrasonography
   c. perform an exploratory laparotomy
   d. apply a compression bandage to the abdomen
   e. transfuse 1 unit of fresh whole blood and observe the patient

46. Concerning trypanosomiasis in dogs in the United States, which statement is most accurate?

   a. Clindamycin is the preferred treatment.
   b. Stupor and somnolence are the most characteristic signs.
   c. The most common means of diagnosing this disease is by finding the organism in a capillary blood smear.
   d. Myocarditis and right-sided heart failure are the most common signs.
   e. This disease is principally limited to the Pacific northwest portion of the United States.

47. The most appropriate treatment for a 5-month-old dog with mild, acute diarrhea of 2 days' duration and of unknown origin is:

   a. oral rehydration solution
   b. a bland, easily digested diet
   c. oral neomycin
   d. loperamide
   e. methscopolamine

48. Concerning coccidioidomycosis in dogs, which statement is most accurate?

   a. Osseous disease tends to occur within 1-3 weeks of exposure.
   b. Disseminated coccidioidomycosis is almost always preceded by an obvious respiratory phase.
   c. Osseous coccidioidomycosis is often easy to distinguish from neoplasia because it tends to exclusively cause osteolysis.

d. Acute, primary coccidioidomycosis is often self-limiting.

e. Infection is primarily via inoculation of cutaneous or oral lesions.

49. *A dog with hepatic cirrhosis of unknown origin has been successfully treated conservatively for 8 months. Over the past 24 hours, however, the dog has again begun having severe signs of encephalopathy. Which of the following is **not** a likely cause of this sudden relapse of clinical signs?*

a. infection

b. gastroduodenal ulceration

c. ingestion of a high-protein meal

d. administration of an inappropriate drug

e. accumulation of ascitic fluid

50. *Which type of enema should **not** be administered to a constipated Maltese dog?*

a. warm soapy water

b. warm water

c. hypertonic phosphate

d. mineral oil

e. warm water with dioctyl sodium sulfosuccinate

51. *A 3-year-old mixed-breed male hunting dog has been coughing for 3 months, has lost about 10% of its body weight and has an intermittent fever (39.3-39.5 C). There is mild, generalized lymphadenopathy, and respiratory sounds are dry and harsh. The disease is slowly getting worse. The most likely cause of these signs is:*

a. pasteurellosis

b. cryptococcosis

c. bordetellosis

d. blastomycosis

e. distemper

52. *A 3-year-old Bedlington Terrier with congenital hepatic disease unrelated to a vascular anomaly would benefit most from treatment with:*

a. lactulose

b. prednisolone

c. surgery

d. trientine

e. a low-protein diet

53. *Which symptomatic treatment is most likely to be effective for acute, severe hepatic encephalopathy causing coma in a dog?*

a. nothing per os, systemic antibiotics, and intravenous fluid therapy with lactated Ringer's solution supplemented with potassium and dextrose

b. nothing per os, warm-water enemas containing neomycin, and intravenous fluid therapy with half-strength saline solution supplemented with potassium and dextrose

c. nothing per os, intravenous phenobarbital, and intravenous fluid therapy with 5% dextrose in water supplemented with potassium

d. lipotropic agents (inositol, methionine), intramuscular amoxicillin, and intravenous fluid therapy with 5% dextrose in water supplemented with potassium

e. diazepam, lactulose, and intravenous fluid therapy with lactated Ringer's solution supplemented with potassium and dextrose

54. *An 8-year-old male dog has had bright red blood on the surface of its stools for the past 3 weeks. The stool is otherwise normal. Blood is occasionally found on the floor where the dog has been lying. Grossly, the perineal region appears normal and there is no obvious evidence of a rectal mass or ulcer on digital rectal examination. Which statement concerning this dog is most accurate?*

a. The dog should be fed a high-fiber diet.

b. Coagulopathy is a likely cause of the hematochezia.

c. Anal sac disease is a likely cause of the hematochezia.

d. The dog should be treated with systemic amoxicillin.

e. The pelvic and anal areas should be radiographed.

Correct answers are on pages 154-179.

Dogs, continued

55. *A 4-year-old, 17-kg male Miniature Schnauzer is presented for a routine checkup. You determine that the dog has marked lipemia, even after fasting for 29 hours. Which statement concerning this dog is most accurate?*

    a. This dog probably now has or will soon develop diabetes mellitus.

    b. This dog probably has hypothyroidism.

    c. This dog is at risk for developing hepatic failure.

    d. This dog probably has hyperadrenocorticism.

    e. This dog is at risk for developing acute pancreatitis.

56. *Concerning perineal hernia in dogs, which statement is **least** accurate?*

    a. Rectal examination is usually diagnostic.

    b. The most common presenting signs include difficulty in defecation and/or perianal swelling.

    c. It is primarily found in older intact male dogs.

    d. German Shepherds, Bulldogs and Labrador Retrievers are commonly affected breeds.

    e. Dyschezia or fecal incontinence are occasional presenting signs.

57. *Concerning salmonellosis in dogs, which statement is most accurate?*

    a. Gentamicin is a preferred therapy for acute gastroenteritis due to salmonellosis.

    b. Cytologic examination is often diagnostic in animals with diarrhea.

    c. Acute salmonellosis typically causes high mortality.

    d. Most animals carrying *Salmonella* are asymptomatic.

    e. Infected dogs usually have a short period of fecal shedding of *Salmonella* organisms.

58. *Concerning oral administration of a hypertonic water-soluble iodinated contrast solution for contrast radiography of canine intestines, which statement is **least** accurate?*

    a. It can cause vomiting in some animals.

    b. It is usually progressively diluted, resulting in poor contrast.

    c. It can occasionally be seen entering the kidneys.

    d. It is the preferred contrast agent for severely dehydrated animals.

    e. It tends to move through the intestinal tract faster than barium sulfate.

59. *A 4-month-old puppy was obtained 10 days previously and has had diarrhea for the past 8 days. The stool is soft but does not contain mucus or blood. The problem has not worsened. The dog is otherwise normal and is fed a commercial brand of puppy chow. Which statement concerning this dog is most accurate?*

    a. Dietary intolerance is a likely cause of the diarrhea.

    b. A parasympatholytic drug is the preferred therapy.

    c. Increased dietary fiber is the preferred therapy.

    d. A barium contrast radiographic study of the intestines is indicated.

    e. A first-generation cephalosporin should be given.

60. *A 2-year-old Great Dane that has traveled throughout the United States is anorectic and acutely lame in its right rear leg. The dog has a slight fever (39.4 C) and a slightly swollen but painful stifle. The animal is otherwise normal. The most likely cause of this dog's disease is:*

    a. nocardiosis

    b. osteosarcoma

    c. chlamydiosis

    d. borreliosis

    e. histoplasmosis

61. *Concerning benign adenomatous polyps in dogs, which statement is most accurate?*

    a. One may easily distinguish benign polyps from malignant growths by their gross appearance.

    b. They principally cause hematochezia coupled with constipation.

c. They usually become malignant if not promptly resected.

d. They principally occur in the rectum.

e. Most rectal polyps arise from chronically inflamed anal sacs.

62. *Concerning lymphocytic-plasmacytic colitis in dogs, which statement is most accurate?*

a. Untreated affected dogs often develop lymphosarcoma.

b. Prednisolone is the preferred therapy.

c. The milder forms often respond to appropriate dietary therapy.

d. Most affected dogs have hematochezia despite otherwise normal stools.

e. Azathioprine is typically needed to control signs in mildly to moderately affected animals.

63. *In a 7-month-old dog with acute onset of fever, anorexia and coughing, what is the best way to help confirm your presumptive diagnosis of acute distemper?*

a. finding enamel hypoplasia on oral examination

b. finding chorioretinitis on ophthalmoscopic examination

c. finding lymphopenia on the complete blood count

d. finding inclusion bodies in white blood cells

e. watching for development of "chewing gum" seizures

64. *A 3-year-old Weimaraner has had diarrhea for 19 months. The diarrhea occurs 2-4 times daily, and is soft and brown. No mucus, blood or straining has been noted. The animal has lost 9% of its body weight despite a good appetite. The dog is otherwise normal. Three fecal flotations have been negative. A complete blood count and serum chemistry profile, including creatinine, urea nitrogen, total protein, albumin, glucose, alanine aminotransferase and alkaline phosphatase, are normal. The most likely cause of these signs is:*

a. small intestinal bacterial overgrowth

b. granulomatous enteritis

c. salmonellosis

d. lymphangiectasia

e. lymphosarcoma

65. *Concerning coccidioidomycosis in dogs, which statement is most accurate?*

a. Ketoconazole is the recommended therapy for dogs with central nervous system involvement.

b. Cytologic examination of lesions is often diagnostic because there are usually numerous organisms present.

c. Culture of exudates is recommended if cytologic and serologic examinations are not diagnostic.

d. Disseminated coccidioidomycosis is usually cured with amphotericin B therapy.

e. Hilar lymphadenopathy is a common radiographic finding in pulmonary coccidioidomycosis.

66. *Concerning dogs that regurgitate or vomit, which statement is most accurate?*

a. Most dogs with esophageal disease regurgitate food in a tubular form.

b. Vigorous retching suggests vomiting and would not be expected in dogs with esophageal disease.

c. Most dogs that regurgitate have grossly evident dilatations in their neck, caused by an enlarged cervical esophagus.

d. Most dogs that regurgitate expel food mixed with green or yellow foam.

e. Regurgitation due to esophageal disease invariably occurs within 1-15 minutes of eating.

67. *Concerning protein-losing enteropathy in dogs, which statement is **least** accurate?*

a. Histoplasmosis can cause this syndrome.

b. Gastrointestinal ulceration can cause this syndrome.

c. The prognosis is very poor.

d. Affected dogs often have panhypoproteinemia.

e. A low-fat diet plus medium-chain triglycerides is often useful in treating one of the causes of this syndrome.

Correct answers are on pages 154-179.

Dogs, continued

68. The **least** appropriate treatment for a dog with vomiting due to gastrointestinal disease of unknown origin is:

    a. intravenous physiologic saline
    b. intravenous fluids with sodium bicarbonate added
    c. intravenous fluids with potassium chloride added
    d. intravenous fluids with dextrose added
    e. intravenous Ringer's solution

69. In a 7-year-old mixed-breed dog with intestinal lymphangiectasia of unknown origin, the most appropriate **initial** therapy is:

    a. a trial elimination (hypoallergenic) diet
    b. prednisolone plus azathioprine
    c. an ultralow-fat diet plus medium-chain triglycerides
    d. oral antibiotics (eg, tylosin or tetracycline)
    e. a high-fiber diet plus azulfidine

70. A 7-year-old male German Shepherd is constipated. The dog has been obviously uncomfortable when defecating during the past 7 weeks. Now it cannot defecate at all. The colon is full of hard feces. The rectal area seems somewhat swollen, but you cannot examine the area well because the dog is extremely painful there. The dog refuses to allow you to perform a rectal examination. The most likely cause of these signs is:

    a. a chronic, healed pelvic fracture
    b. perianal fistulae
    c. ingestion of difficult-to-digest trash (popcorn, hair, plastic wrappings)
    d. rectal polyps
    e. a low-fiber diet

71. Which of the following best describes the radiographic appearance of diffuse infiltrative disease as seen on barium contrast radiographs of the intestines?

    a. flat mucosa, with small linear fissures
    b. "feathering" of the mucosa
    c. drastically decreased passage of barium through the intestines
    d. "thumb printing" or scalloped margins
    e. inconsistent width of the bowel lumen

72. Concerning Ehrlichia canis infection in dogs, which statement is most accurate?

    a. Doxycycline is very effective in treating ehrlichiosis, but this drug is more nephrotoxic than tetracycline.
    b. Epistaxis is very common in affected dogs.
    c. A 7-day course of therapy with tetracycline is effective in acute ehrlichiosis.
    d. Clinical signs of acute ehrlichiosis are often mild and include fever and anorexia.
    e. Chronically infected dogs serve as an important reservoir of the disease for other dogs.

73. Concerning esophageal foreign bodies in dogs, which statement is **least** accurate?

    a. Many foreign bodies can be removed endoscopically.
    b. The cricopharyngeal sphincter is the most common site at which foreign bodies lodge.
    c. Animals with a partial obstruction often regurgitate solids but not liquids.
    d. Some animals with esophageal obstruction become anorectic and drool excessively.
    e. Esophageal perforation is often accompanied by fever, depression and anorexia.

74. A 9-year-old dog has been straining on defecation for the past 3 weeks. The dog had bright red blood on the surface of the feces for 2-4 weeks before that time. At physical examination, the anus seems constricted by a circumferential band of tissue. Which statement concerning this dog is most accurate?

    a. You should treat the dog with a drug that is effective against anaerobic bacteria.
    b. You should perform surgery and try to resect this band of tissue.
    c. You should perform proctoscopy and obtain a deep biopsy of this band of tissue.

d. The dog probably has benign adenomatous rectal polyps.

e. The dog probably has severe anal sac disease.

75. *Concerning acquired esophageal weakness in older dogs, which statement is most accurate?*

a. Myopathies, neuropathies and junctionopathies are important causes.

b. The condition resolves in most affected dogs with conservative dietary management for 3-8 weeks.

c. Esophageal perforation is a major cause of death in affected dogs.

d. Cimetidine is often useful in alleviating clinical signs.

e. Affected dogs should receive prophylactic antibiotics as long as they have the condition.

76. *A 3-year-old male Miniature Schnauzer began having bloody vomiting and bloody diarrhea 3 hours previously. The dog is now somewhat depressed and has a packed cell volume of 64% (normal, 35-55%). The most likely cause of these signs is:*

a. gastrointestinal ulceration

b. hemorrhagic gastroenteritis

c. parvoviral enteritis

d. food allergy

e. arsenic intoxication

77. *Concerning distemper in dogs, which statement is most accurate?*

a. Distemper is one of the most common causes of convulsions in dogs less than 6 months of age.

b. The distemper virus's marked resistance to the environment is the reason this disease is so easily spread from animal to animal.

c. Definitive antemortem diagnosis of acute distemper is best accomplished with serologic testing.

d. Distemper may be differentiated from ehrlichiosis because the latter causes thrombocytopenia.

e. The fluorescent antibody tect on conjunctival scrapings is most useful in dogs with chronic distemper encephalitis.

78. *A 9-month-old dog has* Toxocara *and* Ancylostoma *ova plus* Isospora *oocysts in the feces. The dog appears normal and has normal stools. The best treatment for this dog is:*

a. sulfadimethoxine

b. metronidazole

c. fenbendazole

d. piperazine

e. quinacrine

79. *What observation on a lateral radiograph best indicates an increase or decrease in liver size?*

a. gastric silhouette

b. cranial extent of the duodenal silhouette

c. cranial extent of the left kidney silhouette

d. size of the fat pad under the liver

e. cranial extent of the jejunal silhouette

80. *Concerning diagnosis of gastric dilatation/ volvulus, which statement is most accurate?*

a. Successful passage of a stomach tube rules out volvulus as a diagnostic consideration.

b. Right lateral recumbency is the position of choice for radiographic diagnosis.

c. Contrast radiographs should be obtained to distinguish dilatation with torsion from dilatation without torsion.

d. Chronic, intermittent bloating rules out gastric torsion as a diagnostic consideration.

e. Torsion is usually diagnosed by observing the pylorus on the right side of the abdomen on the ventrodorsal radiographic projection.

81. *Concerning* Ehrlichia canis *infection in dogs, which statement is most accurate?*

a. *Ehrlichia* morulae are commonly found in peripheral white blood cells during the first 3 weeks of infection.

b. Antibody titers ≥1:128 are needed for a definitive diagnosis.

c. Thrombocytopenia is a common hematologic finding in acute and chronic ehrlichiosis.

d. Successful therapy is documented by an undetectable *Ehrlichia* titer 3-5 months after therapy.

e. Pancytopenia associated with ehrlichiosis is due to replacement of the bone marrow with plasma cells.

Correct answers are on pages 154-179.

Dogs, continued

82. *Concerning perianal fistulae in dogs, which statement is **least** accurate?*

    a. Fecal incontinence is a concern after aggressive, wide resection of lesions.

    b. Topical therapy with antibiotics and corticosteroids is often curative.

    c. Recurrence after surgery is a major concern.

    d. High tail amputation has been helpful in halting disease progression and eliminating the fistulae in some dogs.

    e. Mild cases can be confused with anal sac abscesses.

83. *At weaning, a 5-month-old dog begins to regurgitate at every meal. There are no prodromal signs; the dog simply puts its head down and gags up food and mucus. The dog is otherwise normal. The most likely cause of these signs is:*

    a. a vascular ring anomaly

    b. pyloric stenosis

    c. a portosystemic shunt

    d. a gastric foreign body

    e. food intolerance

84. *The drug most likely to control severe vomiting of unknown origin is:*

    a. metoclopramide

    b. bismuth subsalicylate

    c. misoprostol

    d. diphenhydramine

    e. methscopolamine

85. *A 7-year-old dog has had diarrhea consistently for the past 4 months. The diarrhea occurs 2-4 times per day, does not contain mucus or blood, and is not associated with straining. The dog has lost 4% of its body weight. Which statement concerning this dog is most accurate?*

    a. The dog has signs of chronic large intestinal diarrhea.

    b. The dog has signs of chronic small intestinal diarrhea.

    c. The dog has signs of chronic large and small intestinal diarrhea.

    d. One cannot reasonably predict whether the large or small intestine is involved.

    e. The dog probably has a chronic helminth infection.

86. *Concerning initial (immediately after admission) management of a dog with gastric dilatation/volvulus, which statement is most accurate?*

    a. Trocarization is the preferred means of relieving gastric distention before surgery.

    b. Large doses of flunixin meglumine and dexamethasone should be administered initially as part of treatment for shock.

    c. Intravenous lidocaine or intramuscular quinidine should be used in initial management to prevent cardiac arrhythmias.

    d. Potassium chloride (50 mEq/L) should be added to the fluids initially infused to treat shock.

    e. Aggressive intravenous fluid therapy with crystalloids (administered through multiple catheters if needed) is indicated in initial management.

87. *A 5-year-old dog has been apparently normal at home and is normal on physical examination, but its serum alkaline phosphatase activity is 8 times normal. There are no significant abnormalities on a complete blood count. Serum glucose, alanine aminotransferase, total protein, albumin, bilirubin, calcium, sodium and potassium values are within normal limits. These findings are most likely caused by the animal's exposure, in the past 2-3 weeks, to:*

    a. a third-generation cephalosporin

    b. furosemide

    c. triamcinolone

    d. fenbendazole

    e. ivermectin

88. *A mature mixed-breed castrated dog has become increasingly depressed during the past 12 hours and is now vomiting repeatedly. The abdomen seems painful on palpation. A plain abdominal radiograph reveals poor serosal contrast and free gas in the peritoneal cavity. What is the most appropriate course of action?*

  a. perform an exploratory laparotomy as soon as symptomatic therapy improves the dog's condition for anesthesia
  b. perform a positive-contrast radiographic study of the intestines, using iodide contrast medium
  c. collect samples for a complete blood count, urinalysis and serum chemistry profile, and administer intravenous fluids while awaiting these test results
  d. perform abdominocentesis and culture any fluid collected; treat with broad-spectrum antibiotics until culture results are known
  e. administer flunixin meglumine, antibiotics and intravenous fluids and lavage the abdominal cavity with warm crystalloid solution via catheter

89. *Concerning infectious canine hepatitis, which statement is most accurate?*

  a. Corneal edema is most commonly seen in the most severely and acutely affected dogs.
  b. Icterus is common in dogs with acute disease.
  c. Dogs can become ill and die within hours of the onset of signs.
  d. Lack of thrombocytopenia helps differentiate this disease from ehrlichiosis.
  e. The causative virus is very labile.

90. *Which of the following is **least** likely to occur in a dog with severe septic peritonitis associated with spontaneous small intestinal rupture?*

  a. metabolic acidosis
  b. septic shock
  c. regurgitation
  d. disseminated intravascular coagulation
  e. azotemia

91. *Concerning perineal hernia in dogs, which statement is most accurate?*

  a. Recurrence is uncommon in patients that have been treated surgically.
  b. Fecal softeners and occasional enemas are useless in controlling signs.
  c. Retroflexion of the urinary bladder into the hernia can cause acute postrenal uremia.
  d. Dogs with testicular tumors (interstitial-cell tumors, seminomas) have a much lower likelihood of developing perineal hernia.
  e. Colonoscopy or positive-contrast radiographs are needed for definitive diagnosis.

92. *Concerning hepatozoonosis in dogs, which statement is most accurate?*

  a. Acute right-sided heart failure is the main cause of death in affected animals.
  b. Most affected dogs have mild to moderate thrombocytopenia.
  c. Radiography of the lumbar vertebrae and pelvis is the best method of diagnosing this disease.
  d. Intermittent fever and emaciation are the most common presenting complaints.
  e. Marked eosinophilia is the most common and most suggestive hematologic abnormality in affected dogs.

93. *Which of the following would you expect to find in a dog with an acquired hepatic portosystemic shunt due to severe cirrhosis, but only rarely find in a dog with congenital portosystemic shunt?*

  a. vomiting
  b. hypoalbuminemia
  c. ascites
  d. microhepatia
  e. decreased blood urea nitrogen level

Correct answers are on pages 154-179.

Dogs, continued

94. *A 10-year-old dog has been vomiting yellow phlegm and material resembling "coffee grounds" 2-4 times per week for the past 3 weeks. On physical examination, the dog appears normal. Which statement concerning this dog is most accurate?*

   a. The dog should be treated with intravenous fluids.

   b. The dog likely has gastric mucosal hyperplasia.

   c. The dog should be treated with metoclopramide.

   d. The dog likely has a gastric malignancy.

   e. The dog should be treated with a beta-lactam antibiotic.

95. *Concerning herpesvirus infection in dogs, which statement is most accurate?*

   a. Hepatomegaly is the primary gross necropsy finding in fatally affected animals.

   b. Viral inclusions may often be found in circulating white blood cells.

   c. Most puppies are infected via the dam's milk.

   d. Chloramphenicol is the preferred therapy for affected puppies.

   e. Affected puppies often die between 1 and 3 weeks of age.

96. *The drug that most effectively prevents motion sickness in dogs is:*

   a. kaolin-pectin (Kaopectate)

   b. atropine

   c. acepromazine

   d. cimetidine

   e. misoprostol

97. *Concerning histoplasmosis in dogs, which statement is most accurate?*

   a. Subclinical infections are rare in dogs.

   b. Skin testing is inaccurate, but serologic examination is useful in diagnosing disseminated histoplasmosis.

   c. Dogs with disseminated histoplasmosis often have concurrent ocular and osseous lesions.

   d. Large bowel diarrhea is common in dogs with disseminated histoplasmosis.

   e. Cytologically, it is difficult to distinguish *Histoplasma capsulatum* from *Cryptococcus*.

98. *An 8-year-old West Highland White Terrier has been vomiting for 4 months. On exploratory laparotomy, the distal gastric antrum is filled with enlarged folds of gastric mucosa. The wall of the antrum and the pylorus is not thickened. There are no other abnormalities. The most likely cause of these signs is:*

   a. histoplasmosis

   b. gastric adenocarcinoma

   c. gastric lymphosarcoma

   d. hypertrophic mucosal hypertrophy

   e. *Physaloptera* infection

99. *On a plain abdominal radiograph of a constipated dog, you note that the colon is filled with feces and appears to be displaced dorsally at the pelvic inlet. The most likely cause of these findings is:*

   a. colonic foreign body

   b. enlarged sublumbar lymph nodes

   c. rectal tumor

   d. megacolon

   e. prostatomegaly

100. *You are presented with a dog that has been depressed and febrile (39.4-40 C) for the past 3 days. The dog also has marked lymphadenopathy (all lymph nodes are 4-5 times normal size) and severe bilateral uveitis. The most likely cause of these signs is:*

   a. coccidioidomycosis

   b. blastomycosis

   c. cryptococcosis

   d. sporotrichosis

   e. histoplasmosis

101. *The drug that is **least** useful to treat gastrointestinal ulceration in dogs is:*

   a. chlorpromazine

b. cimetidine

c. sucralfate

d. misoprostol

e. ranitidine

102. *It is the middle of summer and you are presented with a 3-year-old mixed-breed hunting dog that travels throughout the southern United States. The dog has been sick for 2 days. It is febrile (39.2-39.4 C), depressed and anorectic, and has a dry cough, moderate generalized lymphadenopathy, and some pitting edema of the extremities. The most likely cause of these signs is:*

a. leptospirosis

b. blastomycosis

c. histoplasmosis

d. borreliosis

e. Rocky Mountain spotted fever

103. *Which signs are most common in dogs with acute ileocolic intussusception?*

a. profuse watery diarrhea, abdominal distention

b. hematochezia, vomiting

c. vomiting, bowel mucosa protruding from the anus

d. abdominal pain, abdominal distention

e. hypoproteinemia, diarrhea

104. *Which findings are most suggestive of a congenital portosystemic shunt in a 15-month-old dog?*

a. microhepatia, hypoalbuminemia and increased postprandial serum bile acid levels

b. hepatomegaly, hypoalbuminemia and hypocholesterolemia

c. markedly increased serum alkaline phosphatase and gamma glutamyltransferase activity, and increased preprandial serum bile acid levels

d. hyperbilirubinemia, decreased blood urea nitrogen level, and increased postprandial serum bile acid levels

e. hypoproteinemia, decreased serum gamma glutamyltransferase and alanine aminotransferase activity, and decreased serum bilirubin level

105. *The most common side effect of ketoconazole use in dogs is:*

a. renal disease

b. hepatic disease

c. fever and depression

d. gastric ulceration

e. cardiac disease

106. *Concerning gastrointestinal ulceration in dogs, which statement is most accurate?*

a. A positive-contrast barium radiographic study is insensitive for diagnosis.

b. Ultrasonographic examination is a sensitive diagnostic method.

c. Most affected dogs die from this disease.

d. Almost all affected dogs have very low serum iron concentrations.

e. Almost all affected dogs have markedly increased white blood cell counts due to inflammation associated with the ulcer.

107. *On a plain lateral radiograph of a dog with abdominal distention, you see excellent serosal detail, and the intestines are pushed into the dorsal aspect of the abdominal cavity. Radiographic findings are otherwise normal. Which statement concerning this dog is most accurate?*

a. The dog probably has hepatic failure.

b. A peritoneal effusion is displacing the intestines dorsally.

c. Mesenteric lymphadenopathy is displacing the intestines dorsally.

d. There is probably a lot of fat in the abdomen.

e. The dog probably has an intestinal foreign body.

Correct answers are on pages 154-179.

Dogs, continued

108. *Concerning leptospirosis in dogs, which statement is most accurate?*

a. Most cases that are diagnosed antemortem are acute or peracute.

b. Peracute leptospirosis is usually manifested as renal failure and icterus.

c. The most reliable way to diagnose acute leptospirosis is by culturing urine on blood agar plates.

d. Renal biopsy is the most sensitive and specific means of diagnosing acute leptospirosis.

e. Treatment with penicillin and dihydrostreptomycin offers the best chance of a cure.

109. *Concerning a dog with its first episode of moderate anal sacculitis (no abscessation), which statement is most accurate?*

a. The gland should be expressed and an antibiotic-corticosteroid solution instilled.

b. Systemic antibiotic therapy is often needed.

c. Anal sac ablation is the most practical and desirable way to treat this problem.

d. Systemic corticosteroids are often needed.

e. Dietary therapy is of no benefit.

110. *Concerning use of azulfidine in dogs, which statement is most accurate?*

a. It is probably effective because of its sulfa moiety.

b. It may cause keratoconjunctivitis sicca as a side effect.

c. It is most useful for chronic small bowel diarrhea.

d. It should be used concurrently with corticosteroids.

e. It should never be used in cats.

111. *Concerning treatment and/or prevention of gastrointestinal ulceration in dogs, which statement is most accurate?*

a. Affected dogs should be fed milk and other bland foods to facilitate healing.

b. Injectable histamine-2 antagonists are effective in preventing ulceration due to any cause.

c. Oral kaolin-pectin (Kaopectate) is an effective treatment for most ulcers.

d. Oral sucralfate is an effective treatment for most ulcers.

e. Metoclopramide aids healing of ulcers by increasing gastric blood flow.

112. *A 2-year-old dog has had episodes of behavioral change for the past 6 months. These episodes occur at any time and tend to develop gradually. Typically, the dog becomes anorectic and unaware of its surroundings, walking into walls and furniture. The episodes usually last 12-96 hours and then slowly resolve spontaneously. On physical examination, the dog is normal except that it is noticeably small as compared with its littermates. A complete blood count, urinalysis and serum chemistry profile are normal, except that the blood urea nitrogen level is 3 mg/dl (normal, 6-20 mg/dl). The most appropriate course of action is to:*

a. obtain preprandial and postprandial serum bile acid determinations

b. perform an electroencephalographic examination and cerebrospinal fluid analysis

c. determine the serum glucose:insulin ratio

d. perform an intravenous glucose tolerance test and serum insulin determination

e. perform an 8-hour fasting serum glucose determination

113. *The treatment that is **least** likely to benefit a dog with gastric ulceration of unknown origin is:*

a. misoprostol and chlorpromazine

b. sucralfate and metoclopramide

c. nothing per os, intravenous fluids and famotidine

d. aminopentamide and flunixin meglumine

e. cimetidine and chlorpromazine

114. *A young male mixed-breed dog has had a fever (39.5 C) and has been vomiting bile for 3* *days. Today the dog is slightly icteric. The most likely cause of these signs is:*

a. chronic active hepatitis
b. distemper
c. blastomycosis
d. leptospirosis
e. bacterial endocarditis

115. *A 5-year-old obese Miniature Schnauzer has been anorectic and vomiting food and/or phlegm for 1 day. These signs began after the dog got loose and roamed the neighborhood for 2 days. Today the dog seems to have cranial abdominal pain when palpated. The sclerae are bright yellow but the mucous membranes are obviously pink. The most likely cause of these signs is:*

a. hepatic cirrhosis
b. chronic active hepatitis
c. extrahepatic bile duct obstruction
d. vacuolar hepatopathy
e. hemolytic anemia

116. *A 5-year-old female Shih Tzu has a painful, inflamed, swollen area to the left of the anus, with a small amount of exudate over the area. The dog has a rectal temperature of 39.7 C. The most appropriate course of action is to:*

a. make plain radiographs of the perineal area
b. perform a proctoscopic examination to look for neoplasia and/or fistulous tracts
c. immediately resect the affected anal sac
d. widely resect the perianal fistulae causing these signs
e. give systemic antibiotics, apply warm compresses to the area, and eventually lance and flush the anal sac abscess

117. *Concerning* Neospora caninum *infection in dogs, which statement is most accurate?*

a. Most clinically evident infections are self-limiting and do not require therapy.
b. Chronic fever of unknown origin is the most common presenting complaint.
c. The diagnosis is best made by multiple fecal examinations.
d. Doxycycline is the preferred therapy.

e. Clinical findings may mimic those seen with toxoplasmosis.

118. *Concerning vascular ring anomalies in dogs, which statement is most accurate?*

a. German Shepherds seem to be predisposed to these anomalies.
b. Substantial congenital esophageal weakness is usually also identified.
c. Aspiration pneumonia is rare in affected animals.
d. Most affected dogs recover completely after appropriate surgery.
e. Most affected dogs have significant concurrent congenital cardiac anomalies.

119. *Which laboratory findings are most consistent with chronic active hepatitis in a Doberman Pinscher (assuming that cirrhosis has not developed)?*

a. serum alanine aminotransferase activity 6 times normal, serum alkaline phosphatase activity 8 times normal, hypoalbuminemia
b. normal serum alanine aminotransferase activity, serum alkaline phosphatase activity 20 times normal, serum bilirubin level 5 times normal
c. normal serum alanine aminotransferase activity, normal serum alkaline phosphatase activity, decreased blood urea nitrogen level
d. normal serum alanine aminotransferase activity, normal serum alkaline phosphatase activity, normal serum bilirubin level, hypoalbumenemia
e. serum alanine aminotransferase activity 18 times normal, normal serum alkaline phosphatase activity, hypocholesterolemia

120. *Which set of laboratory findings is most suggestive of gastric outlet obstruction?*

a. hypochloremia, hypokalemia, metabolic alkalosis
b. hyponatremia, hypochloremia, metabolic acidosis
c. hyponatremia, hyperkalemia, metabolic alkalosis
d. hypokalemia, metabolic acidosis
e. hyperchloremia, metabolic acidosis

Correct answers are on pages 154-179.

Dogs, continued

121. *Concerning nocardiosis in dogs, which statement is most accurate?*

    a. Infected animals with a copious effusion are a human health hazard.

    b. Culture of materal for *Nocardia* requires anaerobic transport and culture conditions.

    c. Not all *Nocardia* species produce so-called "sulfur granules."

    d. Penicillin and enrofloxacin are the drugs of choice.

    e. Culture of infected material typically produces growth of the organism within 3-5 days.

122. *A plain lateral abdominal radiograph reveals that the small intestines are in the cranial abdomen, crowded against the liver and stomach. This finding is most likely related to extreme enlargement of the:*

    a. mesenteric lymph nodes

    b. left kidney

    c. spleen

    d. urinary bladder

    e. right adrenal gland

123. *A 5-year-old Schnauzer that is kept in the house or in a fenced backyard has been anorectic and vomiting bile for 2 days. The dog shows discomfort on palpation of the cranial abdomen. Laboratory findings include a packed cell volume of 57% (normal, 35-55%), white blood cell count of 27,690/μl (normal, 6000-14,000/μl), and urine specific gravity of 1.045. The dog's serum is too lipemic for blood chemistry assays. Which statement concerning this dog is **least** accurate?*

    a. Intravenous fluids are warranted at this time.

    b. Abdominal surgery is inappropriate at this time.

    c. Plain abdominal radiographs are warranted.

    d. Exocrine pancreatic insufficiency is a likely diagnosis.

    e. The dog should not be given food or water per os for at least the next 24-72 hours.

124. *Concerning paragonimiasis in dogs, which statement is most accurate?*

    a. A Baermann concentration technique is required to demonstrate larvae in the feces.

    b. Thiabendazole is the treatment of choice.

    c. Thoracic radiographs often demonstrate air-filled cysts or small masses in the lungs.

    d. This parasite has a direct life cycle and can be spread from animal to animal within a kennel.

    e. The most common result of infection is collapse.

125. *Concerning dogs with esophageal disease causing regurgitation, which statement is most accurate?*

    a. Esophagitis is one of the more common causes of such esophageal disease.

    b. Aspiration pneumonia is a common cause of death.

    c. Distal esophageal myotomy is often useful if there is acquired esophageal weakness.

    d. Surgical plication of redundant esophageal tissue is reasonable therapy if the esophagus is greatly dilated.

    e. Histamine-2 antagonists are recommended to alleviate clinical signs.

126. *The best treatment for moderately severe, symptomatic, biopsy-confirmed, chronic active hepatitis in a dog is:*

    a. neomycin

    b. lactulose

    c. tetracycline

    d. prednisolone

    e. trientine

127. *Concerning parvoviral infection in dogs, which statement is most accurate?*

    a. A positive-contrast barium radiographic study usually reveals intestinal ulcers.

    b. Myocarditis is common in animals affected before 14 weeks of age.

c. Finding severe lymphopenia is a good way to diagnose this disease.

d. Fecal enzyme-linked immunosorbent assay is a sensitive test for 12-15 days after the onset of signs.

e. Many infections probably are clinically mild.

128. Concerning gastrointestinal ulceration in dogs, which statement is most accurate?

a. Purebred dogs are more commonly affected with ulceration.

b. Severe pancreatitis is often associated with ulceration.

c. Severe hepatic failure is often associated with ulceration.

d. Athletic or working dogs are more commonly affected with ulceration.

e. Dogs that chew bones are more often affected with ulceration.

129. What is the best antimicrobial treatment for a dog with fulminating abdominal sepsis associated with leakage of colonic contents?

a. cephalothin and amoxicillin

b. enrofloxacin and gentamicin

c. amikacin, ampicillin and metronidazole

d. clindamycin and metronidazole

e. enrofloxacin, amikacin and trimethoprim-sulfadiazine

130. Concerning pythiosis in dogs, which statement is most accurate?

a. Most animals with disseminated disease have marked monocytosis.

b. Serologic examination is useful for diagnosis.

c. The subcutaneous tissues of the legs are typically swollen.

d. The stomach and intestines are the most commonly affected sites.

e. Amphotericin B is an effective treatment.

131. The *least* likely postoperative complication of surgery to correct gastric dilatation/volvulus in dogs is:

a. disseminated intravascular coagulation

b. cardiac arrhythmias

c. gastric motility disorders

d. renal failure

e. recurrence of dilatation and/or volvulus

132. The drug that most effectively controls diarrhea in dogs is:

a. loperamide

b. atropine

c. methscopalamine

d. kaolin-pectin (Kaopectate)

e. aminopentamide

133. Concerning rabies in dogs, which statement is most accurate?

a. One of the first signs of the paralytic stage of rabies is incoordination.

b. Death occurs from purulent meningoencephalitis, usually 11-14 days after clinical signs are first seen.

c. Immunologic exmination of skin biopsies (especially the sensory vibrissae) allows reliable antemortem diagnosis.

d. Rabies virus is relatively resistant and the area around an infected dog should be disinfected repeatedly with phenolic disinfectants.

e. Rabies is invariably fatal within 2-3 weeks of infection.

134. For the past 8 days, a 4-year-old female Bedlington Terrier has been depressed, anorectic and vomiting bile. The dog's serum alanine aminotransferase activity is 9 times normal and serum alkaline phosphotase activity is 10 times normal. The most likely cause of these signs is:

a. cholangitis-cholangiohepatitis

b. vacuolar hepatopathy

c. chronic active hepatitis

d. hepatic lipidosis

e. copper storage disorder

Dogs, continued

135. *Concerning Rocky Moutain spotted fever in dogs, which statement is most accurate?*

a. The major vector in the United States is *Rhipicephalus sanguineus*.
b. Rocky Mountain spotted fever rarely causes thrombocytopenia, while ehrlichiosis commonly causes thrombocytopenia.
c. Tetracycline is clearly superior to chloramphenicol for treatment.
d. Dogs with acute disease typically have a titer ≥1:128.
e. Many infections in dogs probably are inapparent.

136. *A 3-year-old spayed Miniature Schnauzer that is kept in the house has been depressed, anorectic and vomiting bile for 36 hours. The dog shows discomfort on palpation of the cranial abdomen. Laboratory findings include a packed cell volume of 58% (normal, 35-55%), white blood cell count of 29,390/μl (normal, 6000-14,000/μl) and urine specific gravity of 1.055. The serum is moderately lipemic and assays show a blood urea nitrogen level of 64 mg/dl (normal, 6-20 mg/dl), serum creatinine level of 2.8 mg/dl (normal, 0.1-1.9 mg/dl), serum alanine aminotransferase activity of 145 IU/L (normal, <120 IU/L), serum alkaline phosphatase activity of 245 IU/L (normal, <147 IU/L) and serum lipase activity of 145 IU/L (normal, 30-150 IU/L). The most likely cause of these findings is:*

a. uremia
b. hepatitis
c. acute pancreatitis
d. inflammatory bowel disease
e. gastroenteritis from ingestion of garbage

137. *The **least** effective treatment to decrease gastric acidity is:*

a. famotidine administered once daily
b. cimetidine administered 3 times daily
c. ranitidine administered twice daily
d. omeprazole administered once daily

e. aluminum hydroxide administered twice daily

138. *Concerning salmon poisoning in dogs, which statement is most accurate?*

a. Detection of *Nanophyetus salmincola* ova in the feces is diagnostic.
b. Oxytetracycline and chloramphenicol are reasonable therapeutic choices.
c. Diagnosis is best made by finding a titer for *Neorickettsia helmintheca*.
d. This disease does not cause lymphadenopathy as consistently as does ehrlichiosis.
e. Most clinically affected dogs recover spontaneously.

139. *A Walker Hound that has traveled throughout the United States has had diarrhea containing specks of red blood for the past 4 weeks. There is no straining at defecation and the dog has not lost weight. The dog is normal on physical examination and rectal palpation. The complete blood count shows neutrophilic leukocytosis (14,500 segs/μl; normal, 4000-14,000/μl). The serum chemistry profile and urinalysis findings are normal. No parasites or ova are noted on a single fecal flotation. The most likely cause of these signs is:*

a. rectal adenocarcinoma
b. giardiasis
c. protothecosis
d. salmonellosis
e. trichuriasis

140. *Which radiographic technique is most sensitive and specific for diagnosing ileocolic intussusception?*

a. plain standing lateral projection of the abdomen
b. upper gastrointestinal contrast series
c. barium enema
d. pneumoperitoneography
e. plain abdominal radiographs

141. *Concerning sporotrichosis in dogs, which statement is most accurate?*

a. Serologic examination is the most reliable means of diagnosis.
b. Cytologic examination of material from lesions is the most sensitive means of diagnosis.
c. Cutaneous and cutaneolymphatic lesions are the most common forms.
d. Griseofulvin is the treatment of choice for cutaneous sporotrichosis.
e. Amphotericin B is the treatment of choice for cutaneous sporotrichosis.

142. *A 2-year-old German Shepherd has had diarrhea for 8 months. The diarrhea occurs 1-3 times daily, and is soft and brown. No mucus, blood or straining has been noted. The dog has lost 8% of its body weight despite a good appetite. Five fecal flotations performed with zinc sulfate solution have been negative. The dog is otherwise normal. The most appropriate course of action is to:*

a. examine a direct fecal smear and perform another fecal flotation
b. perform a serum trypsin-like immunoreactivity determination
c. obtain plain abdominal radiographs
d. perform gastroduodenoscopy and obtain an intestinal biopsy
e. obtain contrast abdominal radiographs

143. *Concerning tetanus in dogs, which statement is most accurate?*

a. The incubation period ranges from days to months, in part depending upon how far the wound is from the central nervous system.
b. Definitive diagnosis requires electromyographic analysis.
c. As compared with other animals and people, dogs are relatively susceptible to tetanus.
d. Such drugs as diazepam and methocarbamol are ideal for treatment, while phenobarbital and acepromazine are not useful.

e. Large doses of antitoxin are effective in neutralizing toxin that has reached peripheral nerve fibers or passed through the blood-brain barrier.

144. *At weaning, a 5-month-old dog begins regurgitating at every meal. There are no prodromal signs; the dog simply puts it head down and gags up food and mucus. The dog is otherwise normal. The most appropriate course of action is to:*

a. obtain plain thoracic radiographs
b. perform a complete blood count and serum chemistry profile
c. obtain plain abdominal radiographs
d. perform a positive-contrast barium study of the intestines
e. perform liver function tests

145. *Concerning tuberculosis in dogs, which statement is most accurate?*

a. Dogs are more likely to acquire the infection from people than people are to acquire the infection from dogs.
b. Affected dogs usually have gastrointestinal signs.
c. Dogs usually are infected with *Mycobacterium bovis*.
d. Affected dogs should be treated with a combination of gentamicin, ampicillin and isoniazid.
e. Intradermal testing is the preferred method of diagnosis.

146. *A 2-year-old dog has been vomiting digested blood daily for 1 week. The dog is also somewhat anorectic. The most likely cause of these signs is:*

a. gastric foreign body
b. use of corticosteroids
c. parvoviral enteritis
d. salmonellosis
e. use of nonsteroidal antiinflammatory drugs

Correct answers are on pages 154-179.

Dogs, continued

147. *Concerning cryptococcosis in dogs, which statement is most accurate?*

   a. On cytologic preparations, *Cryptococcus* is best distinguished from other yeasts by its small size and intracellular location.
   b. Dogs are generally affected more commonly than cats.
   c. It is the most common mycosis affecting the canine nasal cavity.
   d. The latex agglutination test for cryptococcal antigen is very sensitive and specific.
   e. Ketoconazole is the treatment of choice for central nervous system involvement.

148. *Concerning congenital esophageal weakness in dogs, which statement is most accurate?*

   a. Most affected dogs can be successfully managed with conservative dietary therapy plus antiemetics.
   b. Endoscopic examination is the best and most precise means of diagnosis.
   c. Metoclopramide stimulates esophageal motility and lessens clinical signs.
   d. Surgery is a useful adjunct to dietary therapy in many affected dogs.
   e. Barium contrast radiographs demonstrate retention of barium throughout the esophagus.

149. *Which laboratory finding is **least** likely to be observed in a dog with severe acute pancreatitis?*

   a. hypercalcemia
   b. neutrophilic leukocytosis
   c. increased serum alkaline phosphatase and/or alanine aminotransferase activities
   d. azotemia
   e. hyperglycemia

150. *Of the following drugs, which is the most effective antiemetic for dogs with severe vomiting?*

   a. aminopentamide
   b. kaolin-pectin (Kaopectate)
   c. atropine
   d. chlorpromazine
   e. cimetidine

151. *Concerning chronic, complete jejunal obstruction in dogs, which statement is most accurate?*

   a. Dilated intestinal loops can often be seen on plain abdominal radiographs.
   b. Endoscopic examination is the most sensitive means of diagnosis.
   c. Contrast radiographs are indicated if you suspect such an obstruction.
   d. Abdominal palpation is usually all that is required for diagnosis.
   e. If a positive-contrast radiographic study is performed, an iodide contrast agent is preferred.

152. *A 9-month-old Boxer has had diarrhea for 4 months. The problem waxes and wanes, but has persisted. The stool is soft, without mucus or blood, and is passed 2-4 times per day without straining. The dog has lost 3-4 lb in the past 4 weeks and is fed a high-quality commercial diet. A direct fecal examination reveals numerous, rapidly motile, pear-shaped protozoa. Which statement concerning this dog is most accurate?*

   a. The dog should be treated with loperamide.
   b. The dog should be treated with sulfadimethoxine.
   c. The dog should be treated with metronidazole.
   d. The protozoa are probably not significant; you should recommend a dietary change.
   e. The dog should be treated with azulfidine.

153. *A 9-year-old mixed-breed dog suddenly begins to regurgitate its food without warning 0-3 times daily. The dog has also developed a soft, moist cough that began 2 weeks before the regurgitation was noted. The dog is otherwise normal, except that the moist cough can easily be elicited by rubbing the trachea. Which statement concerning this dog is most accurate?*

   a. Neuromuscular disease is a likely cause of the signs in this dog.

b. Gastric neoplasia is a likely cause of the signs in this dog.

c. A positive-contrast barium radiographic series of the stomach and intestines should next be performed.

d. A complete blood count and serum chemistry profile should next be performed.

e. Plain abdominal radiographs should next be made.

154. *A 4-year-old Basenji is emaciated and has hypoalbuminemia (1.3 g/dl; normal, 2.5-4.4 g/dl) and hyperproteinemia (7.7 g/dl; normal, 5.5-7.0 g/dl). The most likely cause of these findings is:*

a. hepatic insufficiency

b. lymphosarcoma

c. multiple myeloma

d. immunoproliferative enteropathy

e. lymphangiectasia

155. *On cytologic preparations of lymph node aspirates from dogs with histoplasmosis, Histoplasma organisms appear as:*

a. small (2-4 μ) round organisms with a basophilic center, often found within the host's cells

b. large (10-80 μ) round organisms containing numerous smaller structures

c. moderate-sized round yeast bodies with an obvious capsule around them

d. pleomorphic, cigar-shaped organisms

e. nonseptate hyphae without obvious spores

156. *Gastric outlet obstruction due to benign pyloric stenosis associated with hypertrophy of the circular muscle fibers of the pylorus principally occurs in:*

a. young Doberman Pinschers and old Great Danes

b. old dogs of giant breeds

c. young dogs of brachycephalic breeds

d. old Miniature Schnauzers and Yorkshire Terriers

e. deep-chested dogs of any age

157. *A dog with moderately severe large intestinal diarrhea for 6 weeks has lost 2% of its body weight during this time. The dog has traveled throughout the United States, and has been in Montana for the past 2 months. The client has declined any diagnostic tests. Given this dog's history, the most appropriate treatment is with:*

a. prednisolone

b. a trial elimination diet with added fiber

c. azulfidine

d. pyrantel pamoate

e. azathioprine

158. *A 7-year-old Dachshund has had diarrhea for 4 weeks. The problem waxes and wanes, but has persisted. The stool is soft, without blood or mucus, and is passed 2-4 times per day without straining. The dog has lost 5% of its body weight in the past week and is fed a high-quality commercial diet. Three fecal flotations reveal a few oocysts. Which statement concerning this dog is most accurate?*

a. A barium contrast radiographic study of the intestines is warranted.

b. The dog should be treated with fenbendazole.

c. The dog should be treated with trimethoprim.

d. The dog should be treated with loperamide.

e. The parasite represented by the oocysts is probably not responsible for the diarrhea.

159. *A 7-year-old mixed-breed dog has had marked hepatomegaly but is otherwise normal on physical examination. Serum alkaline phosphatase activity is 13 times normal and serum alanine aminotransferase activity is 1.2 times normal. Serum glucose, total protein, albumin, urea nitrogen, creatinine and electrolyte values are normal. A complete blood count reveals lymphopenia. The urine specific gravity is 1.028. The most likely cause of the increased serum alkaline phosphatase value is:*

a. copper storage disease

b. histoplasmosis

c. hepatic cirrhosis

d. vacuolar hepatopathy

e. portosystemic shunt

Correct answers are on pages 154-179.

Dogs, continued

160. *An undersized 8-month-old Yorkshire Terrier that was the "runt of the litter" is presented for ovariohysterectomy. The surgery goes without problem, but the dog does not awaken from anesthesia for 28 hours. The most likely cause of delayed recovery from anesthesia in this dog is:*

a. inappropriate anesthetic agent
b. anesthetic overdose
c. a portosystemic shunt
d. hypoglycemia
e. congenital renal amyloidosis

161. *Shortly after you give a dog several swallows of a liquid barium suspension, you note barium pooling in the pyloric antrum on the first radiograph made in the series. This observation indicates that the dog probably:*

a. is in left lateral recumbency
b. is in right lateral recumbency
c. has significant gastric outflow obstruction
d. has significant gastric paresis
e. is normal

162. *The drug most likely to be effective in treating acute diarrhea in a dog is:*

a. sucralfate
b. bismuth subsalicylate
c. barium sulfate
d. atropine
e. cimetidine

163. *Five mature dogs in your clinic have developed diarrhea in the past 6 days. Each dog acutely develops profuse, bloody diarrhea but is otherwise normal. You have treated each dog with some combination of kaolin-pectate, aminopentamide, amoxicillin and/or loperamide. The diarrhea usually resolves within 2-4 days, regardless of which treatment you use. The most likely cause of this outbreak of diarrhea is:*

a. salmonellosis
b. clostridial enteritis

c. parvoviral enteritis
d. coronaviral enteritis
e. giardiasis

164. *You perform a positive-contrast barium gastrogram in a dog with a history of vomiting bile. The next day, radiographs reveal that all of the barium is in the colon, except for 2 small, discrete "spots" in the gastric antrum, in which barium is retained. Which statement concerning this dog is most accurate?*

a. The dog probably has gastric antral ulcers.
b. The dog probably has a gastric foreign body.
c. The dog should be treated with metoclopramide.
d. The dog should be treated with chlorpromazine.
e. The dog will probably die from this illness.

165. *Concerning exocrine pancreatic insufficiency in dogs, which statement is most accurate?*

a. It can be reliably diagnosed by oral fat absorption and fecal film digestion tests.
b. It is often accompanied by small intestinal bacterial overgrowth.
c. It is usually caused by chronic or relapsing pancreatitis.
d. It reliably responds to pancreatic enzyme supplementation.
e. It typically causes severe weight loss associated with marked hypoproteinemia.

166. *You are presented with a dog that has ingested a noncorrosive toxic substance. The most reliable emetic for use in this dog is:*

a. apomorphine
b. xylazine
c. syrup of ipecac
d. salt water
e. hydrogen peroxide

167. *A litter of 2-week-old Corgi puppies suddenly becomes ill. The dogs are weak and have very pale oral mucosae and scant, dark diarrhea. These dogs:*

a. should immediately be treated with pyrantel pamoate

b. should immediately be treated with metronidazole

c. should be examined by direct fecal smears and fecal flotation

d. should be tested by enzyme-linked immunosorbent assay for parvoviral enteritis

e. probably have infectious viral diarrhea and should be isolated

168. *A 4-year-old female Great Dane has had diarrhea for 6 weeks. The stools are soft (especially toward the end of defecation) and covered with mucus. There is no blood or straining associated with defecation, but the animal occasionally defecates in the house when it cannot get outside quickly enough. The dog is otherwise normal. Which statement concerning this dog is most accurate?*

a. The dog should be treated with loperamide for up to 1 week before any tests are performed.

b. The dog should be treated with pyrantel pamoate before any tests are performed.

c. The dog probably has chronic large intestinal diarrhea.

d. The dog probably has protein-losing enteropathy.

e. A complete blood count and serum chemistry profile should next be performed.

169. *Concerning* Ehrlichia platys *infection in dogs, which statement is most accurate?*

a. Concurrent infections with *Ehrlichia canis* are probably rare.

b. Finding inclusion bodies in platelets during periods of severe thrombocytopenia is the easiest and most reliable means of diagnosis.

c. Infected animals typically are ill with fever and epistaxis.

d. The pancytopenia caused by this rickettsia tends to be more severe than that caused by *Ehrlichia canis.*

e. The serologic test for antibodies to *Ehrlichia canis* does not cross react with antibodies to *Ehrlichia platys.*

170. *Concerning radiographic demonstration of esophageal foreign bodies, which statement is most accurate?*

a. If a foreign body is seen on plain thoracic radiographs, one should perform contrast esophagography with an iodide contrast agent to determine if perforation has occurred.

b. Use of barium sulfate is generally contraindicated if a foreign body may be present.

c. Metoclopramide should be administered during the procedure to ensure even distribution of the contrast agent.

d. Most foreign bodies can be seen on plain radiographs of the thorax, eliminating the need for contrast studies.

e. Parasympatholytics may be given to reduce esophageal spasm and produce more accurate radiographs.

171. *A 9-month-old mixed-breed dog has had episodes of abnormal behavior during the past 5 months. These episodes principally occur after meals and tend to develop and resolve gradually. The dog becomes ataxic and stumbles into walls and furniture. In addition, the dog seems to drink and urinate excessive amounts, and is much smaller than its littermates. The urine specific gravity is 1.011, serum phosphorus concentration is 7.7 mg/dl (normal, 2.5-5.5 mg/dl), serum alkaline phosphatase activity is 201 IU/L (normal, <145 IU/L) and serum albumin concentration is 2.3 g/dl (normal, 2.5-4.4 g/dl). The most likely cause of these findings is:*

a. ingestion of toxins

b. idiopathic epilepsy

c. renal disease

d. intermittent hypoglycemia

e. hepatic insufficiency

Correct answers are on pages 154-179.

Dogs, continued

172. A 3-month-old mixed-breed dog has peracute onset of severe depression, fever, anorexia, vomiting and diarrhea. The vomitus consists of food and yellow phlegm, while the diarrhea is dark brown and watery. The most likely cause of these signs is:

   a. salmonellosis
   b. coronaviral diarrhea
   c. parvoviral diarrhea
   d. gastrointestinal foreign body
   e. gastroenteritis from ingestion of garbage

173. The finding most indicative of hemorrhagic gastroenteritis in dogs is:

   a. degenerative left shift in peripheral white blood cells on a complete blood count
   b. platelet count <100,000/μl
   c. dilated small intestinal loops on abdominal radiographs.
   d. packed cell volume of 70%
   e. bacterial spores in feces

174. An obese 62-kg mixed-breed dog is retching unproductively and has had a painful cranial abdomen for 2 hours. Findings of the physical examination are otherwise unremarkable except that the dog is clearly depressed. The most appropriate course of action is to:

   a. perform a complete blood count and serum chemistry profile
   b. administer metoclopramide
   c. perform a positive-contrast barium radiographic study of the abdomen
   d. administer flunixin meglumine
   e. make plain abdominal radiographs

175. A 1-year-old male Boxer has severe large intestinal diarrhea unrelated to parasites or diet. Considering the dog's age and breed, the most likely cause of diarrhea is:

   a. cecocolic intussusception
   b. eosinophilic enteritis
   c. intestinal adenocarcinoma
   d. pythiosis
   e. histiocytic ulcerative colitis

176. A sign **rarely** observed in dogs with congenital portosystemic shunt is:

   a. seizures
   b. ascites
   c. stunted growth
   d. polyuria/polydipsia
   e. vomiting

177. Concerning tapeworm infection in young dogs, which statement is most accurate?

   a. *Taenia* species are the most common tapeworms in dogs in the United States.
   b. Most affected animals have soft stools and show a decline in physical condition.
   c. Vomiting of proglottids is often the first sign of infection with *Spirometra*.
   d. Large doses of fenbendazole are effective as treatment for infection with the types of tapeworms found in the United States.
   e. Fleas and lice are intermediate hosts for the most common species.

178. Concerning viral enteritis in dogs, which statement is most accurate?

   a. Severe coronaviral infections cause intestinal crypt necrosis.
   b. Severe parvoviral infections cause widespread loss of villi.
   c. Severe rotaviral infections cause intestinal crypt necrosis.
   d. Coronavirus is very resistant to the environment and most disinfectants.
   e. Rotaviral infections often result in concurrent aspiration penumonia.

179. A 4-year-old dog has been sick for the past 2 weeks. It vomits food every 2-3 days and has a diminished appetite. Yesterday it began passing black, tarry diarrhea. The dog has lost about 5% of its body weight and has pale mucous membranes. The most likely cause of these signs is:

a. chronic large intestinal diarrhea
b. chronic pancreatitis
c. exocrine pancreatic insufficiency
d. gastroduodenal ulceration
e. large intestinal neoplasia

180. *During a positive-contrast barium radiographic study of the esophagus, which drug would probably cause significant artifacts on the esophagogram and make it appear that a normal dog had generalized esophageal weakness?*

a. xylazine
b. acepromazine
c. metoclopramide
d. cimetidine
e. sucralfate

181. *After a normal dog is given liquid barium sulfate per os, the barium solution typically reaches the area of the ileocolic valve within:*

a. 15-45 minutes
b. 30-90 minutes
c. 90-120 minutes
d. 180-240 minutes
e. 240-300 minutes

182. *You examine a 23-week-old mixed-breed dog that appears to have 2-3 inches of bowel mucosa protruding from its anus. The dog has been somewhat depressed and losing weight for the past week, and the protruding segment of bowel was noticed 4 days previously. The most appropriate course of action is to:*

a. resect the prolapsed tissue
b. replace the mucosa and keep it in place with a pursestring suture
c. perform a rectal examination to see if there is a cul-de-sac between the mucosa and rectal wall
d. perform a colonopexy
e. replace the mucosa and administer a lidocaine enema before placing a pursestring suture

183. *A 3-year-old German Shepherd has severe flatulence. Which statement concerning this dog is most accurate?*

a. The gas is probably due to malabsorbed carbohydrates reaching the colon.
b. The gas is probably due to aerophagia.
c. A dietary fiber supplement should be fed.
d. Metoclopramide should be given.
e. Endoscopic biopsy of the colon is indicated as the next step.

184. *Which of the following is **least** likely to cause vomiting in a dog?*

a. uremia
b. hypercalcemia
c. diabetic ketoacidosis
d. hepatic failure
e. hyperadrenocorticism

185. *A 4-month-old Doberman Pinscher puppy developed acute diarrhea this morning. This afternoon, the puppy is severely depressed, anorectic and febrile (40.2 C), and has profuse, odiferous diarrhea, with occasional vomiting of bile. A complete blood count shows a packed cell volume of 32% (normal, 35-53%) and a white blood cell count of 6000/μl (normal, 5000-14,000/μl), with 94% neutrophils and 5% lymphocytes. A direct fecal examination reveals numerous hookworm and roundworm eggs, plus motile pentatrichomonad trophozoites. The most likely cause of these signs is:*

a. bacterial infection
b. food intolerance
c. endoparasitism
d. viral infection
e. reaction to ingestion of garbage

186. *In a dog with suspected ehrlichiosis, the most appropriate course of action is to:*

a. examine a peripheral blood smear for morulae
b. treat the dog with gentamicin for 10 days
c. aspirate and examine a bone marrow sample
d. treat the dog with chloramphenicol for 21 days
e. perform an ophthalmologic examination

Correct answers are on pages 154-179.

Dogs, continued

187. Which radiographic finding is **least** likely
to be observed in a dog with acute pancreatitis?

   a. mass obstructing the mid-descending
      duodenum
   b. poor serosal detail in the cranial right
      quadrant
   c. displacement of descending duodenum to the
      right
   d. widening of the angle between the pyloric
      antrum and proximal duodenum
   e. an air-filled duodenum that is somewhat
      dilated relative to the rest of the intestinal
      tract

188. Which dog is **least** likely to have gastric or
intestinal disease?

   a. 1-year-old dog that vomits food, mucus and
      what appears to be "coffee grounds," 1-3
      hours after eating
   b. 3-year-old dog that looks obviously sick and
      salivates for 5-10 minutes before vomiting
      apparently undigested food
   c. 5-year-old dog that throws up copious
      amounts of yellow foam daily, especially in
      the morning
   d. 2-year-old dog with vigorous retching and
      then projectile vomiting of food, shortly
      after eating
   e. 4-year-old dog that unexpectedly gags up
      food and mucus, not associated with eating

189. Concerning hyperbilirubinemia of 3 mg/dl
(normal, <1.0 mg/dl) and icterus in dogs,
which statement is most accurate?

   a. Exocrine pancreatic insufficiency is a
      relatively common cause.
   b. Icterus is to be expected in nearly every case
      of significant hepatic disease.
   c. Hemolysis may cause this finding.
   d. Gallstones commonly cause extrahepatic
      obstruction with this magnitude of
      bilirubinemia.
   e. This finding is often due to vacuolar
      hepatopathy.

190. Which statement best describes the position
and course of the canine duodenum as seen in
a ventrodorsal projection on a positive-contrast
barium radiograph of the abdomen?

   a. It originates at the pylorus, courses caudally
      to the root of the mesentery, turns cranially
      and then ascends.
   b. It originates at the pylorus, then crosses to
      the left side of the abdomen and courses
      caudally to the root of the mesentery.
   c. It originates at the pylorus, courses caudally
      to about the level of the 7th lumbar
      vertebra, and then crosses to the other side
      of the abdomen.
   d. It originates at the pylorus, courses caudally
      to about the level of the 7th lumbar
      vertebra, turns cranially and ascends on the
      left side.
   e. It originates at the pylorus, courses caudally
      to about the level of the sacrum, and then
      turns cranially.

191. Concerning serum gamma glutamyltransferase activity in dogs, which statement is most
accurate?

   a. It is a more sensitive indicator than serum
      bile acid levels for detecting portosystemic
      shunts.
   b. Serum gamma glutamyltransferase activity
      does not increase in response to
      corticosteroid administration.
   c. Gamma glutamyltransferase is a "leakage"
      enzyme and should always be assayed in
      conjunction with serum alkaline
      phosphatase activity.
   d. It is a less sensitive indicator than serum
      alkaline phosphatase activity for detecting
      hepatic disease.
   e. It is invariably increased in icteric dogs and
      therefore is not useful in them.

192. A 3-year-old Yorkshire Terrier has had
repeated bouts of ataxia and depression. The
episodes began 14 months previously and have
gradually gotten worse. The episodes principally occur after the dog is fed table scraps and
can last hours to days. On physical examination (including rectal and ophthalmologic
examinations), the dog seems normal except

that it is clearly smaller than expected for its age and breed. The owner declines a diagnostic workup. Considering the dog's history and clinical signs, the most appropriate treatment is with:

a. a low-protein, low-salt diet and oral aluminum hydroxide
b. a trial period of several small feedings per day of a high-protein diet
c. lactulose, a low-protein diet and oral neomycin
d. oral phenobarbital
e. oral prednisolone and amoxicillin

193. What is the best treatment for a dog with moderately severe, acute pancreatitis?

a. intravenous balanced electrolyte fluids plus sodium bicarbonate, analgesics and small amounts of a bland diet
b. intravenous balanced electrolyte fluids, and small amounts of a bland low-fat diet
c. nothing per os and intravenous balanced electrolyte fluids
d. antibiotics, analgesics and nothing per os
e. intravenous balanced electrolyte fluids, corticosteroids, antibiotics and small amounts of a low-fat diet

194. The expected location of the cecum on a ventrodorsal radiograph of a dog's abdomen is in the:

a. cranial half, to the right of midline, near the 6th lumbar vertebra
b. cranial half, to the left of midline, near the 2nd lumbar vertebra
c. cranial half, to the right of midline, near the 2nd lumbar vertebra
d. cranial half, to the left of midline, near the 6th lumbar vertebra
e. cranial half, on the midline, near the 6th lumbar vertebra

195. A 5-month-old mixed-breed dog has a fever (40 C), diarrhea, anorexia and depression that began 1 day previously. It is now vomiting bile-stained fluid, even when fasting. The most likely cause of these signs is:

a. gastric ulceration

b. intestinal intussusception
c. gastrointestinal parasites
d. parvoviral enteritis
e. food intolerance

196. A plain ventrodorsal radiograph of a dog's abdomen reveals that the pylorus is markedly displaced caudally and medially. No other abnormalities are noted radiographically. The most likely cause of this finding is:

a. nonlinear alimentary foreign body
b. lymphosarcoma
c. hemangiosarcoma
d. hepatoma
e. linear alimentary foreign body

197. During the past 3 days, a 5-year-old dog has been anorectic and vomiting green phlegm 4-6 times per day. Initial (first day) management of this dog should include all of the following except:

a. a central-acting antiemetic
b. a serum chemistry profile
c. plain abdominal radiographs
d. intravenous fluids
e. endoscopic examination of the stomach and duodenum

198. After a normal dog is given liquid barium sulfate per os, the barium solution typically begins to pass from the stomach into the duodenum within:

a. 0-30 minutes
b. 30-45 minutes
c. 45-60 minutes
d. 60-90 minutes
e. 90-120 minutes

199. Which clinical sign is least likely to be observed in a dog with severe, acute pancreatitis?

a. severe vomiting
b. moderate abdominal pain
c. slight fever
d. marked ascites
e. moderate dehydration

Correct answers are on pages 154-179.

Dogs, continued

200. *You inject an iodinated contrast agent into a jejunal vein and immediately make abdominal radiographs. Which radiographic observation is most suggestive of a congenital portosystemic shunt?*

a. several small vessels exiting the portal vein and coursing cranially, anastomosing with vessels near the esophagus

b. several small vessels exiting the portal vein before entering the liver, anastomosing with the azygos vein or caudal vena cava

c. a single vessel exiting the portal vein before entering the liver and coursing caudally, anastomosing with the renal vein or caudal celiac vein

d. the portal vein entering the liver and branching into many smaller vessels within the hepatic parenchyma

e. a single vessel exiting the portal vein before entering the liver, anastomosing with the azygos vein or caudal vena cava

Cats

S.K. Fooshee, R.G. Sherding

> *Practice answer sheets are on pages 341-344.*

201. *Hypokalemic polymyopathy is a neuromuscular disorder of cats that appears related to decreased dietary intake of potassium, as well as excessive renal wasting of potassium. The classic presenting sign for this polymyopathy is:*

a. urinary incontinence
b. nystagmus
c. ventroflexion of the neck
d. opisthotonus
e. hypalgesia of the extremities

202. *A common biochemical finding in cats with hypokalemic polymyopathy is:*

a. increased serum alkaline phosphatase activity
b. decreased serum alkaline phosphatase activity
c. decreased serum creatine phosphokinase activity
d. increased serum creatine phosphokinase activity
e. increased serum alanine aminotransferase activity

203. *Beta-blockers, such as propranolol, are potentially indicated in treatment of all of the following* **except**:

a. systemic hypertension
b. asthmatic bronchitis
c. hypertrophic cardiomyopathy
d. cardiac arrhythmias
e. tachycardia

204. *Which breed is well recognized for a familial predisposition to renal amyloidosis?*

a. Abyssinian
b. Domestic Shorthair
c. Siamese
d. Burmese
e. Himalayan

205. *How do the pathologic findings of renal amyloidosis in cats differ from those of renal amyloidosis in dogs?*

a. in cats, the amyloid deposits are more severe than in dogs

b. in cats, the proteinuria is more marked than in dogs

c. in cats, the amyloid deposits are medullary, whereas, in dogs, the deposits are glomerular

d. in cats, the prognosis is better than for dogs

e. in cats, renal amyloidosis is usually subclinical, whereas, in dogs, it is usually clinical

206. A geriatric cat has moderate azotemia, unilateral renomegaly, abdominal effusion and vomiting. The cat tests negative for feline leukemia virus by serum enzyme-linked immunosorbent assay (ELISA) and has essentially normal urine. The most likely cause of these findings is:

a. feline immunodeficiency virus infection

b. hemangiosarcoma

c. pancreatic adenocarcinoma

d. metastatic prostatic adenocarcinoma

e. lymphosarcoma

207. Which clinicopathologic finding is consistent with feline infectious peritonitis?

a. increased serum globulin level

b. decreased serum globulin level

c. monoclonal gammopathy

d. Bence-Jones proteinuria

e. decreased serum albumin level

208. Cats are immunologically distinct from dogs. What immunoglobulin has been recognized in dogs but has **not** yet been identified in cats?

a. IgA

b. IgD

c. IgM

d. IgE

e. IgG

209. Both cats and dogs are frequently treated for hypovolemic shock as a result of trauma. Intravenous fluids must be more cautiously administered to cats than dogs, however, because cats have a smaller blood volume. The

blood volume of cats (as a percentage of body weight) is approximately:

a. 1-2%

b. 2-3%

c. 3-4%

d. 4-5%

e. 5-6%

210. Which disease causes ventroflexion of the neck?

a. spinal cord lymphoma

b. thiamin deficiency

c. hepatic lipidosis

d. ischemic encephalopathy

e. cerebellar hypoplasia

211. Concerning the biologic behavior of osteosarcoma in cats, which statement is **least** accurate?

a. It most commonly occurs in the hind limbs.

b. Pulmonary metastasis is less common in cats than in dogs.

c. It is the most common bone tumor of cats.

d. Affected cats generally have a shorter survival time than affected dogs.

e. It tends to occur in older, female domestic shorthair cats.

212. Which test is most specific for evaluation of liver function in cats?

a. fasting and postprandial serum bile acid levels

b. serum albumin level

c. BSP (sulfobromophthalein) clearance

d. indocyanine green clearance

e. serum alanine aminotransferase activity

213. The most common primary brain tumor of cats is:

a. neuroglioblastoma

b. meningioma

c. astrocytoma

d. lymphoma

e. malignant melanosarcoma

Correct answers are on pages 154-179.

Cats, continued

214. *A thin, 15-year-old cat is presented to your clinic with acute onset of hind limb paresis. The owner is hysterical, as the cat appears to be in a great deal of pain. You cannot elicit spinal reflexes in the rear limbs and do not feel any pulses in the femoral arteries. The footpads appear cyanotic. The most likely cause of these signs is:*

   a. trauma
   b. spinal cord tumor, with vascular disruption
   c. coagulation disorder associated with hypertrophic cardiomyopathy
   d. bleeding into the spinal cord associated with an anticoagulant rodenticide
   e. intervertebral disk rupture

215. *Anisocoria is commonly associated with a spinal cord lesion at the level of:*

   a. C1
   b. C5
   c. T1
   d. T10
   e. L1

216. *A cat that has just been struck by an automobile is in extreme respiratory distress. On thoracic auscultation you cannot discern heart sounds or lung sounds. The most likely cause of these findings is:*

   a. diaphragmatic hernia
   b. peritoneopericardial hernia
   c. chylothorax
   d. pericardial tamponade
   e. pulmonary contusions

217. *Prolonged urethral obstruction in male cats can cause life-threatening metabolic derangements. These cats require immediate medical treatment to correct:*

   a. increased serum urea nitrogen and potassium levels, with metabolic alkalosis
   b. increased serum urea nitrogen and potassium levels, with metabolic acidosis
   c. increased serum urea nitrogen and decreased potassium levels, with metabolic alkalosis
   d. increased serum urea nitrogen and decreased potassium levels, with metabolic acidosis
   e. increased serum urea nitrogen and decreased potassium levels, with normal acid-base balance

218. *In cats, a deficiency of which coagulation factor is commonly recognized yet rarely causes clinical bleeding?*

   a. Factor III
   b. Factor VII
   c. Factor VII
   d. Factor X
   e. Factor XII

219. *Transfusion reactions are rare in cats. What is the most common manifestation of transfusion with incompatible blood?*

   a. hemolytic anemia
   b. respiratory arrest
   c. vomiting
   d. hemoglobinuria
   e. seizures

220. *Deficiency of which essential amino acid may lead to hepatic encephalopathy?*

   a. methionine
   b. leucine
   c. tryptophan
   d. arginine
   e. valine

221. *Which drug is **contraindicated** for treatment of hypertrophic cardiomyopathy in cats?*

   a. furosemide
   b. captopril
   c. digoxin
   d. diltiazem
   e. propranolol

222. *The worldwide distribution of various feline blood groups appears to vary with geographic locale. For this reason, reactions to initial blood transfusion are uncommon in some regions. However, severe transfusion reactions almost invariably occur when a:*

   a. type-A recipient receives type-B blood
   b. type-B recipient receives type-A blood
   c. type-A recipient receives type-C blood
   d. type-B recipient receives type-C blood
   e. type-C recipient receives type-B blood

223. *Giardiasis may cause chronic or acute diarrhea in cats. The life cycle of this parasite may involve all parts of the gastrointestinal tract* **except** *the:*

   a. stomach
   b. ileum
   c. duodenum
   d. jejunum
   e. large intestine

224. *The cause of leprosy in cats is:*

   a. *Mycobacterium lepraemurium*
   b. *Mycobacterium fortuitum*
   c. *Mycobacterium stenti*
   d. *Mycobacterium paratuberculosis*
   e. *Mycobacterium avium*

225. *In cats, mast-cell tumors most frequently involve the:*

   a. brain and eyes
   b. conjunctivae and gingivae
   c. mucous membranes and heart base
   d. abdominal viscera and skin
   e. lymph nodes and lung

226. *One of the more commonly recognized clinical manifestations of acromegaly in cats is:*

   a. dwarfism
   b. blindness
   c. severe insulin-resistant diabetes mellitus
   d. hyperadrenocorticism
   e. nephrogenic diabetes insipidus

227. *What is the most common systemic fungal infection of cats?*

   a. coccidioidomycosis
   b. cryptococcosis
   c. histoplasmosis
   d. blastomycosis
   e. mycosis fungoides

228. *Latent infections with feline leukemia virus can only be detected by:*

   a. radioallergosorbent testing (RAST) of serum
   b. enzyme-linked immunosorbent assay (ELISA) of serum
   c. indirect fluorescent antibody (IFA) testing of bone marrow
   d. bone marrow culture and cell reactivation
   e. enzyme-linked immunosorbent assay (ELISA) of tears

229. *In cats, bradycardia is generally defined as a heart rate less than:*

   a. 250 beats/minute
   b. 200 beats/minute
   c. 160 beats/minute
   d. 120 beats/minute
   e. 80 beats/minute

230. *Benzocaine is a topical anesthetic frequently sprayed into the larynx during endotracheal intubation of cats. Why should this practice be avoided in cats?*

   a. the force of the spray aggravates laryngospasm
   b. the drug can cause methemoglobinemia
   c. the drug can cause cardiac arrhythmias
   d. the drug lowers the seizure threshold
   e. the spray can cause irreversible reflex apnea

Correct answers are on pages 154-179.

Cats, continued

231. *Which drug is most useful in treatment of acetaminophen toxicosis?*

   a. xylazine
   b. diazepam
   c. aspirin
   d. acetylcysteine
   e. ketoconazole

232. *Neuromuscular blockade and respiratory failure may occur with use of:*

   a. chloramphenicol
   b. enrofloxacin
   c. amoxicillin
   d. gentamicin
   e. metronidazole

Questions 233 and 234

233. *The most common dermatophyte isolated from cats is:*

   a. *Microsporum gypseum*
   b. *Microsporum canis*
   c. *Trichophyton mentagrophytes*
   d. *Candida albicans*
   e. *Pseudoallescheria boydii*

234. *Cats infected with the dermatophyte described in Question 233 can be effectively treated with any of the following* **except***:*

   a. lime-sulfur dip
   b. captan rinse
   c. chlorhexidine shampoo
   d. amitraz dip
   e. chlorhexidine dip

235. *The cause of acromegaly in cats differs from that in dogs. Essentially all reported cases of acromegaly in cats have been attributed to:*

   a. progestagen induction of growth hormone-mediated insulin resistance
   b. primary brain tumor

   c. adrenal tumor
   d. pituitary tumor
   e. fluctuating progestagen levels caused by the reproductive cycle

236. *The renal threshold for glucose in cats is approximately:*

   a. 120 mg/dl
   b. 180 mg/dl
   c. 200 mg/dl
   d. 240 mg/dl
   e. 290 mg/dl

237. *In cats, the term "walking dandruff" refers to infestation with:*

   a. *Notoedres cati*
   b. *Ctenocephalides felis*
   c. *Rhipicephalus sanguineus*
   d. *Cheyletiella blakei*
   e. *Otodectes cynotis*

238. *Cerebellar hypoplasia in kittens may be caused by* in-utero *infection with:*

   a. feline leukemia virus
   b. feline infectious peritonitis virus
   c. feline panleukopenia virus
   d. feline rhinotracheitis virus
   e. feline immunodeficiency virus

Questions 239 and 240

You are presented with a mature adult cat with severe facial excoriations. The cat appears intensely pruritic and is constantly clawing itself about the face, neck and ears. The cat was previously seen by another veterinarian and given glucocorticoids, with no apparent response.

239. *What is the most likely cause of this pruritus?*

   a. flea-allergy dermatitis
   b. otitis interna
   c. food allergy

---

d. sarcoptic mange

e. contact hypersensitivity

240. *How can the cause of pruritus be definitively diagnosed?*

a. skin biopsy

b. trial feeding of a hypoallergenic diet

c. necropsy

d. trial course of antihistamine therapy

e. isolation of the cat for 2 weeks in your clinic

241. *Which of the following is an exceedingly rare (some say even nonexistent) intestinal parasite of cats?*

a. *Trichuris* species

b. *Ancylostoma tubaeformae*

c. *Toxoplasma gondii*

d. *Dipylidium caninum*

e. *Taenia taeniaeformis*

242. *Which cardiovascular drug should **not** be used in cats?*

a. propranolol

b. diltiazem

c. digoxin

d. digitoxin

e. nitroglycerin

243. *All of the following are useful in management of constipated cats **except**:*

a. dioctyl sodium sulfosuccinate

b. canned pumpkin pie filling

c. psyllium

d. providing fresh water and a clean litterbox

e. phosphate-containing enemas (*eg*, Fleet)

244. *All of the following can cause polyphagia and weight loss in cats **except**:*

a. hyperthyroidism

b. exocrine pancreatic insufficiency

c. diabetes mellitus

d. inflammatory bowel disease

e. hepatic lipidosis

Questions 245 and 246

245. *In a white cat that spends time indoors and outdoors, ulcerated lesions on the nasal planum and ear margins are most likely associated with:*

a. dermatophytosis

b. eosinophilic granuloma complex

c. squamous-cell carcinoma

d. pemphigus foliaceus

e. mast-cell tumor

246. *If the cat in Question 245 were a strictly indoor cat and, in addition to the aforementioned lesions, also had thick, hardened footpads and a low-grade fever, what would be the most likely cause?*

a. dermatophytosis

b. eosinophilic granuloma complex

c. squamous-cell carcinoma

d. pemphigus foliaceus

e. mast-cell tumor

247. *In cats, basophilic stippling of erythrocytes is pathognomonic for:*

a. lead poisoning

b. regenerative anemia

c. disseminated intravascular coagulation

d. feline leukemia virus infection of bone marrow

e. no particular disease

248. *In a living cat, how is feline infectious peritonitis best diagnosed?*

a. serologic testing for coronavirus

b. detailed history and careful physical examination

c. indirect antibody testing of conjunctival scrapings

d. histopathologic examination of organ biopsies

e. analysis of pleural or peritoneal fluid

Correct answers are on pages 154-179.

Cats, continued

249. *Cats are renowned for their sensitivity to many chemical compounds. Which of the following can produce profound neurologic disturbances that frequently result in death of the animal?*

    a. benzyl alcohol
    b. fenbendazole
    c. pyrethrin-based flea products
    d. third-generation cephalosporins
    e. gentamicin

250. *Effusions from cats with feline infectious peritonitis are characterized by their:*

    a. high protein content, lack of bacteria, and relatively high cellularity
    b. high protein content, large numbers of bacteria, and relatively low cellularity
    c. low protein content, lack of bacteria, and relatively low cellularity
    d. low protein content, large numbers of bacteria, and relatively high cellularity
    e. high protein content, lack of bacteria, and relatively low cellularity

251. *The most important source of feline leukemia virus in transmission to susceptible uninfected cats is:*

    a. urine from an infected cat
    b. saliva from an infected cat
    c. contaminated food and water bowls used by an infected cat
    d. bites of infected fleas
    e. sexual contact with an infected cat

252. *Hyperthyroidism is common in older cats and is frequently accompanied by several characteristic electrocardiographic changes. These include all of the following **except**:*

    a. sinus tachycardia
    b. increased R wave amplitude
    c. electrical alternans
    d. atrial premature complexes
    e. ventricular tachycardia

253. *In cats, bacterial endocarditis most commonly affects:*

    a. the mitral valve
    b. the pulmonic valve
    c. the aortic valve
    d. the tricuspid valve
    e. all valves equally

254. *Pleural effusion is not normally detectable on radiographs until the fluid volume reaches approximately:*

    a. 10 ml
    b. 25 ml
    c. 50 ml
    d. 100 ml
    e. 200 ml

255. *A cat is presented to your clinic for evaluation of a lesion on the toe. Histopathologic examination identifies the mass as a squamous-cell carcinoma. Of the following statements, which is **least** appropriate for educating the client about this lesion?*

    a. This tumor is likely to respond to a combined chemotherapy protocol.
    b. This tumor is likely to respond to local irradiation.
    c. This tumor is likely to manifest invasive behavior.
    d. In the absence of clinically demonstrable metastasis, local excision or limb amputation may be warranted to prolong life.
    e. Squamous-cell carcinoma of the digit has a tendency of metastasize early.

256. *Concerning the insulin molecule of cats, which statement is most accurate?*

    a. It is nearly identical to the insulin of cattle.
    b. It is nearly identical to the insulin of pigs.
    c. It is nearly identical to the insulin of fish.
    d. It is nearly identical to the insulin of people.
    e. Its structure has not been defined.

257. *Heartworm infection may go undiagnosed in cats because of vague, nonspecific signs. Which of the following is considered a useful test for feline heartworm infection?*

   a. profound eosinophilia on a complete blood count
   b. concentrating techniques, such as the Knott's test
   c. diagnostic imaging (radiography, ultrasonography, nonselective angiography)
   d. serologic tests for heartworm antibody
   e. response to thiacetarsamide therapy

258. *Concerning neoplasia in cats, which statement is **least** accurate?*

   a. Lymphoma is the most common tumor of cats of all ages.
   b. Lymphoma is a common hepatic neoplasm in cats of any age, regardless of feline leukemia virus status.
   c. Squamous-cell carcinoma is the most common oral neoplasm of cats.
   d. Colonic adenocarcinoma is the most common gastrointestinal neoplasm of cats.
   e. Mammary tumors in cats are usually malignant.

259. *You work in a small animal practice in the midwestern United States and are presented with an adult indoor/outdoor intact male cat. The cat is in profound shock and has a low-grade fever. The cat soon dies despite your efforts. On necropsy, you find blood pooled in the abdomen and petechial hemorrhages on the serosal surfaces of the organs. Some mesenteric vessels contain small thrombi. You evaluate a cytologic specimen obtained from the spleen and find small ring-like parasites in virtually all of the macrophages. The most likely cause of disease in this cat is infection with:*

   a. *Ehrlichia platys*
   b. *Hemobartonella felis*
   c. *Histoplasma capsulatum*
   d. *Trypanosoma cruzi*
   e. *Cytauxzoon felis*

260. *In cats, infectious conjunctivitis is **least** likely to be caused by:*

   a. feline rhinotracheitis virus
   b. feline calicivirus
   c. *Mycoplasma*
   d. *Chlamydia*
   e. *Mycobacterium lepraemurium*

261. *Propylthiouracil had traditionally been the drug of choice for treatment of hyperthyroidism in cats. It has fallen into disfavor because of increasing recognition of its association with:*

   a. immune-mediated hemolytic anemia
   b. hypocalcemia
   c. urolithiasis
   d. congestive heart failure
   e. diabetes insipidus

262. *The most common cause of lymphadenomegaly in cats is:*

   a. lymphosarcoma
   b. feline leukemia virus infection
   c. extramedullary hematopoiesis in response to anemia
   d. lymphoid hyperplasia
   e. metastatic adenocarcinoma

263. *An apparently healthy young adult cat is brought to your clinic for ovariohysterectomy. Preoperative clinicopathologic screening tests reveal hyperglycemia and glucosuria. The most likely cause of these findings is:*

   a. diabetes mellitus
   b. Fanconi syndrome (proximal tubular resorptive defect)
   c. hypoadrenocorticism
   d. hyperadrenocorticism
   e. stress

Correct answers are on pages 154-179.

Cats, continued

264. Which viral antigen of the feline leukemia virus is associated with glomerulonephritis in some infected cats?

   a. gp 70
   b. p27
   c. feline oncornavirus-associated cell membrane antigen (FOCMA)
   d. p15e
   e. reverse transcriptase enzyme

265. Concerning feline immunodeficiency virus, which statement is most accurate?

   a. It is most common in the cattery setting.
   b. It is more common in older cats.
   c. It is known for rapid and aggressive tumor induction.
   d. It is transmitted to people and can cause AIDS in people.
   e. It is transmitted to kittens *in utero* or through the milk.

266. Concerning the teeth of cats, which statement is **least** accurate?

   a. The deciduous incisors are the first teeth to erupt and are usually present in kittens by 2 weeks of age.
   b. Full deciduous dentition is present by 7-8 weeks of age.
   c. Full permanent dentition is present by 7 months of age.
   d. Cats are diphyodont animals.
   e. The upper carnassial tooth is the first molar.

267. Exocrine pancreatic insufficiency is not commonly recognized in cats. However, practitioners should be aware that the best means of diagnosis is:

   a. serum trypsin-like immunoreactivity
   b. 24-hour total fecal fat passage
   c. para-aminobenzoic acid (PABA) absorption
   d. fecal proteolytic enzyme activity
   e. x-ray film digestion

268. Which drug is most likely to cause ototoxicity in cats?

   a. tetracycline
   b. erythromycin
   c. acetaminophen
   d. gentamicin
   e. cefazolin

Questions 269 and 270

A cat is presented to you for evaluation of a coagulation defect. You find that the prothrombin time and partial thromboplastin time are about 2.5 times longer than in control samples. Serum fibrin degradation product values are normal.

269. This coagulopathy is most likely related to:

   a. disseminated intravascular coagulation
   b. deficiency of Factor XII
   c. deficiency of Factor VIII
   d. deficiency of Factors II, VII, IX and X
   e. von Willebrand's disease

270. The most likely underlying cause for the hemostatic defect in this cat is:

   a. toxicity from an anticoagulant rodenticide
   b. toxicity from a cholecalciferol rodenticide
   c. aspirin intoxication
   d. thrombotic disease due to antithrombin III deficiency
   e. a hereditary defect

271. You suspect cryptococcosis in a cat but cannot isolate the organisms. What is the best test to confirm your diagnosis?

   a. agar-gel immunodiffusion
   b. indirect fluorescent antibody test
   c. electrophoresis of cerebrospinal fluid
   d. latex agglutination
   e. trypsin-like immunoreactivity

272. A colleague asks you for advice concerning a problem in a cattery. During the previous 6 months, 3 adult cats in the cattery have died. Histopathologic examination identified the cause of death as feline infectious peritonitis. Of 18 cats remaining in the cattery, 6 have positive titers for coronavirus. What is the most appropriate interpretation of this situation?

 a. The seropositive cats probably have feline infectious peritonitis and should be euthanized.
 b. The seropositive cats have been exposed to feline infectious peritonitis virus, and should be isolated for 6 weeks and then retested.
 c. The seropositive cats probably are also infected with feline leukemia virus, in addition to feline infectious peritonitis virus.
 d. The antibodies in the seropositive cats are not necessarily antibodies to the coronavirus of feline infectious peritonitis.
 e. Feline infectious peritonitis is enzootic in this cattery, and the establishment should be closed.

273. Which of the following represents the formula for permanent dentition in adult cats?

 a. $\frac{(3I\ 1C\ 3P\ 1M)\ x\ 2}{(3I\ 1C\ 2P\ 1M)\ x\ 2}$ = 30 total teeth
 b. $\frac{(3I\ 1C\ 2P\ 2M)\ x\ 2}{(3I\ 1C\ 2P\ 2M)\ x\ 2}$ = 36 total teeth
 c. $\frac{(3I\ 1C\ 3P\ 2M)\ x\ 2}{(3I\ 1C\ 3P\ 2M)\ x\ 2}$ = 36 total teeth
 d. $\frac{(4I\ 1C\ 3P\ 1M)\ x\ 2}{(4I\ 1C\ 3P\ 1M)\ x\ 2}$ = 36 total teeth
 e. $\frac{(3I\ 1C\ 2P\ 1M)\ x\ 2}{(3I\ 1C\ 3P\ 1M)\ x\ 2}$ = 30 total teeth

274. Which of the following should **not** be used in cats with heart failure associated with decompensated hypertrophic cardiomyopathy?

 a. oxygen
 b. intravenous fluids
 c. nitroglycerin
 d. aspirin
 e. diltiazem

275. Which of the following is the **least** likely clinical finding in a cat with lymphoma?

 a. cranial mediastinal mass
 b. unilateral renomegaly
 c. small bowel diarrhea with weight loss
 d. multicentric (generalized) lymphadenopathy
 e. mesenteric lymphadenopathy

276. Giardiasis in cats is effectively treated with:

 a. metronidazole, quinacrine or furazolidone
 b. ketoconazole, methylene blue or polymixin B
 c. methimazole, fenbendazole or ivermectin
 d. quinidine, atipamezol or diltiazem
 e. sucralfate, cimetidine or ceftiofur

277. What is the most common clinical sign of overly rapid intravenous infusion of blood products to cats?

 a. ataxia
 b. bradycardia
 c. vomiting
 d. opisthotonus
 e. diarrhea

278. Acute blindness with bilateral retinal hemorrhage and detachment in a geriatric cat is most likely to be caused by:

 a. chronic renal disease
 b. toxoplasmosis
 c. coagulopathy
 d. acute hepatitis
 e. snake bite

279. The most commonly reported arrhythmia in cats is:

 a. sinus bradycardia
 b. ventricular tachycardia
 c. atrial tachycardia
 d. sinus tachycardia
 e. sinus arrest or block

Correct answers are on pages 154-179.

Cats, continued

280. *Recognized forms of feline cardiomyopathy include all of the following **except**:*

   a. excessive moderator band cardiomyopathy
   b. hypertrophic cardiomyopathy
   c. dilative cardiomyopathy
   d. excessive chordae tendinae/papillary muscle cardiomyopathy
   e. restrictive cardiomyopathy

281. *The most common cause of death in feline leukemia virus-infected cats with persistent viremia is:*

   a. lymphosarcoma
   b. myeloproliferative disease
   c. nonregenerative anemia
   d. immunosuppression and secondary infectious disease
   e. squamous-cell carcinoma

282. *Macular melanosis on the lips and nose of orange tabby cats is called:*

   a. vitiligo
   b. chromboblastosis
   c. lentigo simplex
   d. poliosis
   e. melanosarcoma

283. *Which bacterial population is most likely to be found in a cat with septic pleural effusion (pyothorax)?*

   a. predominantly one species of Gram-positive aerobes
   b. mixed population of Gram-positive aerobes
   c. predominantly one species of Gram-negative aerobes
   d. predominantly one species of Gram-negative anaerobes
   e. mixed population of Gram-negative anaerobes

284. *Which of the following is **not** an appropriate part of diagnosis and management of pyothorax?*

   a. culture (aerobic, anaerobic) of the effusion
   b. Gram stain of the effusion
   c. search for an underlying cause
   d. thoracic drainage and lavage
   e. intrathoracic instillation of antibiotics

285. *Which antibacterial is most appropriate for a cat with the typical microbial population found in pyothorax?*

   a. metronidazole
   b. gentamicin
   c. trimethoprim-sulfa
   d. enrofloxacin
   e. amikacin

286. *One of the more common causes of progressive forebrain dysfunction in cats is:*

   a. toxoplasmosis
   b. bacterial meningitis
   c. hydrocephalus
   d. intracranial neoplasia
   e. head trauma

287. *Which test is particularly useful in differentiating hyperthyroid cats from cats with nonthyroidal disease and basal serum thyroxine levels in the high-normal range?*

   a. thyroxine stimulation
   b. combined thyroxine stimulation/ dexamethasone suppression test
   c. thyroxine suppression
   d. triiodothyronine suppression
   e. thyroid-stimulating hormone stimulation

288. *Which flea species most commonly infests cats?*

   a. *Pulex irritans*
   b. *Ctenocephalides felis*
   c. *Ctenocephalides canis*
   d. *Echidnophaga gallinacea*
   e. *Leptopsylla segnis*

289. Which of the following is the **least** appropriate method of resolving hypothermia in the postoperative period?

a. recirculating warm-water blanket
b. warm inspired air
c. intravenous fluids at normal body temperature
d. warm blankets
e. electric heating pad

290. Which feline viruses are most difficult to destroy by disinfection with chlorhexidine?

a. herpesvirus and leukemia virus
b. sarcoma virus and immunodeficiency virus
c. calicivirus and parvovirus
d. rabies virus and infectious peritonitis virus
e. immunodeficiency virus and herpesvirus

291. What is the most efficient means of transmission of Toxoplasma gondii to cats?

a. congenital *(in utero)*
b. predation on another host infected with cysts
c. inhalation of aerosolized oocysts
d. ingestion of feces
e. contamination of a bite wound by oocysts

292. What is the best available test to detect active toxoplasmosis in cats?

a. paired serum IgG titers
b. single serum IgM titer
c. indirect fluorescent antibody test of blood for *Toxoplasma* antibodies
d. fecal examination for oocysts
e. necropsy and histologic examination

293. Which drug is **not** appropriate for treatment of cats with toxoplasmosis?

a. pyrimethamine
b. clindamycin
c. methylene blue
d. sulfamethazine
e. sulfadiazine

294. One of your clients is pregnant and plans to get rid of her cat because her doctor has mentioned problems associated with toxoplasmosis. She did hear, however, that periodic cleaning of the litterbox can minimize the risk of human infection. To prevent oocyst sporulation, how often must the litterbox be cleaned?

a. every 72 hours
b. every 24 hours
c. every 96 hours
d. every 48 hours
e. once a week

295. Portosystemic shunts are being diagnosed with increasing frequency in cats. Surgical repair of these shunts is generally quite complicated and is usually a referral procedure. However, the practitioner should be aware that most portosystemic shunts in cats are:

a. multiple, extrahepatic and acquired
b. multiple, intrahepatic and acquired
c. single, extrahepatic and congenital
d. single, intrahepatic and congenital
e. multiple, intrahepatic and congenital

296. Clinical signs associated with a portosystemic shunt may be exacerbated by any of the following **except**:

a. high-protein diet
b. benzodiazepine tranquilizers
c. gastrointestinal bleeding
d. increased dietary levels of branched-chain amino acids
e. increased dietary levels of aromatic amino acids

297. What form of cardiomyopathy in cats is caused by a dietary deficiency of taurine?

a. hypertrophic cardiomyopathy
b. restrictive cardiomyopathy
c. dilative cardiomyopathy
d. excessive moderator band cardiomyopathy
e. defective endocardial cushion cardiomyopathy

Correct answers are on pages 154-179.

Cats, continued

298. Which drug is most likely to induce fever in cats?

   a. tetracycline
   b. aspirin
   c. clindamycin
   d. gentamicin
   e. vancomycin

299. Ischemic encephalopathy is a well-defined neurologic syndrome in cats. Which of the following is **not** a common clinical finding in affected cats?

   a. seizures
   b. personality change
   c. crossed-extensor reflex
   d. jumping in the air
   e. circling

300. Feline immunodeficiency virus is classified as:

   a. an oncornavirus
   b. a lentivirus
   c. a sarcomavirus
   d. a syncytium-forming virus
   e. a spumavirus

301. Chloramphenicol is a very effective antibiotic in some circumstances but must be used with caution in cats because of the potential for:

   a. delayed hypersensitivity (Type IV)
   b. methemoglobinemia
   c. bronchoconstriction
   d. dose-dependent bone marrow suppression
   e. uncontrollable fever

302. The maximum rate for safe intravenous infusion of potassium to cats is:

   a. 0.25 mEq/kg/hour
   b. 0.5 mEq/kg/hour
   c. 0.75 mEq/kg/hour
   d. 1 mEq/kg/hour
   e. 5 mEq/kg/hour

303. Which of the following is the **least** common congenital heart defect in cats?

   a. patent ductus arteriosus
   b. ventricular septal defect
   c. endocardial cushion defect
   d. pulmonic stenosis
   e. mitral valve dysplasia

304. What is the predominant distribution of the feline liver fluke, Platynosomum concinnum?

   a. northwestern United States
   b. southwestern United States
   c. Great Lakes area of the United States
   d. Puerto Rico and Florida
   e. northwestern United States

305. What is the drug of choice for treatment of liver fluke infection in cats?

   a. thiabendazole
   b. levamisole
   c. praziquantel
   d. mebendazole
   e. pyrantel pamoate

306. All of the following may cause insulin resistance in diabetic cats **except**:

   a. growth hormone-secreting pituitary tumor
   b. hyperadrenocorticism
   c. hypothyroidism
   d. obesity
   e. megestrol acetate

307. Which pathogen is **least** likely to be isolated from abscesses caused by cat bites?

   a. *Pasteurella multocida*
   b. beta-hemolytic streptococci
   c. *Fusobacterium*
   d. coagulase-positive staphylococci
   e. *Clostridium tetani*

308. What is the most appropriate antibacterial for treatment of an abscess caused by a cat bite?

a. amoxicillin
b. chloramphenicol
c. amikacin
d. enrofloxacin
e. trimethoprim-sulfa

a. *Staphylococcus aureus*
b. *E coli*
c. *Streptococcus epidermidis*
d. *Staphylococcus intermedius*
e. no growth

309. What is the most common hepatic neoplasm of cats?

a. hemangiosarcoma
b. hepatocellular carcinoma
c. bile duct carcinoma
d. lymphoma
e. mast-cell tumor

310. The most common adverse reaction to griseofulvin is:

a. bone marrow disturbance
b. fever
c. diarrhea
d. methemoglobinemia
e. Heinz-body hemolytic anemia

Questions 311 and 312

An adult female cat is presented to you for examination and treatment. The owner has observed the cat attempting to urinate frequently for the past 3 or 4 days. The cat appears to be straining. On physical examination, the cat is alert and has normal vital signs. The urinary bladder is small and firm. On abdominal palpation, the cat appears quite uncomfortable and immediately voids about 3 ml of serosanguineous urine.

311. What is the most likely cause of these signs?

a. obstructive feline urologic syndrome
b. bladder tumor
c. renal tumor
d. nonobstructive feline urologic syndrome
e. bacterial vaginitis

312. You obtain a urine sample by cystocentesis and submit it for culture and sensitivity tests. What is most likely to be found on culture?

313. In cats, stomatitis and gingivitis frequently indicate underlying:

a. general immunosuppression
b. heartworm disease
c. nasopharyngeal polyps
d. pyelonephritis
e. oral cancer

314. In 1982, 5 cases of an apparently "new" disease of cats were reported. The illness was characterized by weight loss, depression, persistent pupillary dilatation, constipation, decreased tear production, prolapsed nictitating membranes and megaesophagus. This disease is now recognized as:

a. feline dysautonomia
b. feline AIDS
c. Chediak-Higashi syndrome
d. Hashimoto syndrome
e. Maroteaux-Lamy syndrome (mucopolysaccharidosis VI)

Questions 315 and 316

Your practice is located in California near the coastline. You are presented with an adult male cat that is quite depressed. In obtaining the history, you learn that the cat is owned by a fisherman and eats primarily fresh fish, especially tuna. The cat is febrile and hyperesthetic, and greatly resents handling. You find a large, painful subcutaneous nodule in the inguinal area.

315. What is the most likely cause of these signs?

a. hypokalemic myopathy
b. immune-mediated myositis
c. subcutaneous foreign body
d. steatitis
e. aberrant dirofilariasis

Correct answers are on pages 154-179.

Cats, continued

316. The most appropriate treatment for this cat is:

   a. vitamin A
   b. vitamin E
   c. thiamin
   d. potassium
   e. taurine

317. Normal cats no longer have any deciduous teeth by what age?

   a. 2 months
   b. 3 months
   c. 4 months
   d. 6 months
   e. 10 months

318. Thromboembolism associated with hypertrophic cardiomyopathy:

   a. should be surgically treated (embolectomy) as soon as possible
   b. may occur anywhere in the body and is nearly always fatal
   c. should not be treated with propranolol, as it may cause vasoconstriction
   d. responds well to heparin therapy
   e. occurs in more than 75% of all cardiomyopathic cats

319. Concerning gastrointestinal lymphoma in cats, which statement is **least** accurate?

   a. It is commonly a B-cell lymphoma.
   b. It is more commonly associated with negative feline leukemia virus status than positive status.
   c. It may cause signs attributable to malabsorptive or obstructive disease.
   d. It is commonly associated with peripheral eosinophilia.
   e. It is generally seen in older cats.

320. Hyperthyroidism in cats is most commonly associated with:

   a. thyroid carcinoma
   b. thyroid adenoma
   c. thyroid adenocarcinoma
   d. thyroid and parathyroid adenoma
   e. Spirocerca lupi infection

321. Tyzzer's disease is caused by:

   a. Francisella tularensis
   b. Yersinia pestis
   c. Dermatophilus congolensis
   d. Mycobacterium avium
   e. Bacillus piliformis

322. Which paraneoplastic syndrome may be associated with an aggressive mast-cell tumor in cats?

   a. hypercalcemia
   b. hypoglycemia
   c. hyponatremia
   d. gastric ulceration due to hyperacidity
   e. insulin secretion by the tumor

323. What is the most appropriate fluid to administer intravenously to a ketoacidotic diabetic cat?

   a. 5% dextrose in water
   b. 2.5% dextrose in water
   c. 0.9% saline
   d. 0.45% saline
   e. 7% saline

324. One of the more commonly reported findings in cats with hepatic encephalopathy is:

   a. extensor rigidity
   b. ptyalism
   c. glucosuria
   d. increased serum urea nitrogen level
   e. weight gain

325. Which antimetabolite chemotherapeutic agent is extremely dangerous to cats and should **never** be given under any circumstance?

   a. bleomycin

b. cyclophosphamide
c. cytosine arabinoside
d. methotrexate
e. 5-fluorouracil

326. *Cats differ significantly from most other mammals in their ability to metabolize certain compounds. In large part, this is due to a greatly diminished ability to conjugate drugs to make them more water soluble and, thus, more easily eliminated from the body. A relative deficiency of which enzyme is responsible for this?*

a. glucuronyl transferase
b. methemoglobin reductase
c. myeloperoxidase
d. hepatic phosphofructokinase
e. pyruvate kinase

327. *Concerning alkaline phosphatase in cats, which statement is **least** accurate?*

a. It has a shorter half-life than in dogs.
b. It may be induced by glucocorticoid administration.
c. It has a low sensitivity but relatively good specificity for liver disease in the cat.
d. It is found in relatively lower concentrations in the feline liver as compared with the canine liver.
e. It may be induced by cholestatic disease.

328. *The anticonvulsant of choice for long-term control of seizures in cats is:*

a. phenobarbital
b. phenytoin
c. diazepam
d. acepromazine
e. valproic acid

329. *In the process of bile acid metabolism in cats, bile acids are conjugated with:*

a. valine
b. leucine
c. tryptophan
d. methionine
e. taurine

330. *The most common cause of lower-lip swelling ("pouting cat") is:*

a. eosinophilic plaque
b. eosinophilic linear granuloma
c. eosinophilic ulcer
d. food allergy
e. squamous-cell carcinoma

331. *Which of the following is **least** likely to cause splenomegaly in cats?*

a. lymphoma
b. myeloproliferative disease
c. hemobartonellosis
d. mast-cell tumor
e. hemangioma

332. *The most common louse found on cats is:*

a. *Hematopinus eurysternus*
b. *Linognathus pedalis*
c. *Linognathus setosus*
d. *Heterodoxus spiniger*
e. *Felicola subrostrata*

333. *The underlying cause of acute conjunctivitis is best diagnosed by:*

a. detailed history and thorough physical examination
b. culture of conjunctival sac specimens
c. fluorescein staining of corneal specimens
d. cytologic examination of conjunctival scrapings
e. response to treatment

334. *Cats are less susceptible to urinary tract infections than dogs because:*

a. cats have a higher urinary pH than dogs
b. cats have a lower urinary pH than dogs
c. cats have a higher urine osmolality than dogs
d. cats have a lower urine osmolality than dogs
e. cats urinate more frequently than dogs

Correct answers are on pages 154-179.

Cats, continued

335. The drug of choice for treating hemobartonellosis is:

a. prednisone
b. tetracycline or oxytetracycline
c. ketoconazole
d. thiacetarsamide
e. chloramphenicol

336. A classic sign of acetaminophen intoxication in cats is:

a. pulmonary edema
b. icterus due to acute hepatic necrosis
c. cyanosis
d. acute renal failure
e. heart failure due to toxic myocardial damage

337. Removal of the spleen in cats favors the appearance of which organism in the peripheral blood?

a. Eperythrozoon felis
b. Hemobartonella felis
c. Ehrlichia platys
d. Anaplasma marginale
e. Babesia microti

338. Use of megestrol acetate in cats is associated with all of the following side effects **except**:

a. diabetes mellitus
b. hyperthyroidism
c. mammary hypertrophy
d. mammary tumors
e. cystic endometritis

339. In cats, there is a strong association between left ventricular hypertrophy and:

a. diabetes mellitus
b. uremic pericarditis
c. inflammatory bowel disease
d. hyperthyroidism
e. multicentric lymphosarcoma

340. Common clinical signs of dilative or hypertrophic cardiomyopathy in cats include all of the following **except**:

a. gallop rhythym
b. ascites
c. pleural effusion
d. pulmonary edema
e. heart murmur

341. Which tissue is most commonly affected by cryptococcosis?

a. skin
b. nasal passages
c. cervical lymph nodes
d. lungs
e. central nervous system

342. A positive indirect fluorescent antibody test for feline leukemia virus indicates:

a. release of p15e from ruptured viral particles into the serum
b. p15e in the cytoplasm of bone marrow-derived cells
c. p27 in the cytoplasm of bone marrow-derived cells
d. FOCMA on the surface of bone marrow-derived cells
e. p27 on the surface of lymphoid-derived cells

343. Concerning notoedric mange, which statement is **least** accurate?

a. It is contagious to other cats.
b. It is caused by a mite of the Sarcoptidae family.
c. It is a nonpruritic skin condition.
d. It may be safely treated with lime-sulfur dips.
e. Early lesions appear mostly on the head, neck and ears.

344. Hepatic lipidosis is a common liver disorder in cats. What is a common predisposing cause?

a. liver entrapment in a diaphragmatic hernia
b. acetaminophen administration

c. chemotherapy with alkylating agents

d. stress and anorexia in an obese cat

e. exposure to organophosphates

345. *Miliary dermatitis has been associated with all of the following* **except**:

a. flea-bite hypersensitivity
b. dermatophytosis
c. atopy
d. *Cheyletiella* infestation
e. mycosis fungoides

346. *Feline leukemia virus is classified as:*

a. an oncornavirus
b. a spumavirus
c. a lentivirus
d. a sarcoma virus
e. a syncytium-forming virus

347. *Which of the following is* **least** *appropriate for intravenous fluid therapy in a hypovolemic hypotensive cat?*

a. 0.9% saline
b. lactated Ringer's solution
c. Ringer's solution
d. 5% dextrose in water
e. citrated Ringer's solution

348. *The most common clinical sign in cats with inflammatory bowel disease is:*

a. vomiting
b. increased appetite
c. decreased appetite
d. weight loss
e. diarrhea

349. *External odontoclastic resorptive lesions (cervical line lesions or neck lesions) are found in the teeth of many cats. Concerning these lesions, which statement is most accurate?*

a. The lesion is painless when touched by a dental probe.

b. The lesion is treated by subgingival curettage.

c. The lesion may be treated by glass ionomer restoration, copal varnish applications, fluoride application or tooth extraction.

d. Once the lesion has been located with the dental probe, dental radiographs are unnecessary.

e. The lesion is associated with chronic morbillivirus infection of the gingivae.

350. *Which finding is always considered abnormal in feline urine?*

a. lipid droplets
b. bilirubinuria
c. proteinuria
d. glucosuria
e. urobilinogen

351. *Which antineoplastic drug is uniformly fatal when given to cats?*

a. doxorubicin
b. vincristine
c. cisplatin
d. cyclophosphamide
e. vinblastine

352. *A major postoperative complication of bilateral thyroidectomy is:*

a. hypercalcemia
b. hypocalcemia
c. hypermagnesemia
d. hyperbilirubinemia
e. hyponatremia

353. *Insecticide toxicity is relatively common in cats. Toxicity with which of the following is responsive to treatment with atropine?*

a. lindane
b. pyrethrin
c. carbamate
d. lime-sulfur
e. chlordane

Correct answers are on pages 154-179.

Cats, continued

Questions 354 and 355

354. In cats, long-term ingestion of a diet consisting predominantly of organ meats may lead to:

a. hyperphosphatemia
b. hypercalcemia
c. vitamin A toxicosis
d. vitamin D toxicosis
e. vitamin B₁ (thiamin) toxicosis

355. Clinical signs of the condition described in Question 354 include all of the following *except*:

a. exostoses of the cervical vertebrae
b. steatitis
c. loss of the incisor teeth
d. lameness
e. pain in long bones

356. Concerning pseudorabies, which statement is most accurate?

a. In cats it begins with excitement, and in dogs with depression.
b. In cats it begins with depression, and in dogs with excitement.
c. Affected cats usually die much later in the course of the disease than dogs.
d. Affected cats are usually much less pruritic than dogs.
e. There is no variation between the clinical presentation in affected dogs and cats.

357. Concerning rabies, which statement is most accurate?

a. Rabid cats are usually very aggressive.
b. Rabid cats are less of a public health risk than rabid dogs.
c. It is definitively diagnosed by lack of response to supportive care.
d. Rabies is caused by a paramyxovirus.
e. Prodromal signs of miosis and subnormal body temperature last 10-12 days.

Questions 358 through 360

You are presented with an adult cat that is extremely anemic. You place a drop of blood on a slide for microscopic examination, but the blood agglutinates before you can make a smear.

358. What is a likely cause of such agglutination?

a. immune-mediated hemolytic anemia
b. hypoproteinemia
c. hemobartonellosis
d. hypereosinophilic syndrome
e. von Willebrand's disease

359. What is the most appropriate course of action?

a. perform direct and indirect Coombs' tests for antibodies to red blood cells
b. apply a drop of saline to look for clot dispersion
c. obtain a bone marrow aspirate to evaluate the erythroid precursors
d. administer a blood transfusion if the hematocrit is less than 20%
e. perform an antithrombin III test

360. You apply a drop of saline to the slide and the cells do not disperse. What is the most appropriate course of action?

a. perform direct and indirect Coombs' tests for antibodies to red blood cells
b. obtain a bone marrow aspirate to evaluate the erythroid precursors
c. initiate heparin therapy
d. initiate aspirin therapy
e. initiate corticosteroid therapy

361. The anemia of chronic disease is usually:

a. macrocytic hypochromic
b. microcytic hypochromic
c. normochromic normocytic
d. macrocytic hyperchromic
e. microcytic hyperchromic

362. Which of the following typifies iron metabolism in the anemia of chronic disease?

a. serum iron levels and bone marrow iron stores are both decreased
b. serum iron levels and bone marrow iron stores are both increased
c. serum iron levels are increased and bone marrow iron stores are decreased
d. serum iron levels are decreased and bone marrow iron stores are increased
e. serum iron levels and bone marrow iron stores vary, depending on the particular disease

363. Which of the following is **least** likely to cause generalized seizures in a 2-year-old male cat?

a. idiopathic epilepsy
b. feline infectious peritonitis
c. trauma
d. ischemic encephalopathy
e. primary brain tumor

364. In cats, the most common cause of a pleural effusion containing neoplastic cells is:

a. metastatic pancreatic adenocarcinoma
b. bronchoalveolar carcinoma
c. chemodectoma
d. cranial mediastinal lymphoma
e. mesothelioma

365. You are presented with a kitten that has been ataxic since birth. The kitten has a wide-based stance and its head bobs up and down. What is the most likely site of the neurologic lesion causing these signs?

a. spinal cord segments C7-T3
b. cerebellum
c. cerebral ventricles
d. forebrain
e. spinal cord segments T4-T13

366. How many pairs of mammary glands are normally found in cats?

a. 3
b. 4
c. 5
d. 6
e. 2

367. Concerning mammary tumors in cats, which statement is **least** accurate?

a. They are usually malignant.
b. They are best treated with early excision.
c. Most cats with mammary tumors die from metastatic disease.
d. They are responsive to hormonal treatment.
e. Most feline mammary tumors are adenocarcinomas.

368. When the triiodothyronine (T3) suppression test is performed on a normal cat, the serum thyroxine (T4) level:

a. increases
b. remains unchanged
c. decreases
d. may increase or decrease
e. first decreases, then increases

369. Which ocular disorder is associated with taurine deficiency in cats?

a. retinal detachment
b. glaucoma
c. central retinal degeneration
d. anterior uveitis
e. iris bombe

370. What is the drug of choice to manage a hyperthyroid cat until thyroidectomy or radiation therapy?

a. propylthiouracil
b. methimazole
c. thyroxine
d. antithyroglobulin antiserum
e. cisplatin

Correct answers are on pages 154-179.

Cats, continued

e. sneezing

371. Which drug may be used to enhance bladder tone in a cat with bladder atony after lower urinary tract obstruction has been relieved?

a. diazepam
b. phenylpropanolamine
c. phenoxybenzamine
d. bethanechol
e. acepromazine

372. Which part of the eye is most likely to show a granulomatous response to feline infectious peritonitis virus?

a. lens
b. sclera
c. conjunctiva
d. cornea
e. uvea

373. The average life span of an adult heartworm in a cat is:

a. 6 months
b. 1 year
c. 2 years
d. 3 years
e. 5 years

374. Which type of aggression against a person is most likely to be exhibited by a cat in a single-cat household?

a. play
b. territorial
c. epileptic
d. fear
e. sexual

375. What is the most significant complicating factor of viral upper respiratory tract infection in kittens?

a. pneumonia
b. ulcerations in the oral cavity
c. secondary bacterial infection
d. serous nasal discharge

376. The normal depth of the gingival sulcus in adult cats is:

a. 0-1 mm
b. 1.5-3 mm
c. 3-4 mm
d. 4-4.5 mm
e. 5-5.5 mm

377. What is the most common nutritional disorder of cats?

a. vitamin A deficiency
b. thiamin deficiency
c. protein deficiency
d. obesity
e. calcium deficiency

378. Concerning hypereosinophilic syndrome in cats, which statement is **least** accurate?

a. Adult cats are usually affected.
b. The bone marrow is frequently involved.
c. Vomiting, diarrhea and weight loss result from bowel infiltration.
d. Clinical signs are well controlled with long-term prednisone therapy.
e. The prognosis for recovery is guarded.

379. The most common cause of death in cats falling from heights (high-rise syndrome) is:

a. cranial trauma
b. spinal cord trauma
c. rupture of abdominal viscera
d. open fractures of long bones
e. thoracic trauma

380. Of the following veins, which is **least** likely to be used for intravenous catheterization in cats?

a. jugular vein and cephalic vein
b. cephalic vein
c. lateral saphenous vein
d. medial saphenous vein

e. jugular vein and medial saphenous vein

381. In cats, which drug is teratogenic when used at any stage of pregnancy?

a. cimetidine
b. propylene glycol
c. griseofulvin
d. pyrantel pamoate
e. fenbendazole

382. Most cases of uveitis in cats are associated with:

a. feline infectious peritonitis, cryptococcosis, rhinotracheitis viral infection or pneumonitis
b. feline infectious peritonitis, toxoplasmosis or feline immunodeficiency virus infection
c. rhinotracheitis, calicivirus infection, feline immunodeficiency virus infection or feline leukemia virus infection
d. feline infectious peritonitis, toxoplasmosis, feline immunodeficiency virus infection, feline leukemia virus infection, cryptococcosis, histoplasmosis or blastomycosis
e. feline infectious peritonitis, feline leukemia virus infection, feline immunodeficiency virus infection or upper respiratory viral infection

383. Hemobartonellosis is caused by Hemobartonella felis. To which order does this organism belong?

a. Rickettsiales
b. Mycoplasmatales
c. Chlamydiales
d. Eubacteriales
e. Pseudomonales

384. Which drug is **least** likely to exacerbate liver disease in a cat?

a. diazepam
b. dioctyl sodium sulfylsuccinate
c. acepromazine
d. methionine
e. tetracycline

385. Which nematode may inhabit the stomach and cause gastritis in cats?

a. Toxascaris leonina
b. Ollulanus tricuspis
c. Ancylostoma tubaeformae
d. Strongyloides stercoralis
e. Trichinella spiralis

386. Adequate urine-concentrating ability is signified by a urine specific gravity greater than:

a. 1.025
b. 1.030
c. 1.010
d. 1.020
e. 1.035

387. An adult male cat has a peculiar plantigrade stance of the pelvic limbs. The hocks are dropped down and the cat appears to be walking "flat footed." The owner reports that the cat has a healthy appetite but continues to lose weight, and has been drinking a bit more water than as a young adult. What is the most likely cause of these signs?

a. hyperthyroidism
b. hypothyroidism
c. diabetes insipidus
d. diabetes mellitus
e. myasthenia gravis

388. You are presented with a 5-month-old kitten found near a garbage container. The kitten appears malnourished and debilitated. Physical examination reveals 2 small holes in the skin, one behind the ear and the other under the neck. The holes are well-circumscribed and exude a small amount of serosanguineous fluid. You can see a small brown speck in the middle of each hole. What is the likely cause of this peculiar finding?

a. wasp or bee sting
b. bite wounds that have abscessed and drained
c. cuterebriasis
d. aberrant migration of heartworm microfilariae
e. paragonimiasis

Correct answers are on pages 154-179.

Cats, continued

389. Which of the following is **least** likely to produce icterus in cats?

    a. toxoplasmosis
    b. feline infectious peritonitis
    c. diabetes mellitus
    d. hepatic lipidosis
    e. cholangiohepatitis complex

390. The "fading kitten" syndrome is generally attributed to:

    a. T-lymphocyte hyperplasia
    b. B-lymphocyte deficiency
    c. acute lymphoblastic leukemia
    d. thymic atrophy
    e. neutrophil function defect

391. The drug of choice for treatment of nocardiosis in cats is:

    a. trimethoprim-sulfa
    b. chloramphenicol
    c. ampicillin
    d. enrofloxacin
    e. dexamethasone

392. All of the following are normal findings on the hemogram of cats **except**:

    a. Heinz bodies
    b. Howell-Jolly bodies
    c. spherocytes
    d. smaller mean corpuscular volume than in dogs
    e. platelet numbers equal to those in dogs

393. The most common tapeworm in cats is:

    a. *Echinococcus granulosus*
    b. *Echinococcus multilocularis*
    c. *Dipylidium caninum*
    d. *Taenia taeniaeformis*
    e. *Anoplocephala perfoliata*

394. The cause of feline viral rhinotracheitis is a:

    a. herpesvirus
    b. calicivirus
    c. retrovirus
    d. parvovirus
    e. paramyxovirus

395. Which organism is most commonly isolated from the uterus of cats with pyometra?

    a. *E coli*
    b. *Pseudomonas aeruginosa*
    c. *Pasteurella multocida*
    d. *Proteus vulgaris*
    e. *Fusobacterium necrophorum*

396. What is the most common oral tumor in cats?

    a. squamous-cell carcinoma
    b. malignant melanoma
    c. lymphoma
    d. fibrosarcoma
    e. mast-cell tumor

397. Accumulation of oily exudate over the tailhead and on the tail of cats is termed:

    a. brushy tail
    b. feline acne
    c. stud tail
    d. grease tail
    e. comedone equinus

398. Which drug combats the adverse metabolic effects of hyperkalemia but does not reduce serum potassium levels?

    a. sodium bicarbonate
    b. glucose
    c. insulin
    d. calcium gluconate
    e. prednisolone

Questions 399 and 400

399. A blue-smoke Persian cat has green irides, red fundic reflections, a propensity to bleed after venipuncture, and intracytoplasmic

inclusions in neutrophils. This combination of findings comprises the:

a. Pelger-Huet anomaly
b. Chediak-Higashi syndrome
c. Hashimoto syndrome
d. Klinefelter's syndrome
e. lentigo simplex syndrome

400. *Concerning the Persian cat in Question 399, which statement is most accurate?*

a. The cat is likely to die of unregulated diabetes mellitus.
b. The cat is likely to be positive for feline leukemia virus on indirect fluorescent antibody testing of bone marrow.
c. The cat is likely to be sterile.
d. The cat is prone to recurrent infections.
e. The cat is likely to develop irreversible blindness.

401. *Which infection is characterized by large intracytoplasmic inclusion bodies within epithelial cells from a conjunctival scraping of a cat?*

a. herpesviral infection
b. coronaviral infectin
c. chlamydial infection
d. mycoplasmal infection
e. caliciviral infection

402. *Ulcerative keratitis is most likely to occur in a cat infected with:*

a. feline herpesvirus
b. feline coronavirus
c. *Chlamydia*
d. *Bordetella*
e. feline calicivirus

403. *Tongue ulceration in cats is most characteristic of infection with:*

a. *Mycoplasma*
b. *Bordetella*
c. feline calicivirus
d. *Chlamydia*

e. feline herpesvirus

404. *Concerning respiratory infections in cats, which statement is most accurate?*

a. Feline calicivirus has a predilection for the epithelium of the upper respiratory tract.
b. Feline caliciviral infection often causes ulceration of the cornea.
c. Chlamydial infection (pneumonitis) typically causes severe pneumonia.
d. Virulent strains of feline calicivirus have an affinity for the lung and often produce primary viral pneumonia.
e. Conjunctival involvement is unlikely in herpesviral infection.

405. *A 4-month-old male domestic shorthair kitten has anorexia, a fever (103.8 F), marked mucopurulent oculonasal discharge, paroxysmal sneezing, a hacking cough and excessive salivation. The most likely cause of these signs is infection with:*

a. feline calicivirus
b. *Mycoplasma*
c. feline herpesvirus
d. *Chlamydia*
e. feline reovirus

406. *Which feline virus, when latent, can be reactivated by stress in chronic carriers?*

a. panleukopenia virus
b. calicivirus
c. feline infectious peritonitis (FIP) virus
d. herpesvirus
e. enteric coronavirus

407. *Which drug is most effective for topical treatment of chlamydial conjunctivitis in cats?*

a. idoxuridine
b. gentamicin
c. polymixin B
d. tetracycline
e. prednisolone

Correct answers are on pages 154-179.

Cats, continued

408. *Which drug is a specific treatment for herpesviral keratitis in cats?*

    a. idoxuridine
    b. levamisole
    c. chloramphenicol
    d. tetracycline
    e. prednisolone

409. *Which form of lymphoma is relatively uncommon in cats as compared with dogs?*

    a. peripheral lymph node
    b. mediastinal
    c. hepatic
    d. splenic
    e. intestinal

410. *A cat tests positive for feline leukemia virus (FeLV) infection by enzyme-linked immunosorbent assay but tests negative by indirect fluorescent antibody testing. Which of the following is **not** a possible explanation of these results?*

    a. early transient FeLV infection
    b. compartmentalized lymphoid infection
    c. FeLV infection without active replication in bone marrow
    d. laboratory error
    e. latent (nonreplicating) FeLV infection

411. *Which of the following is **least** likely to be found in a cat with anemia related to feline leukemia virus infection?*

    a. hematocrit below 12%
    b. concurrent hemobartonellosis
    c. positive Coombs' test
    d. microcytic erythrocytes
    e. hypoplastic bone marrow

412. *The principal cause of false-positive results of enzyme-linked immunosorbent assay for feline leukemia virus is:*

    a. the virus's cross reactivity with feline calicivirus
    b. use of serum instead of whole blood
    c. use of outdated reagents
    d. use of monoclonal antibody reagents
    e. technical error in performing the test

413. *Feline leukemia virus is primarily transmitted via:*

    a. fleas
    b. feces
    c. saliva
    d. respiratory secretions
    e. soil

414. *With which form of feline leukemia virus-induced neoplasia are cats **least** likely to be viremic?*

    a. mediastinal lymphoma
    b. intestinal lymphoma
    c. multicentric lymphoma
    d. nervous system lymphoma
    e. myeloproliferative disorder

415. *In a small animal practice, which measure is **least** likely to reduce the rate of false-positive results of enzyme-linked immunosorbent assay (ELISA) for feline leukemia virus?*

    a. use of the saliva test
    b. use of serum instead of whole blood
    c. use of the filter membrane format instead of the microwell format
    d. use of very thorough washing steps in the procedure
    e. use of ELISA kits with monoclonal instead of polyclonal antibody reagents

416. *Latent (nonreplicating) infection with feline leukemia virus is detected by:*

    a. indirect fluorescent antibody (IFA) test
    b. enzyme-linked immunosorbent assay (ELISA)
    c. antibody titer against feline oncornavirus-associated cell membrane antigen

d. reactivation of virus from cultured bone marrow cells

e. virus-neutralizing antibody titer

417. *Veterinarians often confirm in-office results of enzyme-linked immunosorbent assay (ELISA) for feline leukemia virus by sending a serum sample to a diagnostic laboratory for indirect fluorescent antibody (IFA) testing. Which of the following is the most common discrepancy ("discordancy") between test results?*

a. microwell ELISA negative, IFA positive

b. microwell ELISA positive, IFA negative

c. membrane filter ELISA negative, IFA positive

d. membrane filter ELISA positive, IFA negative

e. saliva ELISA negative, IFA positive

418. *Assuming the tests are performed properly, which statement concerning testing for feline leukemia virus (FeLV) is **least** accurate?*

a. The indirect fluorescent antibody test detects cell-associated viremia.

b. The enzyme-linked immunosorbent assay detects viral antigen in blood, saliva or tears.

c. The enzyme-linked immunosorbent assay is almost always positive if the indirect fluorescent antibody test is positive.

d. The indirect fluorescent antibody test is almost always negative if the enzyme-linked immunosorbent assay is negative.

e. The indirect fluorescent antibody test usually becomes positive before the enzyme-linked immunosorbent assay becomes positive in the early stages of FeLV infection.

419. *Which form of lymphoma is most likely to occur in old cats?*

a. mediastinal

b. intestinal

c. peripheral lymph node

d. cutaneous

e. ocular

420. *Feline immunodeficiency virus is transmitted primarily via:*

a. urine

b. feces

c. saliva

d. milk

e. sexual contact

421. *Concerning the routine enzyme-linked immunosorbent assay for feline immuno-deficiency virus (FIV), which statement is most accurate?*

a. It detects circulating FIV antigen in serum as an indication of current active infection.

b. It detects FIV antigen in circulating lymphocytes as an indication of current active infection.

c. It detects FIV antigen in saliva as an indication of current active infection and viral shedding.

d. It detects circulating anti-FIV antibody as an indication of current and life-long active infection.

e. It detects circulating anti-FIV antibody as an indication of prior exposure and subsequent immune rejection of the virus.

422. *Infection with feline immunodeficiency virus is most commonly manifested as:*

a. diarrhea

b. gingivitis-stomatitis

c. anterior uveitis

d. jaundice

e. urinary tract infection

423. *Which of the following is most compatible with the effusive ("wet") form of feline infectious peritonitis?*

a. suppurative exudate

b. transudate

c. serosanguineous effusion

d. pyogranulomatous exudate

e. modified transudate

Cats, continued

424. *The hallmark of feline infectious peritonitis is widespread vasculitis. Which of the following is most important in the pathogenesis of vasculitis in this disease?*

a. deposition of antigen-antibody complexes in vessel walls
b. direct viral attack on vascular endothelium
c. formation of autoantibodies directed against vessel basement membranes
d. fibrin deposition in the microcirculation, leading to vascular damage and disseminated intravascular coagulation
e. vascular injury caused by toxins released from the virus

425. *The most common ocular manifestation of feline infectious peritonitis is:*

a. ulcerative keratitis
b. anterior uveitis
c. conjunctivitis
d. Horner's syndrome
e. retrobulbar swelling

426. *Concerning feline coronaviral titers (so-called "feline infectious peritonitis antibody test"), which statement is most accurate?*

a. It is rare for a healthy cat to have a positive titer on this test.
b. Because a positive titer is highly specific for feline infectious peritonitis, this test is used to confirm the diagnosis.
c. The major pitfall of this test is a high frequency of false negatives; that is, negative titers in cats that are actually infected with the virus.
d. This test should not be used to cull animals from a cattery on a "test and removal" basis.
e. Intranasal vaccination with the commercial feline infectious peritonitis vaccine consistently produces high serum titers.

427. *Concerning feline coronaviral titers (so-called "feline infectious peritonitis antibody test"), which statement is **least** accurate?*

a. The test also detects cross-reacting antibodies against feline enteric coronavirus, but this virus is very rare in the cat population.
b. Evaluating paired serum samples for a rising antibody titer is not a reliable means of diagnosing feline infectious peritonitis.
c. A few cats with documented feline infectious peritonitis may not have a coronaviral titer.
d. The test should not be used in "test and cull" programs in catteries, as the test for feline leukemia virus is used.
e. The feline infectious peritonitis virus antibody titer does not measure a protective immune response.

428. *What is the most common source of* Toxoplasma *infection in cats?*

a. raw meat
b. cat feces
c. soil
d. transplacental transmission
e. direct contact

429. *Concerning toxoplasmosis in cats, which statement is **least** accurate?*

a. Asymptomatic infection is more common than clinical infection.
b. Ingestion of raw meat containing *Toxoplasma* cysts is the most common source of infection in cats.
c. Shedding of fecal oocysts only occurs in cats.
d. Clindamycin is the drug of choice for treatment.
e. A single high serum IgG *Toxoplasma* antibody titer indicates active infection.

430. *The drug of choice for treating hemobartonellosis in cats is:*

a. ampicillin
b. cephalosporin
c. trimethoprim-sulfa
d. tetracycline
e. erythromycin

431. *Which fungal organism appears in feline cytologic specimens as a budding yeast with a distinctive thick, nonstaining, polysaccharide capsule?*

a. *Cryptococcus neoformans*
b. *Blastomyces dermatitidis*
c. *Coccidioides immitis*
d. *Histoplasma capsulatum*
e. *Aspergillus fumigatus*

432. *Which organism is **not** associated with anterior uveitis in cats?*

a. *Cryptococcus*
b. *Toxoplasma*
c. feline infectious peritonitis virus
d. *Chlamydia*
e. feline leukemia virus

433. *Cerebellar hypoplasia in kittens is caused by perinatal infection with:*

a. panleukopenia virus
b. herpesvirus
c. calicivirus
d. feline infectious peritonitis coronavirus
e. feline leukemia virus

434. *Feline enteric coronavirus is important because of the confusion it causes in laboratory testing for which other organism infecting cats?*

a. *Toxoplasma*
b. herpesvirus
c. feline infectious peritonitis virus
d. feline leukemia virus
e. *Chlamydia*

435. *Which oral antifungal drug is effective for treatment of histoplasmosis in cats?*

a. miconazole
b. amphotericin B
c. clotrimazole
d. 5-fluorocytosine
e. ketoconazole

436. *Hyperglobulinemia is a common clinical finding in cats with:*

a. herpesviral infection
b. cryptococcosis
c. panleukopenia
d. toxoplasmosis
e. feline infectious peritonitis

437. *Concerning feline leukemia virus (FeLV) vaccination, which statement is most accurate?*

a. Vaccine side effects are mostly a reaction to the adjuvants used.
b. Most FeLV vaccines contain live virus, though the virus is attenuated for safety.
c. All FeLV vaccines induce anti-FOCMA (feline oncornavirus cell membrane antigen) antibody titers indicative of antitumor immunity.
d. FeLV testing before vaccination is recommended because vaccination of an FeLV-positive cat hastens progression of the disease.
e. Vaccine trials have shown consistently that nearly 100% of vaccinated cats are protected against FeLV challenge, regardless of the brand of vaccine used.

438. *In a cat with respiratory signs, a history of recent exposure to other cats in a multi-cat household environment is most important relative to increased risk of:*

a. thoracic trauma
b. exposure to fungi causing systemic mycoses
c. exposure to viruses
d. exposure to lungworm eggs or larvae
e. exposure to animal-derived allergens

Cats, continued

439. *Concerning bronchial asthma in cats, which statement is **least** accurate?*

   a. Typical presenting signs include chronic cough, wheezing and dyspnea.
   b. Air bronchograms are the most characteristic radiographic abnormality.
   c. Hematologic examination sometimes reveals eosinophilia.
   d. Effective treatment can include corticosteroids and bronchodilators.
   e. The pathogenesis involves small-airway obstruction from bronchiolar smooth muscle contraction, bronchiolar inflammation, and intraluminal accumulation of mucus and exudate.

440. *Which drug is a sympathomimetic bronchodilator used in treatment of bronchial asthma in cats?*

   a. theophylline
   b. terbutaline
   c. butorphanol
   d. isopropamide
   e. bethanecol

441. *Which drug is indicated for treatment of a cat with acute bronchial asthma?*

   a. aminophylline
   b. furosemide
   c. propranolol
   d. butorphanol
   e. acepromazine

442. *In cats, polyps occur most often at which site?*

   a. external nares
   b. frontal sinus
   c. nasopharynx
   d. larynx
   e. trachea

443. *Chronic granulomatous pulmonary disease with extensive fibrosis in cats is caused by:*

   a. bacterial pneumonia
   b. allergic pulmonary reaction
   c. lungworm infection
   d. mineral oil inhalation
   e. smoke inhalation

444. *Cytologic examination of a transtracheal aspirate (airway washing) in a cat reveals predominantly eosinophils. The most likely cause of this finding is:*

   a. bronchial asthma
   b. nonspecific irritant bronchitis
   c. pulmonary blastomycosis
   d. aspiration pneumonia
   e. bacterial bronchopneumonia

445. *Which bacteria are most consistently associated with pyothorax in cats?*

   a. *Escherichia coli* and *Bacillus pisiformis*
   b. streptococci and staphylococci
   c. *Klebsiella* and *Rhodococcus*
   d. *Pseudomonas* and *Corynebacterium*
   e. anaerobic bacteria

446. *Radiographs of a cat reveal pleural effusion associated with a right middle lung lobe that is completely opaque. The most likely cause of these findings is:*

   a. bronchopneumonia
   b. aspiration pneumonia
   c. chronic obstructive airway disease
   d. lung lobe torsion
   e. chylofibrosis

447. *In cats, thoracic lavage and drainage via chest tube are most appropriate for treatment of:*

   a. pneumothorax
   b. mediastinal lymphosarcoma
   c. feline infectious peritonitis
   d. pyothorax
   e. chylothorax

448. *Most pleural effusions in cats are bilateral. Which disorder is most likely to cause unilateral pleural effusion?*

a. dilative cardiomyopathy
b. feline infectious peritonitis
c. mediastinal lymphoma
d. pyothorax
e. chylothorax

449. *In cats, decreased compliance of the cranial thorax on palpation is most commonly associated with:*

a. pneumomediastinum
b. pleural effusion
c. rib fracture
d. mediastinal lymphoma
e. rib tumor

450. *Increased resonance (increased tympany) on thoracic percussion of a cat typically indicates:*

a. pleural effusion
b. diaphragmatic hernia
c. consolidating pneumonia
d. intrathoracic neoplasia
e. pneumothorax

451. *In a cat, which clinical observation could be described as orthopnea?*

a. abnormal increase in the depth of respiration
b. abnormal increase in the rate of breathing
c. inability to breathe comfortably except in an upright (sitting or sternal) position, which allows maximal caudal excursion of the diaphragm
d. shallow, choppy restrictive breathing usually due to painful breathing from rib fractures, pleuritis, etc
e. difficult or labored breathing

452. *Aspiration pneumonia in cats is most often associated with:*

a. heartworm disease
b. esophageal disease
c. lungworm infection
d. thoracic trauma
e. tracheal collapse

453. *Which of the following is most effective in preventing retention of respiratory secretions and inspissation of airway mucus in an animal with severe pneumonia?*

a. antitussive drugs
b. fluid therapy to maintain systemic hydration
c. diuretics to reduce fluid retention
d. atropine to "dry up" secretions
e. cage rest to restrict exercise

454. *Which fungus has a predilection for the feline nasal cavity?*

a. *Histoplasma*
b. *Blastomyces*
c. *Coccidioides*
d. *Cryptococcus*
e. *Pythium (Hyphomyces)*

455. *In cats, laryngeal paralysis is diagnosed by:*

a. radiography
b. blood gas analysis
c. auscultation
d. direct observation of the laryngeal orifice during breathing
e. cytologic examination of airway aspirates

456. *In a cat, a regimen consisting of a bronchodilator, a diuretic and oxygen is most appropriate for treatment of:*

a. bronchial asthma
b. electrocution injury
c. pyothorax
d. traumatic hemothorax
e. bacterial pneumonia

457. *In which of the following would treatment with a bronchodilator alone be expected to produce the most rapid and pronounced improvement in a cat with respiratory distress?*

a. bronchial asthma
b. aelurostrongylosis
c. tracheobronchial foreign body
d. bacterial bronchopneumonia
e. noncardiogenic pulmonary edema

Correct answers are on pages 154-179.

Cats, continued

458. Respiratory failure associated with paradoxic respirations is most likely to occur in a cat with:

a. intercostal muscle avulsion
b. open pneumothorax
c. flail chest
d. tension pneumothorax
e. diaphragmatic hernia

459. Which clinical manifestation is **least** likely in a cat with a lung tumor?

a. pleural effusion
b. hemoptysis
c. dyspnea
d. stridor
e. cough

460. A cat develops respiratory distress, subcutaneous emphysema and pneumomediastinum after being hit by a car. The most likely injury underlying these signs is:

a. tracheobronchial laceration
b. diaphragmatic hernia
c. rib fracture
d. flail chest
e. rupture of pulmonary alveoli

461. Abrupt onset of unilateral nasal signs is most consistent with:

a. viral rhinitis
b. allergic rhinitis
c. nasal tumor
d. nasal foreign body
e. nasal cryptococcosis

462. Concerning Campylobacter infection, which statement is **least** accurate?

a. Dogs and cats may carry Campylobacter asymptomatically.
b. Because Campylobacter is very species specific, there is minimal chance of animal-to-human transmission.

c. Campylobacter is difficult to isolate in culture and requires specialized selective media.
d. Microscopic examination of feces may be used for presumptive diagnosis of Campylobacter infection.
e. Erythromycin or neomycin is usually an effective treatment.

463. For which feline diarrheal disease is metronidazole **not** an appropriate choice for therapy?

a. giardiasis
b. salmonellosis
c. small intestinal bacterial overgrowth
d. chronic colitis
e. lymphocytic-plasmacytic inflammatory bowel disease

464. Which disease of cats is best treated with sulfasalazine?

a. salmonellosis
b. campylobacteriosis
c. giardiasis
d. chronic colitis
e. small intestinal bacterial overgrowth

465. Which clinical sign is **least** likely to be associated with large bowel diarrhea in a cat?

a. urgency and frequency of defecation
b. melena
c. tenesmus (straining to defecate)
d. abundant mucus in the feces
e. frank red blood in the feces

466. Duodenal ulcers due to gastric hypersecretion of acid have been associated with which nonenteric neoplasm in cats?

a. mastocytoma
b. thyroid adenoma
c. hemangiosarcoma
d. mammary adenocarcinoma
e. pulmonary adenocarcinoma

467. The predominant inflammatory cell found in lesions of inflammatory bowel disease of cats is the:

a. neutrophil
b. eosinophil
c. lymphocyte
d. macrophage
e. mast cell

468. You find a fibrous, stricture-like stenotic lesion in the distal ileum of a 12-year-old cat with anorexia, chronic weight loss and occasional vomiting. The most likely cause of this finding is:

a. intestinal adenocarcinoma
b. intestinal lymphoma
c. intestinal histoplasmosis
d. eosinophilic enteritis
e. salmonellosis

469. Severe life-threatening fluid and electrolyte losses requiring intensive intravenous fluid therapy are most likely to occur in a cat with:

a. acute viral diarrhea
b. exocrine pancreatic insufficiency
c. chronic colitis
d. lymphocytic-plasmacytic enteritis
e. ascarid infection

470. Narcotic analgesic opioids, such as loperamide and diphenoxylate, combat diarrhea by:

a. enhancing intestinal peristalsis
b. inhibiting prostaglandins
c. decreasing rhythmic segmentation contractions of the gut
d. anticholinergic (parasympatholytic) activity
e. prolonging intestinal transit and inhibiting loss of fluid through the gut mucosa

471. Dietary hypersensitivity has been associated with which feline enteropathy?

a. lymphangiectasia
b. regional granulomatous enteritis
c. small intestinal bacterial overgrowth
d. lymphocytic-plasmacytic inflammatory bowel disease
e. lipofuscinosis

472. Concerning lymphocytic-plasmacytic inflammatory bowel disease, which statement is most accurate?

a. Only the small intestine is affected.
b. Dietary management does not play a role in treatment.
c. Endoscopy is not usually adequate for demonstrating lesions; full-thickness biopsies obtained at laparotomy are usually required.
d. The results of upper gastrointestinal barium radiography are usually unremarkable.
e. Corticosteroids should be avoided because of the risk of bacterial overgrowth.

473. In cats, oral lactulose is an effective treatment for:

a. diarrhea
b. urinary tract infection
c. vomiting
d. anorexia
e. constipation

474. Increased fecal mucus in cats is most likely to be associated with:

a. gastric polyps
b. colitis
c. tapeworm infection
d. small intestinal bacterial overgrowth
e. pancreatitis

475. In cats, the most effective treatment for chronic recurrent obstipation associated with idiopathic megacolon is:

a. intermittent phosphate enemas
b. low-fiber diet
c. mineral oil laxatives
d. cholinergic drugs
e. subtotal colectomy

Correct answers are on pages 154-179.

Cats, continued

476. *Which serum chemistry value is most likely to be* **abnormal** *in a cat with a congenital portosystemic shunt?*

    a. alanine aminotransferase
    b. albumin
    c. bile acids
    d. alkaline phosphatase
    e. bilirubin

477. *Which liver disease is* **not** *a cause of jaundice in cats?*

    a. hepatic lipidosis
    b. cholangiohepatitis
    c. hepatic lymphoma
    d. pyogranulomatous hepatitis associated with feline infectious peritonitis
    e. corticosteroid-induced hepatopathy

478. *Concerning serum alkaline phosphatase activity in cats, which statement is the* **least** *accurate?*

    a. Elevated serum alkaline phosphatase activity indicates hepatic cholestasis.
    b. Elevations of serum alkaline phosphatase activity in cats are generally of lesser magnitude than in dogs.
    c. Serum alkaline phosphatase activity is frequently elevated in cats with idiopathic hepatic lipidosis syndrome.
    d. Serum alkaline phosphatase activity is usually normal in cats with congenital portosystemic shunts.
    e. Corticosteroid therapy causes elevated serum alkaline phosphatase activity in cats.

479. *Which anticonvulsant drug should* **not** *be used in cats?*

    a. phenobarbital
    b. phenytoin
    c. diazepam
    d. primidone
    e. lorazepam

480. *Which electrolyte disturbance is most likely to be life threatening in a cat with urethral obstruction?*

    a. hypocalcemia
    b. hypokalemia
    c. hyperkalemia
    d. hyponatremia
    e. hypernatremia

481. *What is the most common cause of dermatophytosis (ringworm) in kittens?*

    a. *Microsporum canis*
    b. *Microsporum gypseum*
    c. *Microsporum audouinii*
    d. *Trichophyton mentagrophytes*
    e. *Trichophyton terrestre*

482. *Concerning acetaminophen toxicosis in cats, which statement is* **least** *accurate?*

    a. Methemoglobinemia with cyanosis and acute respiratory distress may occur.
    b. Heinz-body hemolytic anemia may occur.
    c. An overdosage far exceeding the human dosage is required to produce toxicosis in cats.
    d. Prolonged exposure to the drug may cause liver damage and jaundice.
    e. N-acetylcysteine can be given for treatment of acute toxicosis.

483. *A cat with anorexia, depression and vomiting has a blood urea nitrogen level of 98 mg/dl, serum phosphorus level of 11 mg/dl, serum calcium level of 7.3 mg/dl, total plasma protein level of 8.2 g/dl, and urine specific gravity of 1.066. The most likely mechanism underlying azotemia in this cat is:*

    a. dehydration
    b. acute primary renal failure
    c. urinary tract obstruction
    d. chronic renal failure
    e. renal lymphoma

484. Which of the following is **not** a manifestation of taurine deficiency in cats:

   a. dilative cardiomyopathy
   b. central retinal degeneration
   c. reproductive failure
   d. cirrhosis
   e. growth deformities in kittens

485. Hypokalemia-induced "hanging head syndrome" is most likely to occur in a cat with:

   a. feline leukemia virus infection
   b. hyperthyroidism
   c. chronic renal failure
   d. lower urinary tract disease ("feline urologic syndrome")
   e. inflammatory bowel disease

486. Hyperthyroidism in cats can be successfully controlled with:

   a. cyclophosphamide, vincristine or thyroidectomy
   b. prednisolone, iodine radioisotope or thyroidectomy
   c. methimazole, iodine radioisotope or thyroidectomy
   d. thyroxine, prednisone or iodine radioisotope
   e. somatostatin, cyclosporine or cisplatin

487. In cats, what is the most common cardiac manifestation of hyperthyroidism?

   a. hypertrophic cardiomyopathy
   b. mitral valve insufficiency due to endocardiosis
   c. pericardial effusion
   d. dilative cardiomyopathy
   e. sinus bradycardia

488. Which of the following is **not** a typical manifestation of hyperthyroidism in cats?

   a. polydipsia and polyuria
   b. diarrhea
   c. weight loss
   d. ravenous appetite
   e. hepatic encephalopathy

489. Which of the following is **not** a likely effect of corticosteroid treatment in cats?

   a. polyuria and polydipsia
   b. increased appetite
   c. elevated serum alkaline phosphatase activity
   d. gluconeogenesis
   e. suppression of inflammation

490. Concerning diabetes mellitus in cats, which statement is most accurate?

   a. Diabetes mellitus is most prevalent in female cats.
   b. Diabetic ketoacidosis does not occur in cats.
   c. Diabetic cats always require daily insulin injections to maintain normoglycemia.
   d. Insulin injections in cats typically have a longer duration of action than in dogs.
   e. Cats do not develop diabetic cataracts.

491. In cats, diabetes mellitus may result from treatment with:

   a. tetracycline
   b. azathioprine
   c. aspirin
   d. megestrol acetate
   e. ketoconazole

492. A diabetic cat is given insulin at 8 AM and fed at 8 AM and 6 PM. Blood glucose levels are 425 mg/dl at 8 AM, 225 mg/dl at 11 AM, 140 mg/dl at 2 PM, 260 mg/dl at 5 PM, and 355 mg/dl at 8 PM. What do these blood glucose values indicate?

   a. the cat is being fed at inappropriate times
   b. the cat is being fed excessive amounts
   c. the insulin dosage is too low
   d. the duration of action of this type of insulin is too short
   e. the cat has developed insulin resistance associated with hyperadrenocorticism

Correct answers are on pages 154-179.

Cats, continued

493. *Which type of insulin has the longest duration of action?*

    a. regular insulin
    b. ultralente insulin
    c. semilente insulin
    d. NPH insulin
    e. Lente insulin

494. *In cats, methimazole is used to treat:*

    a. dilative cardiomyopathy
    b. lymphoma
    c. hyperthyroidism
    d. renal secondary hyperparathyroidism
    e. cholangiohepatitis

495. *As compared with dogs, cats have a prolonged half-life of elimination of:*

    a. aspirin
    b. insulin
    c. prednisone
    d. gentamicin
    e. digitalis

496. *Heinz-body hemolytic anemia in cats is associated with:*

    a. administration of aspirin
    b. administration of chloramphenicol
    c. warfarin poisoning
    d. administration of acetaminophen
    e. topical application of organophosphate insecticides

497. *In cats, hyperthyroidism is most often associated with:*

    a. bilateral thyroid adenomas
    b. unilateral thyroid adenoma
    c. bilateral thyroid adenocardinomas
    d. unilateral thyroid adenocarcinoma
    e. pituitary-dependent thyroid hypersecretion

498. *Which feline respiratory parasite causes thick-walled pulmonary cysts and passes yellow-brown single-operculated ova in the feces?*

    a. *Capillaria*
    b. *Paragonimus*
    c. *Toxoplasma*
    d. *Aelurostrongylus*
    e. *Filaroides*

499. *Bilirubinuria is:*

    a. an abnormal finding in both male and female cats
    b. an abnormal finding in male cats only
    c. an abnormal finding in female cats only
    d. a normal finding in both male and female cats
    e. only normal in cats under 4 months of age

500. *Which liver disease is **least** likely to cause jaundice in a cat?*

    a. hepatic lipidosis
    b. cholangiohepatitis
    c. pyogranulomatous hepatitis associated with feline infectious peritonitis
    d. congenital portosystemic shunt
    e. hepatic lymphoma

Dogs and Cats

D.W. Macy, F.W. Scott, C.B. Waters

Practice answer sheets are on pages 341-344.

501. *Concerning polydactylism in cats, which statement is most accurate?*

    a. Affected cats should have any extra toes removed.

b. Owners should be advised that it is an inherited autosomal dominant disorder.

c. It is a random congenital defect; no genetic information is available.

d. It is seen most often in Siamese.

e. It is seen most often in Rex cats.

502. *Passive immunity, derived from colostrum, can interfere with development of active immunity following vaccination for canine distemper. Until what age can this interference last in puppies born to immune bitches?*

a. 4-6 weeks of age

b. 8-10 weeks of age

c. 14-16 weeks of age

d. 18-20 weeks of age

e. 22-24 weeks of age

503. *Concerning serum calcium, which statement is* **least** *accurate?*

a. Approximately 50% is bound to albumin.

b. Acidosis decreases ionized calcium levels.

c. Alkalosis decreases ionized calcium levels.

d. Approximately 5% of serum calcium is in the form of calcium salts.

e. Lipemia may result in increased measured levels.

504. *Progestogens are used for controlling estrus in domestic animals. Which of the following is* **not** *a side effect of exogenous progestogens?*

a. obesity

b. behavior changes

c. mammary gland dysplasia

d. adrenal gland suppression in cats

e. urinary incontinence

505. *Pain at the administration site, urticaria, and occasionally abscessation are most commonly associated with administration of:*

a. bacterins

b. killed-virus vaccines

c. modified-live-virus vaccines

d. genetically engineered vaccines

e. intranasal vaccines

506. *When should the first panleukopenia-rhinotracheitis-calicivirus vaccination be given to a kitten?*

a. 10-12 weeks

b. 15-16 weeks

c. 3-4 weeks

d. 8-9 weeks

e. 5-6 weeks

507. *Which breed of dog should* **not** *be given ivermectin at dosages above 200 µg/kg?*

a. German Shepherd

b. Collie

c. Dachshund

d. Poodle

e. Labrador Retriever

508. *All of the following affect the immune response to vaccination* **except***:*

a. nutritional status

b. concurrent infections

c. concurrent drug therapy

d. diagnostic radiography

e. route of vaccination

509. *Which disease is* **not** *zoonotic?*

a. rabies

b. plague

c. leptospirosis

d. parvoviral enteritis

e. sporotrichosis

510. *With normal nursing behavior, what approximate percentage of a dog's circulating immunoglobulins is derived from absorption of colostrum in the neonatal period?*

a. 50%

b. 75%

c. 65%

d. 95%

e. 15%

Correct answers are on pages 154-179.

Dogs and Cats, continued

511. Which of the following is **not** a round-cell tumor?

   a. mast-cell tumor
   b. lymphosarcoma
   c. squamous-cell carcinoma
   d. histiocytoma
   e. transmissible venereal tumor

512. In cats, the tumor induced by exposure to ultraviolet radiation (sunlight) is the:

   a. melanoma
   b. squamous-cell carcinoma
   c. basal-cell carcinoma
   d. histiocytoma
   e. transmissible venereal tumor

513. Based on the World Health Organization's TNM system of classifying tumors, which tumor has the **poorest** prognosis?

   a. T1, N2, MP
   b. T2, N2, M0
   c. T2, N0, M0
   d. T1, N0, M0
   e. T1, N3, M0

514. Which of the following is the **least** commonly documented result of spaying in dogs?

   a. reduced incidence of mammary tumors if done before 2 1/2 years of age
   b. possible urinary incontinence
   c. reduced incidence of pyometra
   d. no attraction of male dogs
   e. obesity

515. Which anthelmintic is most effective against whipworms in dogs?

   a. fenbendazole
   b. bunamidine
   c. pyrantel pamoate
   d. thenium closylate
   e. praziquantel

516. The daily caloric requirement for a 4-year-old male German Shepherd that is a house pet receiving a moderate amount of exercise is approximately:

   a. 35-40 kcal/lb
   b. 20-30 kcal/lb
   c. 10-15 kcal/lb
   d. 40-45 kcal/lb
   e. 50-55 kcal/lb

517. What is the best fecal flotation solution to use if you suspect Giardia infection?

   a. Smith's sugar solution
   b. zinc sulfate solution
   c. magnesium sulfate solution
   d. saturated sucrose solution
   e. saturated sodium chloride solution

518. Which hormones **decrease** sebaceous secretions in dogs?

   a. L-thyroxine and estrogens
   b. growth hormone and L-thyroxine
   c. androgens and estrogens
   d. corticosteroids and estrogens
   e. androgens and L-thyroxine

519. Which fungal organism causes disease more commonly in cats than in dogs?

   a. *Cryptococcus neoformans*
   b. *Coccidioides immitis*
   c. *Blastomyces dermatitidis*
   d. *Histoplasma capsulatum*
   e. *Trichophyton simii*

520. A 7-year-old intact male German Shepherd has bilateral nonpruritic truncal alopecia. Skin scrapings and dermatophyte cultures are negative. Both testicles are descended and normal on palpation. The resting serum thyroxine (T4) level is 3.5 µg/dl and the resting triiodothyronine (T3) level is 1.50 ng/ml. A skin biopsy reveals an "endocrine pattern." What is the **least** likely cause of this dog's dermatosis?

a. Sertoli-cell tumor
b. pituitary-dependent hyperadrenocorticism
c. cortisol-secreting adrenal tumor
d. hypothyroidism
e. seminoma

521. *Currently, the most accurate test to determine if a dog has hyperadrenocorticism is the:*

a. ACTH stimulation test
b. low-dosage dexamethasone suppression test
c. TSH stimulation test
d. xylazine stimulation test
e. endogenous ACTH assay

522. *The test recommended for diagnosis of hypothyroidism in dogs is:*

a. baseline serum thyroxine (T4) level
b. combination of baseline serum thyroxine (T4) and triiodothyronine (T3) levels
c. TSH response test
d. response to thyroid hormone supplementation
e. skin biopsy

523. *For pruritus to occur in a dog with hyperadrenocorticism, at least 1 of 4 clinical conditions must be present. Which of the following is **not** one of those conditions?*

a. pyoderma
b. seborrhea
c. thin skin
d. calcinosis cutis
e. demodicosis

524. *Which clinical sign is specific for Sertoli-cell tumor?*

a. seborrhea
b. hyperpigmentation
c. pruritus
d. truncal alopecia
e. linear preputial dermatosis

525. *Which of the following is **not** a potential complication of megestrol acetate therapy in cats?*

a. mammary hyperplasia and neoplasia
b. pyometra
c. diabetes mellitus
d. hypoadrenocorticism
e. diabetes insipidus

526. *Based on the causes of pruritic miliary dermatitides of cats in the United States, which of the following is the most rational and effective initial therapy for the problem?*

a. systemic corticosteroids
b. systemic antibiotics
c. topical and systemic antifungal therapy
d. flea control and systemic corticosteroids
e. hypoallergenic diet trial

527. *Concerning feline infectious peritonitis antibody titers, which statement is **least** accurate?*

a. A titer greater than 1:3200 is common in normal cats.
b. Titers do not always correlate with shedding of coronavirus.
c. The titer may be negative in terminally ill cats.
d. The titer is useful in helping detect carrier cats and eliminate coronavirus from catteries.
e. The titer may be positive in 20-40% of the cat population.

528. *Concerning diabetes mellitus in cats, which statement is **least** accurate?*

a. Diabetes mellitus generally develops in cats 6 years of age or older.
b. Stressed cats uncommonly develop blood glucose concentrations above 200 mg/dl.
c. Polyuria, polydipsia, polyphagia and weight loss are common clinical signs in diabetic cats.
d. Hyperbilirubinemia is common in diabetic cats.
e. Protein zinc insulin is preferred for treatment of most diabetic cats.

Correct answers are on pages 154-179.

Dogs and Cats, continued

529. *Concerning the cutaneous manifestations of food allergies in cats, which statement is **least** accurate?*

  a. Pruritus may be quite refractory to systemic corticosteroids.
  b. Food allergies may cause pruritic dermatitis restricted to the head and neck.
  c. Food allergies may cause miliary dermatitis.
  d. Food allergies are commonly associated with gastrointestinal signs (vomition, diarrhea).
  e. Diagnosis is supported by feeding a trial hypoallergenic diet (*eg*, Gerber's lamb baby food) for 3 weeks.

530. *Concerning the skin of dogs and cats, which statement is **least** accurate?*

  a. The supracaudal organ ("tail gland") area of dogs is restricted to the proximodorsal aspect of the tail, while in cats this tissue extends the entire length of the dorsum of the tail.
  b. Feline acne and canine acne are similar in that both only affect young, prepubertal animals.
  c. Stress exacerbates sebaceous-gland hyperplasia ("stud tail") in intact male cats.
  d. Aluminum acetate solution is primarily used for its astringent properties in management of feline acne.
  e. Feline acne is probably a manifestation of a focal, epidermal, keratinizing defect.

531. *Coronaviral vasculitis in cats is best treated with:*

  a. azathoprine and corticosteroids
  b. tylosin
  c. methimazole
  d. vitamin E
  e. penicillin

532. *Concerning skin disease in cats, which statement is **least** accurate?*

  a. Dermatophytosis may be intensely pruritic.
  b. Superficial pyoderma is common in cats.

  c. The Mackenzie toothbrush technique is used for dermatophyte culture in asymptomatic cats.
  d. Intradermal testing can delineate sources of inhalant allergy.
  e. The pruritus associated with inhalant allergy is usually responsive to systemic glucocorticoids.

533. *Which treatment is most likely to prevent permanent scarring in severe cases of juvenile cellulitis in dogs?*

  a. systemic antibiotics
  b. topical wet dressings/astringents
  c. topical corticosteroids
  d. systemic corticosteroids
  e. topical antibiotics

534. *Which of the following is most commonly associated with griseofulvin toxicity in cats?*

  a. diabetes mellitus
  b. myelosuppression
  c. hypertrophic cardiomyopathy
  d. dilative cardiomyopathy
  e. uveitis

535. *Which of the following is **not** a recognized complication of mast-cell tumors?*

  a. shock
  b. hemorrhage
  c. erythema and edema
  d. delayed wound healing
  e. irregular heart rate

536. *Which tumor is **least** likely to spread to regional lymph nodes?*

  a. intracutaneous cornifying epithelioma
  b. anal-sac adenocarcinoma
  c. mast-cell tumor
  d. hemangiopericytoma
  e. malignant melanoma

537. *Which tumor is **least** likely to yield cells on aspiration?*

a. fibrosarcoma

b. mast-cell tumor

c. histiocytoma

d. cutaneous lymphoma

e. transmissible venereal tumor

538. *Concerning diabetes mellitus, which statement is* **least** *accurate?*

a. Diabetes mellitus is a metabolic disorder characterized by disturbances of carbohydrate, lipid and protein metabolism.

b. Diabetes mellitus can result from an absolute or relative lack of insulin.

c. Type-I diabetes mellitus in people is usually insulin dependent.

d. In dogs, the age of onset is 4-14 years, and the disease is not usually insulin dependent.

e. Hyperglucagonemia potentiates the effects of hypoinsulinism by increasing glucose production and by increasing fatty acid oxidation and ketogenesis.

539. *In cats, which of the following tumors is most common?*

a. histiocytoma

b. perianal-gland adenoma

c. ceruminous-gland adenoma

d. trichoepithelioma

e. keratoacanthoma

540. *Excessive bleeding is frequently associated with mast-cell tumors and is thought to be due to release of:*

a. histamine

b. proteolytic enzymes

c. heparin

d. Hageman factors

e. ethylenediamine tetraacetic acid

541. *All of the following are common features of both canine and feline fibrosarcomas* **except**:

a. recurrence following surgical removal

b. caused by a retrovirus

c. spindle-type cells

d. require wide excision

e. occur in many organs

542. *Which tumor is associated with hypercalcemia?*

a. perianal-gland adenocarcinoma

b. keratocanthoma

c. anal-sac adenocarcinoma

d. trichoepithelioma

e. histiocytoma

543. *Which tumor is most likely to undergo spontaneous remission?*

a. mast-cell tumor

b. melanoma

c. transmissible venereal tumor

d. lymphosarcoma

e. plasmacytoma

544. *In dogs, which form of lymphosarcoma is most frequently associated with hypercalcemia?*

a. alimentary

b. mediastinal

c. generalized

d. osseous

e. ocular

545. *Which drug used in treatment of lympho-sarcoma in dogs is limited by its cardiotoxicity?*

a. prednisolone

b. doxorubicin

c. vincristine

d. cyclophosphamide

e. L-asparginase

546. *Which form of lymphosarcoma is most common in dogs?*

a. multicentric

b. alimentary

c. mediastinal

d. osseous

e. ocular

Correct answers are on pages 154-179.

Dogs and Cats, continued

547. Dogs with hypercalcemia commonly demonstrate:

    a. convulsions
    b. hyperactivity
    c. polyuria and polydipsia
    d. ravenous appetite
    e. twitching of facial muscles

548. Which organ is most adversely affected by hypercalcemia?

    a. brain
    b. heart
    c. kidney
    d. bladder
    e. intestine

549. Which breed of dog is most likely to lose its hair following therapy with doxorubicin?

    a. Golden Retriever
    b. Labrador Retriever
    c. Doberman Pinscher
    d. Old English Sheepdog
    e. Dalmatian

550. Which feline virus is **least** contagious?

    a. feline leukemia virus
    b. feline immunodeficiency virus
    c. feline rhinotracheitis virus
    d. feline infectious peritonitis virus
    e. feline calicivirus

551. Which combination of drugs is used most commonly in treatment of lymphosarcoma in dogs and cats?

    a. cyclophosphamide, prednisone, vincristine
    b. mitoxantrone, prednisone, methotrexate
    c. doxorubicin, cyclophosphamide, vincristine
    d. bleomycin, mitoxantrone, prednisone
    e. bleomycin, mitoxantrone, prednisone

552. In the United States, the feline immunodeficiency virus infection rate is half that of feline leukemia virus. What percentage of the clinically healthy, low-risk cat population is infected with feline immunodeficiency virus?

    a. 2%
    b. 5.5%
    c. 10%
    d. 11%
    e. 17%

553. Serologic tests for feline immunodeficiency virus infection detect:

    a. antigen
    b. antibody
    c. antigen-antibody complexes
    d. IgE
    e. P27

554. Which drug used in cancer therapy is termed "phase specific"?

    a. prednisolone
    b. vincristine
    c. cyclophosphamide
    d. doxorubicin
    e. prednisone

555. Which tumor of dogs is curable with chemotherapy alone?

    a. lymphosarcoma
    b. transmissible venereal tumor
    c. fibrosarcoma
    d. mast-cell tumor
    e. mammary carcinoma

556. Which clinical disease has **not** been associated with hypercalcemia?

    a. hypoadrenocorticism
    b. lymphosarcoma
    c. apocrine-gland tumors of the anal sac
    d. parathyroid adenoma
    e. histiocytoma

557. Which fungal disease is most frequently seen in dogs in the southwestern United States?

    a. cryptococcosis

b. blastomycosis

c. coccidioidomycosis

d. histoplasmosis

e. sporotrichosis

558. *Throughout history, plague has killed large numbers of people. Which domestic animal is associated with 10% of the human cases of plague today?*

a. dog

b. cat

c. duck

d. cow

e. horse

559. *In dogs, skin biopsies are most useful in diagnosing:*

a. inhalant allergy

b. food allergy

c. pemphigus foliaceus

d. bacterial dermatitis

e. drug allergy

560. *Concerning eosinophilic ulcers (indolent ulcers, rodent ulcers) in cats, which statement is **least** accurate?*

a. They usually occur on the upper lip.

b. They may undergo malignant transformation to squamous-cell carcinoma.

c. They are typically associated with peripheral blood eosinophilia.

d. They have been associated with food allergies.

e. One recommended therapy is methyl-prednisolone acetate injection.

561. *Which pattern of alopecia suggests a sex hormone imbalance in a dog?*

a. hair loss beginning over the dorsum

b. hair loss beginning over the head and distal extremities

c. hair loss beginning in the perineum or flank

d. hair loss beginning with development of a "rat tail"

e. hair loss beginning in the axillae and ventral thorax

562. *The most consistent and diagnostically relevant laboratory abnormality in cats with feline infectious peritonitis is:*

a. high serum gammaglobulin level

b. anemia

c. leukocytosis

d. *Hemobartonella* in red blood cells

e. feline leukemia virus positive

563. *Which diagnostic procedure is recommended for diagnosis of pemphigus foliaceus in dogs?*

a. direct immunofluorescence testing of formalin-fixed skin biopsies

b. direct immunofluorescence testing of skin biopsies fixed in Bouin's solution

c. indirect immunofluorescence testing of serum

d. direct immunofluorescence testing of skin biopsies fixed in Michel's medium

e. direct immunofluorescence testing of serum

564. *You are presented with a 3-year-old Labrador Retriever with multiple lick granulomas on all of its limbs. Treatment with oral prednisone stops the licking, and the lesions dramatically improve. Unfortunately, the lesions recur after discontinuation of corticosteroid therapy. The most likely underlying cause of the granulomas in this dog is:*

a. psychological problem

b. systemic bacterial infection

c. foreign bodies

d. dermatophytosis

e. inhalant allergy

565. *Which tumor is frequently associated with fragmentation of red blood cells?*

a. fibrosarcoma

b. mast-cell tumor

c. hemangiosarcoma

d. melanoma

e. histiocytoma

Correct answers are on pages 154-179.

Dogs and Cats, continued

566. Which tumor is frequently associated with excessive bleeding during excision?

   a. fibrosarcoma
   b. mast-cell tumor
   c. squamous-cell carcinoma
   d. basal-cell carcinoma
   e. histiocytoma

567. The antigen-presenting cell in the central nervous system is the:

   a. lymphocyte
   b. astrocyte
   c. microglial cell
   d. monocyte
   e. mast cell

568. Blunt trauma to the central nervous system results in swelling that is:

   a. primarily associated with edema
   b. almost completely associated with astrocyte swelling
   c. usually associated with a hematoma
   d. primarily associated with release of histamine from astrocytes
   e. primarily associated with degranulation of mast cells

569. All of the following can cause insulin resistance in dogs **except**:

   a. acromegaly
   b. hyperadrenocorticism
   c. bacterial bronchopneumonia
   d. uremia
   e. heartworm infection

570. The most common primary site of hemangiosarcoma in dogs is the:

   a. left atrium
   b. spleen
   c. lungs
   d. bladder
   e. liver

571. Concerning insulin, which statement is **least** accurate?

   a. Insulin is a two-chain polypeptide.
   b. Insulin is produced by the beta cells of the pancreas.
   c. Entry of glucose into red blood cells is an insulin receptor-dependent process.
   d. Insulin promotes nucleic acid formation into mononucleotides.
   e. Insulin inhibits gluconeogenesis.

572. All of the following tumors may be diagnosed through fine-needle aspiration of the spleen **except**:

   a. keratoacanthoma
   b. hemangiosarcoma
   c. mast-cell tumor
   d. lymphoma
   e. plasmacytoma

573. In dogs, appropriate treatment for cholecalciferol rodenticide toxicity includes all of the following **except**:

   a. saline
   b. furosemide
   c. calcitonin
   d. thiazide diuretic
   e. aluminum hydroxide

574. Concerning hyperosmolar nonketotic syndrome in dogs, which statement is most accurate?

   a. It is relatively common.
   b. Mild hyperglycemia and increased serum osmolality are usually present.
   c. Most affected dogs are ketotic.
   d. Development of cerebral edema during treatment is common.
   e. NPH insulin is the insulin of choice during the initial stages of management.

575. Which agent is **not** appropriate for topical therapy of seborrhea in dogs?

   a. sulfur
   b. salicylic acid

c. tar
d. captan
e. benzoyl peroxide

576. Which drug is **not** acceptable for long-term management of pruritus?

a. prednisolone
b. methylprednisolone
c. dexamethasone
d. diphenhydramine
e. essential fatty acid supplement

577. Impetigo is another name for:

a. superficial pustular pyoderma
b. juvenile pyoderma
c. bacterial hypersensitivity
d. skin-fold pyoderma
e. deep pyoderma

578. The most common dermatophyte of cats is:

a. *Microsporum canis*
b. *Microsporum felis*
c. *Trichophyton mentagrophytes*
d. *Trichophyton felis*
e. *Microsporum gypseum*

579. Copper toxicosis is seen in Bedlington Terriers and other breeds. Copper toxicosis is appropriately treated with all of the following **except**:

a. dietary zinc supplementation
b. dietary restriction of copper
c. penicillamine
d. tetramine
e. dietary supplementation

580. In treating infections of the liver, one should select an antimicrobial that is excreted in the bile. Which drug is **not** appropriate for treatment of liver infections because it is not excreted in bile?

a. ampicillin
b. amoxicillin
c. cephalexin

d. cefadroxil
e. gentamicin

581. Which drug is **not** appropriate in treatment of bile duct infection in dogs with concurrent liver failure?

a. ampicillin
b. chloramphenicol
c. cephalexin
d. cefadroxil
e. amoxicillin

582. All of the following drugs are potentially hepatotoxic in dogs or cats **except**:

a. halothane
b. griseofulvin
c. acetaminophen
d. primidone
e. chloramphenicol

583. Which corticosteroid has the greatest glucocorticoid activity (is most potent)?

a. hydrocortisone
b. prednisone
c. betamethasone
d. triamcinolone
e. prednisolone

584. Which drug is **not** considered potentially toxic to the kidney?

a. amphotericin B
b. gentamicin
c. thiacetarsamide
d. amoxicillin
e. cisplatin

585. All of the following drugs are used to stimulate appetite **except**:

a. diazepam
b. cyproheptadine
c. prednisolone
d. oxazepam
e. naloxone

Correct answers are on pages 154-179.

Dogs and Cats, continued

586. Toxoplasmosis is a zoonotic disease. Cats may play a role in transmission of the disease to people. At what age is a cat most likely to excrete oocysts in its feces?

   a. 3-5 years
   b. 1-2 weeks
   c. 2-12 months
   d. 8-10 years
   e. 5-7 years

587. The recommended treatment for toxoplasmosis in cats is:

   a. ampicillin
   b. amoxicillin
   c. chloramphenicol
   d. clindamycin
   e. gentamicin

588. Large-breed dogs are predisposed to appendicular osteosarcoma. Following amputation of the affected limb, what percentage of dogs survives at least 1 year with no other therapy?

   a. 30%
   b. 50%
   c. 10%
   d. 70%
   e. 90%

589. Which antifungal agent is used primarily for treatment of cryptococcosis and is of limited use for other fungal infections?

   a. amphotericin B
   b. ketoconazole
   c. flucytosine
   d. itraconazole
   e. potassium iodide

590. Left untreated, lymphosarcoma in dogs is typically fatal within 30 days. However, treatment with chemotherapeutic agents, such as doxorubicin, cyclophosphamide, vincristine and prednisone, produces complete remission in approximately what percentage of treated dogs?

   a. 10%
   b. 25%
   c. 50%
   d. 75%
   e. 95%

591. In dogs, chemotherapy for lymphosarcoma allows survival for an average of:

   a. 3 months
   b. 10 months
   c. 20 months
   d. 30 months
   e. 40 months

592. What is the most common infectious cause of nasal discharge in dogs?

   a. cryptococcosis
   b. blastomycosis
   c. viral rhinotracheitis
   d. aspergillosis
   e. coccidioidomycosis

593. Which common feline virus is most difficult to inactivate with disinfectants?

   a. calicivirus
   b. coronavirus
   c. panleukopenia virus
   d. feline immunodeficiency virus
   e. feline leukemia virus

594. Hypokalemic myopathy of cats is most similar in its clinical presentation to:

   a. thiamin deficiency
   b. tetanus
   c. borreliosis
   d. cytauxzoonosis
   e. botulism

595. Which drug is most effective in treatment of hyperthyroidism in cats?

a. cyclophosphamide
b. doxorubicin
c. cisplatin
d. methimazole
e. atropine

a. fasting hyperglycemia
b. glycosuria
c. hypercholesterolemia
d. lipemia
e. hypocalcemia

596. A 12-year-old German Shepherd has a chronic mucohemorrhagic discharge from its right naris. What is the most likely cause, but not necessarily the only possible cause, of this problem?

a. nasal tumor
b. bacterial infection
c. viral infection
d. foreign body
e. allergy

597. You remove a hemangiosarcoma from the spleen of an 8-year-old German Shepherd. The chance that the dog will survive at least 1 year after the surgery is:

a. less than 10%
b. 30%
c. 60%
d. 80%
e. greater than 90%

598. Concerning management of uncomplicated diabetes mellitus in dogs, which statement is most accurate?

a. A glucose curve should be calculated the day diabetes mellitus is diagnosed.
b. NPH insulin IV at 2.2 units/kg is a good starting dosage.
c. Protein zinc insulin is the insulin of choice for initial use in dogs.
d. Semi-moist foods should be avoided due to their high sugar content.
e. NPH insulin SC at 2.2 units/kg is a good starting dosage.

599. Which of the following is **not** commonly associated with uncomplicated diabetes mellitus in dogs?

600. Concerning insulin-producing islet-cell tumors in dogs, which statement is **least** accurate?

a. The amended serum insulin/glucose ratio is the most sensitive test for insulin-producing islet-cell tumors, but the diagnosis should not be based on this test alone.
b. The glucagon tolerance test can be used to help confirm the diagnosis of insulin-producing islet-cell tumor.
c. Insulin-producing islet-cell tumors are most common in older dogs.
d. Insulin-producing islet-cell tumors can be solitary or multiple.
e. Most insulin-producing islet-cell tumors are carcinomas, but metastasis is rare.

601. An adjuvant is a substance that:

a. is used to adhere antibody to a plastic plate used in enzyme-linked immunosorbent assay
b. enhances antigenicity or antibody response when mixed with an antigen
c. enhances the activity of certain antiviral compounds
d. enhances the antigen response in natural viral infections
e. is used to adhere proteins to the nitrocellulose paper in the Western blot assay

602. Which statement best characterizes an attenuated virus?

a. The virulence of the virus has been reduced to an acceptable level for use as a vaccine.
b. The virus multiplies in the host animal but, by definition, cannot produce clinical signs.
c. The virus has been inactivated by chemical or physical means.
d. The virus has been altered by biotechnology.
e. The virus has been adapted to cell culture.

Correct answers are on pages 154-179.

Dogs and Cats, continued

603. *Concerning capsomeres of the feline parvovirus virion, which statement is* **least** *accurate?*

    a. Capsomeres are composed of the gp70 glycoprotein, which stimulates the primary immune response elicited by commercial vaccines against feline panleukopenia.
    b. Capsomeres are morphologic units of the capsid of a virion.
    c. Capsomeres are composed of polypeptides.
    d. Capsomeres are composed of proteins.
    e. Capsomeres contain the primary antigen responsible for stimulation of an immune response in the infected cat.

604. *Concerning the peplomer of the feline leukemia virus, which statement is* **least** *accurate?*

    a. It is a glycoprotein unit that contains the antigen responsible for antigenicity and, hence, protective immunity.
    b. It is the morphologic unit that protrudes from the surface of the viral envelope.
    c. It is inserted into the altered cell membrane, which eventually becomes the envelope of the virus during viral replication.
    d. It contains feline oncornavirus cell membrane antigen (FOCMA).
    e. It contains the gp70 glycoprotein.

605. *After vaccination of a cat, humoral antibody to feline parvovirus generally appears in the serum after approximately:*

    a. 1 day
    b. 2-3 days
    c. 6-7 days
    d. 14 days
    e. 28 days

606. *In kittens, the half-life of passive maternal antibodies is approximately:*

    a. 1-2 days
    b. 3-4 days
    c. 8-10 days
    d. 14-16 days
    e. 20-25 days

607. *A client's kitten has just died from feline panleukopenia (feline parvovirus) and she wants to replace it with an unvaccinated 14-week-old kitten from a neighbor. How long after vaccination of the kitten should she wait before taking it home?*

    a. she can take the kitten home immediately
    b. 3 days
    c. 1 week
    d. 2 weeks
    e. 1 year

608. *In most cases, to diagnose a disease in a cat by serum antibody titer determination, one must demonstrate a significant rise in titer in paired serum samples. What constitutes a "significant" rise in titer?*

    a. a positive titer (>1:10) in both samples
    b. 2-fold increase
    c. 4-fold increase
    d. 10-fold increase
    e. 100-fold increase

609. *You collect paired serum samples 2 weeks apart from a group of 5 dogs with suspected canine distemper and submit the samples to the diagnostic laboratory. Which titers in the acute and convalescent samples, respectively, indicate acute canine distemper?*

    a. 1:80 and 1:160
    b. 1:320 and 1:320
    c. 1:40 and 1:320
    d. 1:320 and 1:40
    e. 1:640 and 1:920

610. *"Blue eye" in dogs is caused by:*

    a. canine adenovirus-1 vaccination
    b. the immunosuppressive effect of canine parvovirus vaccination
    c. parainfluenza virus vaccination
    d. canine adenovirus-2 vaccination
    e. canine distemper vaccination

611. A new antiviral drug has specific action against DNA virus but no effect on RNA virus. Against which canine viruses is this drug likely to be effective?

   a. distemper virus, herpesvirus, parvovirus
   b. infectious hepatitis virus, herpesvirus, parvovirus
   c. distemper virus, infectious hepatitis virus, parainfluenza virus
   d. parainfluenza virus, adenovirus-2, reovirus
   e. distemper virus, reovirus, parvovirus

612. Another new antiviral drug is effective only against RNA viruses. Against which feline viruses is this drug likely to be effective?

   a. panleukopenia virus, calicivirus, rhinotracheitis virus
   b. rhinotracheitis virus, calicivirus, infectious peritonitis virus
   c. infectious peritonitis virus, leukemia virus, panleukopenia virus
   d. calicivirus, infectious peritonitis virus, leukemia virus
   e. immunodeficiency virus, leukemia virus, panleukopenia virus

613. You suspect feline infectious peritonitis (FIP) in a 6-month-old Persian cat because of the severe clinical disease, including a persistent, nonresponsive fever, palpable lumps on the kidney, and progressive weight loss and anorexia. Despite heroic treatment, the cat develops progressive neurologic signs, and you and the owner reluctantly conclude that euthanasia is necessary. What single sample should be collected before euthanasia or at necropsy, and how should the sample be examined to confirm your diagnosis of FIP?

   a. blood smear examined for FIP virus by indirect fluorescent antibody test
   b. serum examined for coronaviruses by indirect fluorescent antibody test
   c. serum examined for FIP antibody titer by serum neutralization test
   d. throat swab cultured for FIP virus
   e. kidney tissue examined microscopically

614. The commercial feline leukemia virus vaccine Leukocell (SmithKline) is a subunit vaccine containing 2 antigens, feline oncornavirus cell membrane antigen and:

   a. p15E
   b. p27
   c. gp70
   d. p70
   e. gp27

615. Which term best describes a group of 2 or more feline caliciviruses that contain the same major antigenic determinants, and that are neutralized to a similar degree by antiserum to each of the separate viruses?

   a. subtype
   b. serotype
   c. isolate
   d. strain
   e. biotype

616. Feline infectious peritonitis is a progressive, debilitating, highly fatal disease of cats caused by a:

   a. parvovirus
   b. retrovirus
   c. rhabdovirus
   d. coronavirus
   e. calicivirus

617. The laboratory test used in most diagnostic laboratories as an aid to diagnosis of feline infectious peritonitis (FIP) is:

   a. direct fluorescent antibody testing of tissues to detect FIP virus
   b. agar gel immunodiffusion of serum to detect coronavirus antigen (Coggins' test)
   c. serum neutralization test to detect antibodies specific for FIP virus
   d. indirect fluorescent antibody testing of serum to detect coronavirus antibodies
   e. enzyme-linked immunosorbent assay of serum to detect coronavirus antibodies

Correct answers are on pages 154-179.

Dogs and Cats, continued

618. *Cloudy, blue corneal edema in a dog 2 weeks after vaccination is due to:*

a. synergistic immunosuppressive effects of distemper virus and parvovirus in the vaccine

b. adenovirus-2 infection of the dog before vaccination

c. replication of vaccine-origin adenovirus-1 in the eyes

d. recrudescence of herpesviral infection because of the immunosuppressive effects of vaccination

e. formation of immune complexes in the cornea from interaction of *Bordetella* in the vaccine and anti-*Bordetella* antibodies

619. *Which antiviral drugs can be used as antiherpetic eye ointments for treatment of cats with ulcerative herpetic keratitis?*

a. ribavirin, adenine arabinoside

b. adenine arabinoside, idoxuridine

c. idoxuridine, ribavirin

d. amantadine, adenine arabinoside

e. amantadine, ribavirin

620. *The most common cause of vaccine failure in dogs and cats is:*

a. interference by maternally derived immunity with vaccine virus

b. loss of immunogenicity from improper handling of vaccines

c. low antigenic mass of vaccines

d. split dosages of vaccine to reduce cost of vaccination

e. inappropriate administration of vaccine (subcutaneous instead of intramuscular)

621. *A client's unvaccinated cat will soon be exposed to panleukopenia virus in a boarding establishment, and you must decide how to best protect the cat against infection. Ranking in order from most rapid to least rapid induction of immunity, what is the protective potential of available products?*

a. antiserum, killed-virus vaccine, modified-live-virus vaccine

b. antiserum, modified-live-virus vaccine, killed-virus vaccine

c. killed-virus vaccine, modified-live-virus vaccine, antiserum

d. modified-live-virus vaccine, killed-virus vaccine, antiserum

e. modified-live-virus vaccine, antiserum, killed-virus vaccine

622. *Which of the following is an example of a heterotypic vaccine?*

a. canine parvovirus vaccine to protect against canine distemper

b. bovine virus diarrhea vaccine to protect against canine distemper

c. measles vaccine to protect against canine distemper

d. rinderpest vaccine to protect against bovine virus diarrhea

e. measles vaccine to protect against canine parvoviral infection

623. *Two caliciviruses are isolated at the state diagnostic laboratory from similar clinical disease outbreaks of upper respiratory disease in 2 breeding catteries. Vaccination of kittens at 8-10 weeks of age does not control the upper respiratory infections within these catteries because most kittens become infected before vaccination. You question whether a "new" virus has evolved, against which currently available vaccines are not effective. Characterization of these 2 viruses in the laboratory reveals that they both have the same major antigenic determinants. Which statement best characterizes the relationship between these 2 viruses?*

a. The viruses belong to the same virus serotype.

b. The viruses are subtypes of the same serotype.

c. The viruses are merely strains of the same virus.

d. The viruses are 2 new viral isolates.

e. The viruses are serotypes of the same subtype.

624. In feline viral rhinotracheitis, herpesvirus-1 is spread from local lesions to sites of latent infection in the central nervous system by:

a. macrophages
b. peripheral nerves
c. cell-free viremia
d. lymphatics
e. cell-associated viremia

625. Concerning feline infectious peritonitis (FIP), which statement is **least** accurate?

a. Clinical FIP is the result of Arthus-like interactions of antigen, antibody and complement across vessel walls, accompanied by virus persistence within mononuclear phagocytes.
b. Coronaviral antibodies contribute to enhancement of the disease process by facilitating uptake of virus into mononuclear phagocytes.
c. A positive coronaviral antibody titer (as determined by immunofluorescence or enzyme-linked immunosorbent assay) in a clinically ill animal is diagnostic of FIP.
d. The mechanism responsible for immunity against FIP is not known but is suspected to be T-cell mediated.
e. The magnitude of the coronaviral antibody titer in a cat with FIP has little relationship to the chronicity of the disease process.

626. Concerning feline leukemia virus (FeLV), which statement is **least** accurate?

a. FeLV-associated diseases include lymphosarcoma, myeloproliferative disorders, nonregenerative anemia, and panleukopenia-like syndrome.
b. The reservoir of FeLV in nature is the chronically viremic carrier cat, which excretes infectious virus in respiratory secretions, feces, urine and, most importantly, saliva.
c. The persistent viremia in FeLV infection is frequently reversible.
d. A negative FeLV test, either by the slide test or enzyme-linked immunosorbent assay, in no way indicates past infection, with integration of FeLV proviral DNA into host cells.

e. An effective FeLV control program begins with testing of all cats in the household and removal or permanent isolation of all persistently infected cats.

627. Feline panleukopenia is caused by a:

a. papovavirus
b. parvovirus
c. herpesvirus
d. calicivirus
e. lentivirus

628. The longest time that feline panleukopenia virus may survive at room temperature in a contaminated environment is:

a. 1 day
b. 1 week
c. 1 month
d. 6 months
e. more than 1 year

629. Chlorhexidine (Nolvasan) has virucidal activity against which feline viruses?

a. panleukopenia virus, herpesvirus-1 and calicivirus
b. herpesvirus-1 but not calicivirus or panleukopenia virus
c. calicivirus but not herpesvirus-1 or panleukopenia virus
d. calicivirus and herpesvirus-1 but not panleukopenia virus
e. panleukopenia virus and calicivirus but not herpesvirus-1

630. To be most effective by aerosol therapy for chronic respiratory tract infections in cats, an antimicrobial should be:

a. rapidly absorbed from the respiratory mucosa, such as kanamycin or gentamicin
b. rapidly absorbed from the respiratory mucosa, such as penicillin or tetracycline
c. slowly absorbed from the respiratory mucosa, such as kanamycin or gentamicin
d. combined with an antiviral compound, such as idoxuridine
e. slowly absorbed from the respiratory mucosa, such as penicillin or tetracycline

Correct answers are on pages 154-179.

Dogs and Cats, continued

631. *In treatment of tracheobronchitis in dogs, aerosol therapy with antibacterials:*

 a. does not reduce numbers of bacteria in the trachea, and reduces clinical signs
 b. reduces numbers of virus particles but not bacteria in the trachea, and reduces clinical signs
 c. reduces numbers of bacteria but not virus particles in the trachea, and does not reduce clinical signs
 d. reduces numbers of bacteria in the trachea and reduces clinical signs
 e. has no local or clinical effect

632. *Feline parvovirus can replicate:*

 a. only in mature enterocytes
 b. only in cells undergoing mitosis
 c. in both mature and mitotic cells
 d. only in the cerebellum of newborn kittens
 e. only if a helper virus is present, such as type-A feline leukemia virus

633. *Feline infectious peritonitis is caused by a:*

 a. gammaherpesvirus
 b. retrovirus
 c. cell-associated reovirus
 d. lentivirus
 e. coronavirus

634. *In the environment, feline infectious peritonitis virus is:*

 a. extremely resistant, surviving for over 1 year at room temperature
 b. moderately resistant, surviving several weeks at room temperature
 c. moderately labile, surviving several days at room temperature
 d. labile, surviving only 1-3 days at room temperature
 e. very labile, and is inactivated in less than 24 hours at room temperature

635. *Passive maternal immunity in kittens:*

 a. persists as long as the kittens are nursing
 b. is transferred to kittens via colostrum during the first 24 hours
 c. is transferred to kittens only *in utero*
 d. is transferred to kittens via colostrum during first 4 weeks of life until they become immunocompetent
 e. protects the kittens against *in-utero* infection but has no protective benefits after birth

636. *Following initial vaccination of a cat against rhinotracheitis (herpesvirus-1), a secondary immune response can occur if a second dose of vaccine is given after:*

 a. 1 day
 b. 4 days
 c. 7 days
 d. 14 days
 e. 21 days

637. *In cats, commercially available rhinotracheitis-calicivirus vaccines should be given:*

 a. only intranasally
 b. only intramuscularly
 c. only subcutaneously
 d. only by conjunctival inoculation
 e. according to the manufacturer's recommendations

638. *In cats, corneal dendritic ulcers are usually caused by:*

 a. feline parvovirus
 b. feline herpesvirus-1
 c. feline calicivirus
 d. feline pneumonitis virus
 e. feline immunodeficiency virus

639. *In cats, lingual ulcers are usually caused by:*

 a. feline parvovirus
 b. feline herpesvirus-1
 c. feline calicivirus
 d. feline pneumonitis virus
 e. feline immunodeficiency virus

640. *In both the wet (effusive) and dry forms of feline infectious peritonitis, the most consistent finding is:*

   a. hypergammaglobulinemia
   b. chorioretinitis
   c. nephritis
   d. low specific gravity of any effusion
   e. hepatitis

641. *In cats, Tyzzer's disease is caused by:*

   a. the protozoan blood parasite, *Eperythrozoon felis*
   b. the bacterium, *Bacillus piliformis*
   c. an unclassified DNA virus
   d. a systemic fungus, *Conidiobolus avis*, which is acquired from birds
   e. the intestinal protozoan parasite, *Giardia lamblia*

642. *In cats, Salmonella typhimurium:*

   a. is nonpathogenic
   b. causes mild, self-limiting gastroenteritis
   c. can cause severe gastroenteritis in some cats, especially after stress, but often produces only subclinical infections
   d. produces severe gastroenteritis in all infected cats, often with associated pyogranuloma formation throughout the abdominal organs
   e. is a common cause of chronic upper respiratory infection, especially in cats with immunosuppression by feline immunodeficiency virus or feline leukemia virus

643. *Ranking in order from most effective to least effective, what is the efficacy of products to protect cats in animal shelters against feline panleukopenia?*

   a. killed-virus vaccine, modified-live-virus vaccine, antiserum
   b. killed-virus vaccine, antiserum, modified-live-virus vaccine
   c. antiserum, modified-live-virus vaccine, killed-virus vaccine
   d. modified-live-virus vaccine, killed-virus vaccine, antiserum
   e. modified-live-virus vaccine, antiserum, killed-virus vaccine

644. *Concerning feline viral rhinotracheitis, which statement is most accurate?*

   a. The serum neutralization titer is directly proportional to the degree of protection.
   b. The minimum protective virus neutralizing antibody titer is 1:10.
   c. The local antibody titer is the only significant protective titer.
   d. Protection is determined by a combination of humoral antibody, local antibody and cell-mediated immunity.
   e. Protection is only provided by T-cell-mediated immunity.

645. *Feline leprosy, a disease characterized by single or multiple skin nodules, some of which may ulcerate, is caused by:*

   a. an acid-fast bacterium
   b. feline leukemia virus
   c. feline papovavirus
   d. *Actinobacillus leprae*
   e. *Leptospira felis*

646. *Under normal environmental conditions, feline rhinotracheitis virus (herpesvirus-1) contaminating a cage or ward is usually inactivated within:*

   a. 1 hour
   b. 1 day
   c. 1 week
   d. 1 month
   e. 3 months

647. *In a cat with rabies, when is rabies virus excreted in the saliva?*

   a. from 1 week before through 1 week after the onset of clinical signs
   b. throughout the course of disease, beginning at the onset of clinical signs
   c. for 1 week after the onset of clinical signs
   d. from 1 day before through 3 days after the onset of clinical signs
   e. from up to 6 months before the onset of clinical signs, throughout the course of disease

Correct answers are on pages 154-179.

Dogs and Cats, continued

648. "Chronic panleukopenia" or
"panleukopenia-like syndrome" is caused by:

   a. *Salmonella typhimurium*
   b. feline leukemia virus
   c. *Bacillus piliformis*
   d. feline panleukopenia virus
   e. feline rotavirus

649. For effective aerosol therapy of lower
respiratory diseases in cats, a nebulizer should
deliver an aerosol with a particle size of:

   a. less than 5 μ
   b. 5-10 μ
   c. 10-20 μ
   d. 20-100 μ
   e. more than 100 μ

650. Concerning feline calicivirus vaccine, which
statement is most accurate?

   a. They have limited value due to the multiple
serotypes of calicivirus.
   b. They protect cats against upper respiratory
disease but not against pneumonia caused
by calicivirus.
   c. They protect cats against pneumonia but not
against upper respiratory disease caused by
calicivirus.
   d. They protect cats against caliciviral enteritis
but not against upper respiratory disease or
pneumonia.
   e. They protect against both upper respiratory
infection and pneumonia caused by
calicivirus.

651. In viral respiratory infection of cats, virus
may be shed from the pharyngeal area
beginning 3 weeks after infection (so-called
"carrier cat"), with virus shedding continuing
for at least a year. Concerning patterns of virus
shedding, which statement is most accurate?

   a. It occurs with rhinotracheitis virus but not
with calicivirus.

   b. It occurs with calicivirus but not with
rhinotracheitis virus.
   c. Both calicivirus and rhinotracheitis are shed
continuously.
   d. Rhinotracheitis virus is shed intermittently,
while calicivirus is shed almost continuously.
   e. Calicivirus is shed intermittently, while
rhinotracheitis virus is shed continuously.

652. The first feline infectious peritonitis vaccine
was produced from a temperature-sensitive
mutant virus. This vaccine virus grows at:

   a. 40 C but not at 37 C
   b. 33 C better than at 37 C
   c. 37 C but not at 40 C
   d. 37 C but not at 33 C
   e. 37 C but not at 35 C or 39 C

653. In production of vaccines, viruses are
frequently modified or attenuated in virulence.
There are advantages and disadvantages to
modified-live-virus (MLV) vaccines. When you,
as a clinician, are faced with certain situations
in practice, you must decide whether to use an
inactivated (killed-virus) vaccine or a MLV
vaccine. Concerning MLV feline vaccines,
which statement is **least** accurate?

   a. MLV vaccines provide protection more
quickly than inactivated vaccines.
   b. MLV vaccines should not be used in a
pregnant cat unless specifically approved
for this use.
   c. MLV vaccines are preferable for use in
contaminated environments, such as animal
shelters.
   d. MLV vaccines can only be given as a
monovalent vaccine because of viral
interference if 2 or more viruses are
combined into one vaccine.
   e. MLV vaccines generally produce higher
antibody titers than inactivated vaccines
and therefore produce longer-lasting
immunity in vaccinated cats.

654. Concerning inactivated (killed-virus) feline
panleukopenia vaccines, which statement is
most accurate?

a. Inactivated panleukopenia vaccines stimulate interferon production because the inactivation process releases nucleic acid, which is an interferon inducer.

b. Inactivated panleukopenia vaccines are usually preferable to modified-live-virus vaccines for vaccination of pregnant cats.

c. Inactivated vaccines are seldom used in veterinary medicine today because of the superior modified-live-virus vaccines.

d. Inactivated panleukopenia vaccines may be given effectively by the oral route.

e. Very effective inactivated vaccines have been developed using recombinant DNA technology, with insertion of the genome into *E coli*.

655. *In feline leukemia (FeLV) infection, a cat is described as persistently viremic if it has 2 or more positive FeLV tests during a period of at least:*

a. 1 week
b. 2 weeks
c. 3 weeks
d. 4 weeks
e. 12 weeks

656. *Concerning viruses you may encounter in your small animal hospital, and the ease with which these viruses can be inactivated by physical and chemical agents, which statement is most accurate?*

a. Rabies virus, canine distemper virus and canine parvovirus are easily inactivated.

b. Feline herpesvirus, feline calicivirus and feline parvovirus are easily inactivated.

c. Feline herpesvirus, canine distemper virus and rabies virus are easily inactivated.

d. Canine distemper virus and feline parvovirus are easily inactivated, but not feline herpesvirus.

e. Feline leukemia virus, feline herpesvirus and canine distemper virus are not easily inactivated.

657. *Following exposure to feline parvovirus (natural or vaccination), circulating antibodies are first detected in the serum of cats after approximately:*

a. 3-4 days
b. 6-7 days
c. 10-11 days
d. 14-15 days
e. 28-30 days

658. *The half-life of circulating antibodies in dogs and cats is approximately:*

a. 1-2 days
b. 3-4 days
c. 8-10 days
d. 20-25 days
e. 30-35 days

659. *Concerning the serum neutralization test, which statement is **least** accurate?*

a. Results of this antibody assay are reported as a "titer."

b. The reaction in a positive serum neutralization test is not detectable, even with the aid of a microscope; therefore, some indicator system, such as inoculation of susceptible cell cultures, embryonated eggs or susceptible animals, must be used to indicate whether or not the infectious virus in an assay has been "neutralized."

c. The serum neutralization test is generally more expensive and more time consuming than enzyme-linked immunosorbent assay.

d. In many viral diseases, such as feline panleukopenia, there is an excellent correlation between positive serum neutralization titer and protection against infection with virus.

e. The serum neutralization test is highly specific but not very sensitive.

Correct answers are on pages 154-179.

Dogs and Cats, continued

660. *Concerning use of electron microscopy in diagnosis of feline viral infections, which statement is most accurate?*

a. Electron microscopy can rapidly identify specific serotypes of viruses based on the morphology of the virion.

b. Electron microscopy is quite sensitive in diagnosing the cause of intestinal infections in that one can observe as few as 1 or 2 viral particles per gram of feces.

c. Electron microscopy can be used with specific antiserum to obtain an immune electron microscopy test by which one can identify serotypes of virus.

d. Electron microscopy is inexpensive and readily available.

e. The most common assay used with electron microscopy is the Western blot.

661. *Concerning enzyme-linked immunosorbent assay (ELISA), which statement is **least** accurate?*

a. An in-clinic ELISA kit is available for diagnosis of canine heartworm disease.

b. KELA is an ELISA that has been standardized and computerized to automatically calculate the titer of the antibody in the test serum.

c. ELISA can only be used to detect serum antibodies and cannot detect antigen.

d. ELISA is a very sensitive test.

e. An in-clinic ELISA kit is available for diagnosis of feline leukemia virus infection.

662. *Canine parvovirus produces severe enteritis in many susceptible dogs. Concerning canine parvovirus, which statement is **least** accurate?*

a. Canine parvovirus and feline parvovirus are antigenically very similar.

b. Canine parvovirus and minute virus of canines cannot be differentiated by electron microscopic examination of fecal samples.

c. Canine parvovirus is readily inactivated by most disinfectants and at normal room temperature within 30 days.

d. Mink enteritis virus cross reacts with canine parvovirus.

e. It is clear from retrospective studies on banks of canine serum samples that canine parvovirus did not exist in the canine population before it was recognized in 1978.

663. *The cause of "cat scratch disease" in people is:*

a. a Gram-positive intracellular coccus, believed to be *Rhodococcus pyocyaneus*

b. *Cytauxzoon felis*

c. *Brugia pahangi*

d. feline leukemia virus

e. a Gram-negative intracellular bacillus, believed to be either *Afipia felis* or *Rochalimaea henselae*

664. *Concerning caliciviruses, which statement is **least** accurate?*

a. The name of the family (Caliciviridae) is derived from the morphology of the capsomeres of the virions, that is, they appear to be "cup-shaped" when examined by electron microscopy.

b. Caliciviruses are enveloped DNA viruses that are almost never shed after infection and are easily inactivated by disinfectants and environmental conditions.

c. Caliciviral infection may cause ulcerative, respiratory or enteric disease.

d. Caliciviruses contain single-stranded RNA.

e. Feline caliciviruses were originally called "feline picornaviruses."

665. *Concerning rabies, which statement is **least** accurate?*

a. Rabies virus can infect most warm-blooded animals, including people.

b. Rabies virus is classified as a Lyssavirus of the Rhabdoviridae.

c. In cats, rabies is routinely diagnosed by identification of Negri bodies in sections of brain.

d. In cats, rabies may be manifested in the furious form or the paralytic (dumb) form.

e. Rabies virus travels to the central nervous system from the original site of infection via nerves.

666. *Parvoviruses of carnivores are similar in that antibodies stimulated against one virus protect against infection by a number of parvoviruses from other species. Concerning parvovirus, which statement is **least** accurate?*

a. The genomes of canine parvovirus-2 and feline parvovirus are similar, but there are slight variations between them.

b. The DNA of feline parvovirus, raccoon parvovirus and mink enteritis are very similar.

c. Raccoon parvovirus is more closely related to feline parvovirus than to canine parvovirus.

d. Mink enteritis virus can be used as a vaccine for preventing feline parvoviral infection in cats.

e. Parvoviruses are extremely resistant to inactivation by chemical and physical agents because of their double-stranded DNA genomes.

667. *An IgG antibody titer against feline parvovirus in the serum of a 6-month-old, nonvaccinated cat indicates:*

a. chronic parvoviral infection

b. recent infection (within 2 weeks) with feline paravovirus or exposure to canine parvovirus-2

c. only that the animal was infected with this virus sometime in the past

d. persistent viremia

e. that the cat has passive immunity acquired from the queen

668. *Concerning enzyme-linked immunosorbent assay (ELISA), which statement is **least** accurate?*

a. ELISA can detect virus antigen if specific antibody is adhered to the test well or membrane.

b. ELISA can detect antibody if viral antigen is adhered to the test well or membrane.

c. ELISA can detect virus and antibody using the membrane technique.

d. ELISA can detect antibody titer if a kinetics test or KELA is used.

e. ELISA can detect antigen or antibody but not antibody titer.

669. *The indirect immunofluorescent assay for feline leukemia (Hardy test) detects antigen of the virus in:*

a. plasma

b. serum

c. peripheral blood leukocytes

d. erythrocytes

e. whole blood, but only after it is first processed in cell cultures

670. *Concerning feline immunodeficiency virus infection, which statement is **least** accurate?*

a. The virus was first called feline T-lymphotropic virus.

b. The virus is not highly contagious within a group of socially stable cats.

c. The first commercial diagnostic test used to detect infected cats measured virus or viral antigen in the serum.

d. Most, if not all, infected cats remain persistently viremic for the remainder of their lives.

e. The primary method of transmission is via cat bites.

Correct answers are on pages 154-179.

Dogs and Cats, continued

Questions 671 through 677

You receive a call from a fellow veterinarian concerning an outbreak of a fatal disease in cats within a local animal shelter. Your colleague wants to know if the state diagnostic laboratory can confirm the diagnosis of a certain disease by serologic tests. Further discussion reveals that kittens come into the shelter, are vaccinated and then develop acute disease consisting of vomiting, diarrhea, dehydration and death. A private home where orphan kittens were taken for rearing also is experiencing the same problems. Necropsy reveals dehydration, evidence of diarrhea, and edematous, hemorrhagic small intestines. Histopathologic changes reported by the local pathology laboratory are consistent with feline panleukopenia.

671. *Which of the following characterizes feline panleukopenia virus (feline parvovirus)?*

    a. RNA virus, double-stranded genome, enveloped, labile
    b. DNA virus, double-stranded genome, enveloped, labile
    c. DNA virus, single-stranded genome, enveloped, labile
    d. RNA virus, double-stranded genome, non-enveloped, resistant
    e. DNA virus, single-stranded genome, non-enveloped, resistant

672. *What rapid diagnostic test could you perform in your office to be reasonably sure of your diagnosis before the results of gross and histopathologic examination are known?*

    a. total plasma protein level
    b. rectal temperature of infected kittens
    c. total leukocyte count
    d. total erythrocyte count
    e. enzyme-linked immunosorbent assay for gp27 antigen

673. *Which virus is **not** antigenically related to feline parvovirus?*

    a. bovine parvovirus
    b. mink enteritis virus
    c. raccoon parvovirus
    d. canine parvovirus-2
    e. feline panleukopenia virus

674. *What disinfectant would you recommend to the director of the shelter for immediate use in contaminated cages, water/feed utensils, and on floors and other surfaces?*

    a. chlorhexidine
    b. povidone-iodine
    c. sodium hypochlorite (household bleach)
    d. ammonia
    e. quaternary ammonium

675. *At what dilution should this disinfectant be used?*

    a. undiluted from the container
    b. diluted 1:10
    c. diluted 1:32
    d. diluted 1:128
    e. diluted 1:640

676. *What type of panleukopenia vaccine should be used in this facility?*

    a. inactivated (killed-virus) vaccine because it is safer
    b. modified-live-virus vaccine because it evokes immunity more quickly
    c. modified-live-virus vaccine for respiratory viruses, combined with an inactivated (killed-virus) vaccine for panleukopenia
    d. intranasal inactivated (killed-virus) vaccine for local protection
    e. an autogenous vaccine because it is specific for the bacteria as well as the viruses involved in this outbreak

677. *At what age should the kittens entering this facility be vaccinated?*

    a. 4 weeks
    b. 6 weeks
    c. 8 weeks

d. 12 weeks

e. immediately upon entry to the shelter

678. *Concerning canine parvovirus (CPV) and CPV infection, which statement is* **least** *accurate?*

a. CPV-1 and CPV-2 are subtypes of the same virus.

b. CPV-1 and CPV-2 are distinct viruses antigenically, with no cross-protection provided by vaccines.

c. Feline parvovirus vaccines will protect against CPV-2 but not CPV-1.

d. CPV-2 exists in the canine population as 2 subtypes, CPV-2a and CPV-2b.

e. Gross and microscopic lesions in dogs infected with CPV-2 are similar to lesions produced in cats with feline parvovirus.

Questions 679 through 687

Feline immunodeficiency virus (FIV) infection is characterized by mild or subclinical infection initially. Clinical disease is associated with immunosuppression, resulting in a variety of secondary infections.

679. *Feline immunodeficiency virus is classified as a:*

a. herpesvirus

b. calicivirus

c. parvovirus

d. morbillivirus

e. retrovirus

680. *To which subfamily of viruses does FIV belong?*

a. Oncovirinae

b. Lentivirinae

c. Spumavirinae

d. Rhabdovirinae

e. Calicivirinae

681. *The enzyme-linked immunosorbent assay for FIV detects:*

a. p27 antigen

b. gp70 antigen

c. antibodies to viral antigen

d. membrane antigen

e. peplomer antigen

682. *The period from original infection with FIV until significant clinical disease develops in infected cats generally is:*

a. less than 1 week

b. between 1 and 2 weeks

c. 2-4 weeks

d. less than 1 year

e. 3-5 years

683. *Concerning the relationship between FIV and human immunodeficiency virus, which statement is most accurate?*

a. There is no similarity at all between these 2 viruses.

b. The 2 viruses belong to different families, but both infect T-cells within the host.

c. Both viruses infect B-cells within the host and impair humoral immune responses.

d. Both are lentiviruses, but there is no known cross infectivity between species (cats, people).

e. The 2 viruses are subtypes of the same virus, and cross infectivity between species (cats, people) occurs.

684. *The primary means of transmission of FIV between infected and uninfected cats is by:*

a. sexual contact

b. direct contact of the queen with kittens

c. cat bites

d. contact with contaminated urine and feces in litter pans

e. aerosol transmission within a contaminated household

Correct answers are on pages 154-179.

Dogs and Cats, continued

685. The primary cells infected by FIV in a cat are:

  a. B-cells
  b. platelets
  c. peripheral blood leukocytes
  d. T-cells
  e. erythrocytes

686. In FIV-infected cats, the pathophysiologic problem underlying clinical disease is:

  a. antibody-dependent enhancement of infection of blood monocytes
  b. immunosuppression due to decreased numbers of CD4+ T-cells
  c. anemia due to cytolysis of bone marrow precursor cells
  d. complement-dependent aggregation of virus and antibody
  e. delayed hypersensitivity reactions to secondary bacterial pathogens

687. A positive enzyme-linked immunosorbent assay for FIV should be confirmed by a different type of test. Which test is the most useful in confirming FIV infection in a cat?

  a. virus neutralization assay for IgM antibodies
  b. Western blot
  c. complement fixation
  d. direct fluorescent antibody test
  e. virus isolation from a throat swab

688. An 8-year-old female Labrador Retriever is presented because of polyuria and polydipsia. In obtaining the history, it is appropriate to ask the owner about all of the following **except** the dog's:

  a. appetite
  b. general attitude and activity level
  c. reproductive history
  d. dental history
  e. drugs given recently and currently

689. A dog is hit by a car and presented to your clinic 10 minutes later, in shock. The illness in this dog is classified as:

  a. acute
  b. peracute
  c. subacute
  d. chronic
  e. subchronic

690. A cat has been coughing intermittently for 4 months. The illness in this cat is classified as:

  a. acute
  b. peracute
  c. subacute
  d. chronic
  e. subchronic

691. A dog with lameness for 1 day is presented for treatment. The illness in this dog is classified as:

  a. acute
  b. peracute
  c. subacute
  d. chronic
  e. subchronic

692. A dog has had diarrhea for 4 days. The illness in this dog is classified as:

  a. acute
  b. peracute
  c. subacute
  d. chronic
  e. subchronic

693. In obtaining an animal's history, routine questions concerning vaccination should include all of the following **except**:

  a. dates of most recent vaccination
  b. date and type of initial vaccinations
  c. if a cat, date and result of feline leukemia virus test
  d. dates and types of annual vaccinations
  e. if a dog, date and result of canine parvovirus test

694. A client complains that his dog has had diarrhea for 4 weeks. To determine if the diarrhea is of small bowel or large bowel origin, questions should include all of the following **except**:

   a. "Does the dog strain to defecate?"
   b. "Does the stool appear bloody?"
   c. "Does the dog eat with a hearty appetite?"
   d. "Is there any mucus on the stools?"
   e. "How many times per day does the dog defecate?"

695. Clients are asked to provide information on their pet's history so you can:

   a. get to know the client better and develop rapport
   b. become acquainted with the pet's personality and determine if the animal is fractious
   c. obtain pertinent information that may help define the animal's presenting problem
   d. learn what the cat or dog likes to eat in the event it must be hospitalized
   e. occupy the client during the examination

For Questions 696 through 701, select the correct answer from the 6 choices below.

   a. ascites
   b. melena
   c. hematochezia
   d. hematuria
   e. icterus/jaundice
   f. dyspnea

696. Frank (red) blood in the stool.

697. Dark, tarry stools containing occult (digested) blood.

698. Accumulation of serous fluid in the abdominal cavity.

699. Bloody urine.

700. Difficulty in breathing.

701. Yellow discoloration of the mucosae and sclerae.

Questions 702 and 703

A 6-year-old male Corgi is rushed to your clinic after the owner finds the dog prostrate at home. You quickly evaluate the dog and observe that the mucous membranes are pale and capillary refill time is 4 seconds. The dog is unable to stand and the abdomen is markedly distended. The dog appears alert.

702. Which of the following best describes this dog's condition?

   a. comatose and overhydrated
   b. demented and cyanotic
   c. weak and in shock
   d. psychotic and polycythemic
   e. semicomatose and dyspneic

703. The dog has a rectal temperature of 37.2 C, a respiratory rate of 45 breaths per minute, a heart rate of 200 beats per minute, and 80 pulses palpated per minute. Which of the following best describes this dog's condition?

   a. hypothermic and eupneic, with pulse deficits
   b. normothermic and eupneic, with pulse deficits
   c. hypothermic and tachypneic, with appropriate pulses
   d. hyperthermic and tachypneic, with pulse deficits
   e. hypothermic and tachypneic, with pulse deficits

704. A 13-year-old cat is presented because of lethargy and anorexia. You notice that the skin remains tented when you pinch it away from the body. The cat's mucous membranes feel very dry. In regard to hydration status, this cat is most likely:

   a. not dehydrated but very emaciated
   b. 2% dehydrated
   c. 4% dehydrated
   d. 6% dehydrated
   e. 8% or more dehydrated

Correct answers are on pages 154-179.

Dogs and Cats, continued

705. Damage to the spinal cord is **least** likely to cause:

   a. paresis
   b. paralysis
   c. loss of proprioception
   d. head tilt
   e. urinary or fecal incontinence

Questions 706 and 707

A client brings his 6-month-old Labrador Retriever to your clinic. The dog vomited twice this morning, but now appears alert and normal.

706. Relevant questions you should ask include all of the following **except**:

   a "What is the dog's current diet?"
   b. "Does the dog receive any table scraps or treats?"
   c. "Does the dog have access to garbage?"
   d. "Has the dog ever limped or exhibited pain in its limbs?"
   e. "What is the dog's deworming history?"

707. You examine this dog and finds no abnormalities. The most appropriate course of action is to:

   a. administer metoclopramide until the vomiting stops
   b. admit the dog to the hospital, perform a complete blood count, serum chemistry assays and urinalysis, administer intravenous fluid therapy, and withhold food and water
   c. advise the owner to withhold food and water for 24 hours and gradually reintroduce water and then foods if the vomiting ceases; if vomiting persists, bring the dog back for reevaluation
   d. make abdominal radiographs to look for a possible foreign body
   e. administer Pepto-Bismol until the vomiting stops

708. Normal puppies are characterized by all of the following **except**:

   a. crawl and right themselves at birth
   b. open eyelids by 1-3 weeks of age
   c. regulate their body temperature by 4 days of age
   d. ear canals open by 13-17 days of age
   e. suckle at birth

709. A client presents a 3-year-old Basset Hound with a 1-week history of a bloody nasal discharge. The clinical sign this dog is displaying is termed:

   a. hematemesis
   b. hemoperitoneum
   c. hemonasum
   d. epistaxis
   e. hemostaxis

710. In dogs and cats, acceptable sites for venipuncture include all of the following **except** the:

   a. jugular vein
   b. cephalic vein
   c. coccygeal (tail) vein
   d. lateral saphenous vein (dog)
   e. medial saphenous vein (cat)

711. Serum values of which constituents are most likely to be increased in an azotemic dog?

   a. alanine aminotransferase and alkaline phosphatase
   b. aspartate aminotransferase and creatine phosphokinase
   c. urea nitrogen and creatinine
   d. unconjugated bilirubin and cholesterol
   e. gamma glutamyltransferase and glucose

712. A 10-year-old dog with chronic renal failure has a blood urea nitrogen level of 90 mg/dl and a serum creatinine level of 4.0 mg/dl. The specific gravity of urine from this dog is most likely to be:

   a. between 1.020 and 1.040
   b. between 1.006 and 1.025
   c. less than 1.006

d. between 1.030 and 1.055

e. greater than 1.050

713. *After a dog is determined to be infected with heartworms, the most appropriate additional diagnostic tests before starting treatment include:*

a. thoracic radiographs and a serum biochemistry panel

b. abdominal radiographs and ultrasonographic examination

c. direct blood pressure measurements and blood gas analysis

d. pulmonary function tests and a liver biopsy

e. ophthalmologic examination and pelvic radiographs

714. *When performing cystocentesis, it is important to:*

a. direct the needle cranially before inserting it into the abdomen

b. aspirate as you withdraw the needle through the bladder and abdominal walls

c. insert the needle to the hub

d. stabilize the bladder before inserting the needle

e. use an 18-gauge, 1 1/2-inch needle

715. *The most common risk associated with bladder catheterization via the urethra is:*

a. damage to the urethra

b. damage to the bladder

c. bacterial infection

d. overinserting the catheter, causing the catheter to knot in the urinary bladder

e. damage to the ureters

Questions 716 and 717

716. *A cat is presented with pinpoint hemorrhages on the skin and mucous membranes. This condition is called:*

a. anemia

b. cyanosis

c. icterus

d. purpura

e. petechiation

717. *In this cat showing hemorrhages, what is the most likely hematologic abnormality?*

a. increased packed cell volume

b. decreased packed cell volume

c. increased platelet count

d. decreased platelet count

e. decreased bleeding time

718. *Concerning shock, which statement is **least** accurate?*

a. Shock is a maldistribution of blood flow, causing decreased delivery of oxygen to tissues.

b. Shock should be considered an emergency situation, warranting immediate treatment.

c. Shock causes a marked parasympathetic response.

d. Shock can be caused by hemorrhage, severe stress, infection or anaphylaxis.

e. An animal in shock can develop tachypnea and tachycardia.

For Questions 719 through 723, select the correct answer from the 5 choices below.

a. constipation

b. obstipation

c. anal sac impaction

d. perianal fistulae

e. rectal prolapse

719. *Eversion of the bowel out through the anus.*

720. *Infected draining tracts around the anal region.*

721. *Difficult evacuation of feces.*

722. *Inability to pass a stool because of long-standing failure to evacuate feces.*

723. *Common cause of "scooting""or rubbing the anal area along the ground.*

Correct answers are on pages 154-179.

Dogs and Cats, continued

724. Regurgitation is:

a. commonly associated with hookworm infection
b. preceded by retching
c. the expulsion of undigested food
d. a definitive sign of lead toxicity
e. almost always seen in old dogs

725. Common cutaneous and subcutaneous tumors of dogs include all of the following **except***:*

a. lipoma
b. mast-cell tumor
c. malignant melanoma
d. malignant fibrous histiocytoma
e. histiocytoma

726. Hip dysplasia:

a. most often affects small breeds of dogs
b. is not hereditary
c. resolves with age
d. is diagnosed by ventrodorsal radiographs of the pelvis
e. is common in cats

727. Concerning osteomyelitis, which statement is **least** *accurate?*

a. Osteomyelitis is a bacterial or fungal infection of the bone.
b. Osteomyelitis may require surgery and long-term medical therapy.
c. Pain, fever and lameness are frequently associated with osteomyelitis.
d. The best way to determine which antibiotic is appropriate for treatment is usually with a Gram-stained preparation.
e. Radiographs can be helpful in making a definitive diagnosis.

728. An 8-week-old Collie puppy has had diarrhea for 3 days and you suspect a parasite infection. Gastrointestinal parasites this puppy is most likely to have include all of the following **except***:*

a. coccidia
b. roundworms
c. whipworms
d. hookworms
e. tapeworms

729. You perform a fecal flotation on a dog's stool and observe whipworm eggs in the sample. The most appropriate anthelmintic for use in treating this dog is:

a. pyrantel pamoate (Nemex, Strongid-T)
b. piperazine citrate
c. praziquantel (Droncit)
d. fenbendazole (Panacur)
e. bunamidine hydrochloride (Scolaban)

730. Enzyme-linked immunosorbent assay (ELISA) on serum from an apparently healthy cat is positive for feline leukemia virus infection. The most appropriate course of action is to:

a. euthanize the cat immediately
b. retest the cat by ELISA in 1 week
c. retest the cat by ELISA or indirect fluorescent antibody test in 1 month or later
d. permanently isolate the cat to prevent infection of other cats
e. administer a broad-spectrum antibiotic at low levels for 6 months

731. A common yeast that often causes otitis in dogs is:

a. *Candida albicans*
b. *Malassezia pachydermatis*
c. *Sporothrix schenckii*
d. *Blastomyces dermatitidis*
e. *Aspergillus flavus*

732. The most common coccidial parasite of the gastrointestinal tract of dogs and cats is:

a. *Eimeria*
b. *Isospora*
c. *Toxoplasma*
d. *Sarcocystis*
e. *Neospora*

733. *All of the following are caused solely by a virus **except**:*

    a. feline infectious peritonitis
    b. canine distemper
    c. kennel cough
    d. rabies
    e. feline panleukopenia

734. *Of the following sets of diseases, which set consists only of zoonotic diseases?*

    a. leptospirosis, ringworm, salmonellosis, toxoplasmosis
    b. leptospirosis, Rocky Mountain spotted fever, feline immunodeficiency virus infection, sarcoptic mange
    c. leptospirosis, canine parvovirus infection, salmonellosis, giardiasis
    d. rabies, brucellosis, canine adenovirus infection, cryptosporidiosis
    e. rabies, salmonellosis, toxoplasmosis, feline immunodeficiency virus infection

735. *If a puppy is infected with heartworm (Dirofilaria immitis) microfilariae on the second day of life, what is the earliest time at which the animal will test positive for microfilariae?*

    a. 2 months of age
    b. 3 months of age
    c. 6 months of age
    d. 8 months of age
    e. 9 months of age

736. *Heartworm infection can be prevented by use of any of the following drugs except:*

    a. ivermectin
    b. milbemycin
    c. fenbendazole
    d. diethylcarbamazine
    e. diethylcarbamazine with oxibendazole

737. *In cats, all of the following diseases may **directly** cause upper respiratory disease **except**:*

    a. rhinotracheitis
    b. calicivirus infection
    c. chlamydial infection
    d. feline leukemia virus infection
    e. bacterial rhinitis

738. *A 55-lb dog develops acute pulmonary edema. You decide to give 5% furosemide intravenously at 2 mg/kg of body weight. What quantity of furosemide should you give?*

    a. 1 ml
    b. 0.5 ml
    c. 1.5 ml
    d. 5 ml
    e. 10 ml

739. *A 28-lb mongrel has been vomiting for 3 days and is estimated to be 8% dehydrated. What approximate fluid volume should you give to rehydrate this dog?*

    a. 500 ml
    b. 1000 ml
    c. 2000 ml
    d. 2240 ml
    e. 1500 ml

740. *When administering intravenous fluids to a cat or dog, care must be taken to monitor for overhydration. The best initial indicator of overhydration is:*

    a. edematous skin
    b. pulmonary edema
    c. polyuria
    d. continued weight gain after the animal has been rehydrated appropriately
    e. tachypnea

741. *You are using a microdrip to administer intravenous fluids to a cat. The cat must receive 360 ml of fluid during a 24-hour period. At what rate should the fluid be infused?*

    a. 15 drops/minute
    b. 15 drops/second
    c. 150 drops/hour
    d. 15 ml/minute
    e. 36 ml/hour

Correct answers are on pages 154-179.

Dogs and Cats, continued

742. An example of an isotonic fluid is:

a. 50% dextrose
b. water
c. 0.9% saline
d. 10% calcium gluconate
e. lactated Ringer's solution with 2.5% dextrose

743. Concerning total parenteral nutrition (intravenous feeding), which statement is most accurate?

a. The solution usually contains equal volumes of B vitamins and dextrose.
b. If a dextrose solution in a concentration of 10% or higher is used, the fluid should be infused into the jugular vein.
c. The catheter should be flushed thoroughly with saline before administering any intravenous medications.
d. Laboratory tests are seldom necessary, as long as asepsis is strictly observed.
e. Solutions can be mixed in a bowl that has been sterilized in a dishwasher.

744. An owner telephones and says her adult Irish Setter had been fine until an hour ago, when the dog began retching. The owner thinks the dog is becoming progressively more uncomfortable. Additionally, she mentions that the dog's abdomen looks markedly distended. What is the most appropriate advice for this client?

a. withhold food and water overnight and bring the dog to the clinic in the morning if the problem persists
b. you will telephone her when you are finished with appointments in 2 hours
c. this could be a life-threatening emergency and she should bring the dog to the clinic immediately

d. induce emesis with syrup of ipecac
e. apply gentle pressure to the abdomen to help relieve the distention

745. The preferred enema solution for cats and dogs is:

a. sodium phosphate
b. soapy water
c. warm tap water
d. mineral oil
e. vegetable oil

*746. Complications of enema administration may include all of the following **except**:*

a. hypothermia
b. vomiting
c. anemia
d. constipation
e. diarrhea

747. The most concentrated source of red blood cells is:

a. fresh plasma
b. packed red blood cells
c. whole blood
d. platelet-enriched plasma
e. fresh-frozen plasma

*748. First aid for a limb fracture should include all of the following **except**:*

a. controlling excessive hemorrhage
b. covering open wounds with a sterile dressing to prevent contamination
c. realigning the bone fragments
d. immobilizing the limb
e. treating for shock, if necessary

Answers

1. **b** Amphotericin is extremely nephrotoxic and must be administered carefully with saline loading and by slow IV infusion.

2. **e** The compression bandage is useless. Intravenous infusion of physiologic saline solution will simply dilute the remaining red

blood cells in the intravascular compartment. Immediate surgery will almost certainly kill the dog. Infusion of 1 unit of packed red blood cells is helpful but not nearly enough in a 57-kg dog. Fresh whole blood would be preferred. Vitamin K3 will not help if there is rodenticide intoxication. Autotransfusion is the best chance of keeping the patient alive until the bleeding slows and either adequate whole blood transfusion plus vitamin K1 therapy or exploratory surgery is possible.

3. **a** The agar gel immunodiffusion test for blastomycosis is one of the few serologic tests for fungal infections with high sensitivity (>90%) and high specificity (>90%). The test is also good for cryptococcosis.

4. **a** The other items listed are used to treat encephalopathy (lactulose, neomycin, low-protein diet) or help control ascites (low-salt diet). Dexamethasone may exacerbate bacterial cholangitis or may further diminish hepatic function due to vacuolar hepatopathy.

5. **d** Barium enemas are rarely indicated.

6. **c** The description of the wound suggests an anaerobic infection. Metronidazole has excellent antianaerobic activity.

7. **a** Preincubation with food does not have a significant impact on the efficacy of powdered pancreatic enzyme supplements.

8. **c** Coagulopathy is a rare cause of hematemesis. If hepatic failure causes hematemesis, it is through gastrointestinal ulceration. Bacterial infection almost never causes ulceration, unless it is through septic shock.

9. **c** The description of the wound (discoloration, crepitus, odor) suggests an infection with anaerobic bacteria as the predominant type, as opposed to aerobic bacteria as the predominant type. *Bacteroides* and *Clostridium* are common anaerobic bacteria.

10. **e** Prostatomegaly, a common cause of tenesmus, would be difficult to diagnose on physical examination of such a large dog. It would be difficult to reach the prostate via the rectum and difficult to isolate it on abdominal palpation. Perineal hernia, perianal fistulae and anal sacculitis should be easy to diagnose

on physical examination. The appearance of the feces makes dietary causes unlikely.

11. **a** Cefazolin is a first-generation bactericidal cephalosporin with a relatively broad antibacterial spectrum. It is relatively safe (nontoxic). Amikacin is nephrotoxic and must be given by injection. Lincomycin has a narrow antibacterial spectrum. Tetracycline would be effective against *Ehrlichia,* but there is no reason to suspect ehrlichiosis in this dog. Also, tetracycline is bacteriostatic. Trimethoprim should not be used alone, but rather in conjunction with a sulfa drug.

12. **e** Polyuria and polydipsia are often seen in dogs with chronic hepatic insufficiency, especially when the blood urea nitrogen level is decreased. This sign is rarely present in dogs with acute, fulminating hepatic failure. All of the other signs may be seen in animals with acute or chronic hepatic insufficiency.

13. **d** Nocardiosis and malignancy can cause pleural effusion. The age and occupation of this dog suggest nocardiosis, as does the inflammatory nature of the exudate.

14. **a** The effusion is a pure (low-protein) transudate, typically seen in hypoproteinemic animals. Lymphangiectasia causes protein-losing enteropathy and often produces a pure transudate due to hypoalbuminemia. Dogs with lymphangiectasia often have minimal or no diarrhea. The other 4 diseases usually cause modified transudates (also called high-protein transudates) or exudates.

15. **e** The "grains" are tapeworm segments. Praziquantel is effective for eliminating cestodes.

16. **e** The dog has a modified transudate (high-protein transudate), which is usually caused by hepatic disease (especially cirrhosis), right-heart failure, or abdominal neoplasia. Serum bile acid concentrations would help determine if hepatic disease (especially cirrhosis) is present. Abdominal radiographs would probably be useless because of the fluid in the abdomen. Intestinal biopsy and a urine protein:creatinine ratio can detect causes of hypoalbuminemia. Culture would detect infection, a cause of an exudate.

17. **b** All dogs with blastomycosis should be treated. Though amphotericin is toxic, it is effective. Ketoconazole can be used if there is substantial kidney disease (*ie,* amphotericin is contraindicated). Current data suggest that

17. **b** All dogs with blastomycosis should be treated. Though amphotericin is toxic, it is effective. Ketoconazole can be used if there is substantial kidney disease (*ie*, amphotericin is contraindicated). Current data suggest that itraconazole may be the preferred therapy. Griseofulvin is used to treat dermatophytosis.

18. **d** The fluid is an exudate. Bile acid determinations are used to diagnose hepatic disease, which is not a serious consideration in this case. Plain radiographs might detect a tumor or spontaneous pneumoperitoneum (note that there is not a large volume of fluid in this dog). Culture might detect an infection (septic peritonitis). Ultrasonography may reveal a tumor. A CBC and serum chemistry profile are needed to ascertain electrolyte balance, renal function and coagulation, which may be seriously disturbed in a dog with septic peritonitis.

19. **a** Corticosteroids and anticonvulsants are common causes of iatrogenic hepatic disease. Arsenicals may also produce this problem (primarily seen in dogs treated for adult heartworms).

20. **b** The fluid is a pure (low-protein) transudate, almost certainly caused by hypoalbuminemia. Thoracic radiographs would be useful in evaluating the heart, but heart failure is not expected in this patient. Urine protein:creatinine ratio, endoscopic biopsy, and serum bile acid concentrations would help determine why the albumin level is decreased. Ultrasonography would help evaluate the liver.

21. **c** While corticosteroids (*eg*, prednisolone) may cause some gastric disease, nonsteroidal antiinflammatory drugs (*eg*, ibuprofen) are the most consistent cause of severe ulceration.

22. **c** The fluid is an exudate. The nondegenerate neutrophils suggest nonseptic peritonitis. Creatinine determinations can detect uroabdomen, a cause of nonseptic exudates. The dog is not icteric, so biliary tract rupture is very unlikely. If there were intestinal leakage, you would see bacteria, food particles and/or degenerate neutrophils on abdominocentesis. You should not perform surgery until you know whether uroabdomen is present. If uroabdomen is present, you should perform a contrast radiographic examination first to determine the location of the leakage.

23. **e** Cirrhosis may result in reduced liver size. Determining the cause of the cirrhosis may allow you to arrest or reverse the process that initiated the disease, and thereby help maintain the animal in remission.

24. **e** The presence of blood clots shows that the hemorrhage is ongoing and is almost certainly iatrogenic. The other choices listed would not cause clots in the abdominal fluid. Abdominal distention does not necessarily mean that an effusion is present. Inability to ballotte a fluid wave makes abdominal effusion less likely.

25. **d** Bordetellosis is a likely cause of this dog's disease. A CBC would not diagnose tracheal infection. Radiographs are not needed because the dog has an acute upper respiratory infection that is not causing systemic disease. Theophylline is a mild antitussive but it would not help resolve the infection. Prednisolone without antibiotics would probably allow the infection to persist.

26. **b** Many dogs with acute Rocky Mountain spotted fever do not have circulating antibodies when signs of disease are first seen. Ampicillin and gentamicin would not be useful in treatment of the 2 common tick-borne diseases, ehrlichiosis or Rocky Mountain spotted fever.

27. **a** The fluid is an exudate and probably septic, based upon the apparent septic shock (hypothermia and injected mucous membranes). The very high WBC count is also suggestive of septic peritonitis. Alimentary tract leakage is a common cause of spontaneous bacterial peritonitis, which often produces septic peritonitis. Cirrhosis causes a modified transudate. Pancreatitis rarely causes peritoneal effusion, and then only in meager amounts. Hemangiosarcoma would probably cause hemoabdomen. Hemangiosarcoma and carcinomatosis rarely cause intestinal perforation, septic peritonitis or septic shock.

28. **c** Chronic aspergillosis often mimics nasal neoplasia in signs and turbinate osteolysis. Occasional fungal hyphae can be found in nasal samples from unaffected dogs. The preferred treatment is enilconazole flushes or oral itraconazole.

29. **e** The dog has signs of small intestinal diarrhea. Colonic adenocarcinoma would produce large bowel signs.

sis, which often causes Coombs'-positive, regenerative anemia. (Indirect fluorescent antibody testing is also useful for diagnosis of babesiosis.) Doxycycline is useful for treatment of rickettsial infection but not babesiosis. There is no appreciable human health hazard.

32. **b** The dog is regurgitating and should have its esophagus evaluated. Acute regurgitation of solids but not liquids may suggest an esophageal foreign body. Therefore, plain films are indicated first. There is no reason to think the dog is dehydrated at this time.

33. **e** This dog obviously has hepatic insufficiency. Doberman Pinschers often develop chronic active hepatitis. Vacuolar hepatopathy and lipidosis are almost never symptomatic in dogs and rarely, if ever, cause cirrhosis. Pancreatitis does not cause hepatic insufficiency. Lymphosarcoma is possible, but it typically causes hepatomegaly due to infiltrative disease.

34. **d** Any organ can be affected. The other 4 systems are commonly affected in dogs with blastomycosis.

35. **e** *Bordetella bronchiseptica* is the most common bacterial cause of infectious tracheobronchitis in dogs. Herpesvirus is a rare cause.

36. **c** The dog appears to be regurgitating because of esophageal disease. Aspiration pneumonia is a major cause of death in these dogs.

37. **c** Vitamin K$_1$ would not prevent bleeding from an ulcer or erosion. Abdominal compression bandages are not effective. You cannot autotransfuse when the blood is entering the stomach. Acepromazine lowers blood pressure and exacerbates shock. In this animal, you must eliminate the source of the hemorrhage by resecting the ulcer.

38. **d** Dogs do not develop the skin lesions typically observed in affected people. Many dogs have high titers but do not have clinical disease. It is very uncertain if kidney disease is caused by borreliosis. Thrombocytopenia is found in rickettsial infections (borreliosis is a bacterial infection).

39. **b** Salmon poisoning requires therapy with tetracycline. Metronidazole is useful for anaerobic infections and intestinal protozoal infections, and as an immunomodulator in inflammatory bowel disease.

40. **c** The feces can be assayed for the causative toxin, but rarely are the causative bacteria isolated. Once the toxin has bound to the nerves, antitoxin will not affect it. Flaccid paralysis and normal pain perceptions are classic findings.

41. **a** Chronic tenesmus and dyschezia suggest inflammation or obstruction of the rectum. The easiest and most sensitive way to detect obstruction (likely in an old German Shepherd) is by digital rectal examination. Urecholine would be contraindicated if obstruction is a possibility.

42. **b** Congenital shunts rarely cause hepatocellular membrane damage; therefore, serum alanine aminotransferase activity is rarely increased.

43. **a** The rapid slide test is not specific (there are many false-positive reactions). Human infections are usually mild. Infected male dogs may shed the bacteria for weeks after infection. The asymptomatic nature of many infections is one reason why the disease can be spread so easily.

44. **c** Campylobacteriosis is an acute enteritis of dogs that is transmissible to people. Salmonellosis is possible but very unlikely. Giardiasis would probably not cause bloody diarrhea. Yersiniosis is very rare in dogs.

45. **b** This dog has chronic hemoabdomen. Compression bandages are useless. Autotransfusion is used in emergencies, but this is a chronic problem. One unit of fresh, whole blood might help in rodenticide intoxication, but this is too chronic for that. Surgery may be useful, but it would be better to perform ultrasonography, looking for areas suggestive of hemangiosarcoma (common in older German Shepherd dogs and often manifested as described). If such a tumor were present and if it were found throughout the abdomen, you might avoid unnecessary surgery.

46. **d** The disease is principally found in and around Texas. There is no effective therapy for most symptomatic dogs. Diagnosis is usually made at necropsy, after the dog dies suddenly from acute heart failure.

47. **b** The dog is not dehydrated and is unlikely to become so; therefore, fluid therapy is not warranted. Most acute diarrhea is caused by the diet, parasites and/or infections. Oral neomycin is rarely useful in acute diarrhea.

48. **d** Osseous coccidioidomycosis has an extremely poor long-term prognosis and often does not have any other obvious disease preceding it. This is in contrast to acute coccidioidomycosis, which is often respiratory in nature and self-limiting.

49. **e** Ascites is common in dogs with severe cirrhosis and does not cause decompensation.

50. **c** Hypertonic enemas should not be administered to cats or small dogs, especially if the animal is obstipated.

51. **d** The other diseases listed do not cause fever, emaciation and lymphadenopathy, and tend not to be so chronic. Cryptococcosis does not usually affect the lungs in dogs.

52. **d** Trientine is used to reduce the body copper concentration.

53. **b** Lactated Ringer's solution can increase the body pH and exacerbate hepatic encephalopathy. Phenobarbital would deepen the coma. "Lipotropic agents" are contraindicated.

54. **c** Chronically inflamed anal sacs can produce such blood on otherwise normal stools. The normal stool consistency suggests that there is not colonic disease; hence, dietary fiber and pelvic radiographs are not needed. Coagulopathy is very unlikely to cause chronic bleeding from the anal region. There is no reason to suspect infection, so amoxicillin is not needed.

55. **e** Schnauzers are at increased risk for idiopathic hyperlipidemia. Fasting hyperlipidemia seems to be a risk factor for acute pancreatitis in dogs.

56. **d** The most commonly affected breeds are Boston Terriers, Boxers, Collies, Pekingese and Welsh Corgies.

57. **d** Cytologic examination is not useful. Mortality is rare, unless the patient is septicemic. Fecal shedding can be protracted, especially if inappropriate antibiotic therapy has been administered (eg, gentamicin).

58. **d** These media produce poor contrast because they draw water from the body into the intestines. Thus, they may further decrease extracellular fluid volume, and should not be used in dehydrated animals.

59. **a** Diet, infection and parasites are the most common causes of diarrhea in young animals. Parasympatholytics are inferior for treatment of diarrhea. Fiber is used for chronic large bowel disease, not for acute diarrhea in a young animal. Barium contrast radiographs are seldom needed in diarrheic animals. Bacterial infection is seldom identified as a cause of such diarrhea. Antibiotics are rarely indicated in these patients.

60. **d** Osteosarcoma is unlikely in a 2-year-old dog. Histoplasmosis rarely affects bone. Borreliosis best fits the signs described.

61. **d** Polyps principally occur in the rectum. They may have a very broad head, and the stalk may be short and difficult to see. Polyps can also be multiple. They rarely cause constipation. Polyps in dogs rarely become malignant, unlike those seen in people.

62. **c** Dietary therapy (a trial elimination diet or a fiber-enriched diet) is often successful in so-called "mild" lymphocytic-plasmacytic colitis. Prednisolsone and azathioprine are rarely needed in such cases. Long-term prednisolone therapy may cause significant side effects in dogs. Diarrhea and/or fecal mucus are the most common signs.

63. **b** Enamel hypoplasia suggests preceding distemper infection. Inclusion bodies are rarely seen. Lymphopenia is nonspecific. Central nervous system signs may occur now, later, much later or never.

64. **a** Lymphangiectasia causes hypoalbuminemia. Salmonellosis is a rare cause of chronic diarrhea. Granulomatous enteritis is very rare. It is doubtful the animal would have lived this long or would be this healthy if it had lymphosarcoma.

65. **e** Respiratory infection is commonly seen in acute coccidioidomycosis. The most common radiographic sign is hilar lymphadenopathy. The organism is often hard to find cytologically, and culture is almost never recommended. Central nervous system involvement is very difficult to treat. Disseminated disease often involves bones and is difficult or impossible to cure.

66. **b** Though tubular forms of regurgitated food suggest esophageal disease, they are rarely seen. Bile indicates that duodenal fluid is present; hence, the animal is vomiting. Animals may vomit or regurgitate anytime after eating. Retching is part of the centrally mediated reflex associated with vomiting, as opposed to regurgitation.

67. **c** Many dogs with lymphangiectasia can be treated for substantial periods. The most common causes of protein-losing enteropathy (lymphocytic-plasmacytic enteritis, lymphosarcoma) do not respond well to a low-fat diet.

68. **b** Vomiting dogs may be significantly alkalotic; therefore, bicarbonate supplementation is inappropriate unless you have strong reason to suspect severe acidosis. Mild acidosis is best treated by volume replacement.

69. **c** This diet would prevent further engorgement of lacteals and subsequent protein loss. Medium-chain triglycerides would allow the animal to assimilate calorie-rich fats.

70. **b** The obvious pain in the perineal area would best be explained by inflammation or a foreign object. Severe inflammation is often caused by perianal fistulae, which are common in German Shepherds. Polyps are an unlikely cause of constipation. The other causes listed would not be likely to cause such pain.

71. **d**

72. **d** Epistaxis is seen in <50% of affected animals. At least 14 days of treatment are needed to effect a cure with tetracycline. Ticks are the major reservoir, and doxycycline is not nephrotoxic.

73. **b** The most common sites of esophageal foreign bodies are the thoracic inlet, base of the heart, and the lower esophageal sphincter.

74. **c** The band should be biopsied, as it may be associated with neoplasia, histoplasmosis, pythiosis or scar tissue. Surgery would probably make the dog incontinent and would not help the dog if it had a malignancy.

75. **a** The esophagus is a muscular tube; therefore, diseases that affect muscular tone may affect the esophagus. Causes of lower motor neuron disease are important causes of acquired esophageal dysfunction. These dogs very rarely recover from this disease spontaneously. Cimetidine and prophylactic antibiotics are not useful in this disease.

76. **b** Acute bloody diarrhea and vomiting in a mature small-breed dog with severe hemoconcentration is almost diagnostic for hemorrhagic gastroenteritis. Parvoviral enteritis does not usually cause such hemoconcentration. Ulceration causes anemia. Arsenic intoxication is very rare in dogs and does not typically cause hemoconcentration.

77. **a** The virus is not particularly resistant to the environment. Serologic examination would be of dubious value. Both distemper and ehrlichiosis may cause thrombocytopenia. Distemper is thought to be a relatively common cause of seizures in young dogs.

78. **c** Finding *Isospora* cysts does not warrant therapy, as there are no clinical signs. The nematode infections should be treated to prevent infection of other dogs and people. Only fenbendazole will eliminate both *Toxocara* and *Ancylostoma*.

79. **a** Intestinal and kidney silhouettes do not help diagnose microhepatia.

80. **b** Radiographs made with the animal in left lateral recumbency sometimes do not allow the clinician to discern the "shelf" of tissue in the dilated stomach that indicates torsion. A stomach tube can often be passed when an animal has gastric torsion. Animals with chronic gastric torsion may bloat intermittently.

81. **c** Thrombocytopenia is the most common clinicopathologic change in dogs with acute ehrlichiosis. Morulae are rarely, if ever, seen. Any titer is significant. You cannot repeat the serologic examination to see if the dog is cured; the titer stays high for some time after successful therapy. Plasma cells are found in the bone marrow, but they do not cause myelophthisis.

82. **b** Surgery is the only therapy that offers a reasonable chance for a cure. Conservative therapy is rarely effective.

83. **a** The dog is regurgitating; therefore, it has esophageal disease as opposed to gastrointestinal dysfunction. A vascular ring anomaly is most likely, as it is the only cause of esophageal disease.

84. **a** Though metoclopramide is not the ideal antiemetic, it is the only central-acting drug listed among the answer choices and, as such, is much more effective than the other drugs listed. Methscopolamine is a parasympatholytic. Bismuth subsalicylate is a local-acting drug. Misoprostol and sucralfate are used for ulceration; they are not antiemetics.

85. **b** The small intestine functions to absorb food. The low frequency of diarrhea plus the absence of blood, mucus and tenesmus (often seen in large intestinal diarrhea) confirms small intestinal diarrhea, as opposed to large intestinal diarrhea.

86. **e** Management of hypovolemic shock is the first concern. Flunixin is used for septic shock. Flunixin plus dexamethasone is likely to cause severe gastric ulceration. Lidocaine is used after arrhythmias occur, not before. This is far too much potassium to add to fluids being infused in large volumes to treat shock.

87. **c** Triamcinolone is a commonly used corticosteroid. Corticosteroids commonly increase serum alkaline phosphatase activity, with less effect on serum alanine aminotransferase activity.

88. **a** Free gas strongly sugggests a ruptured viscus, which would produce septic peritonitis. Peritonitis is consistent with depression, vomiting and abdominal pain. The abdomen must be lavaged and the ruptured viscus repaired to prevent further contamination. This should be done as soon as the patient can withstand anesthesia.

89. **c** Dogs with acute disease often die before they become icteric. Corneal edema is a chronic manifestation. Thrombocytopenia occurs due to disseminated intravascular coagulation associated with acute hepatic failure.

90. **c** Septic shock causes acidosis, disseminated intravascular coagulation and azotemia. Regurgitation is caused by esophageal disease, which is unlikely in this case.

91. **c** Retroflexion of the urinary bladder into the perineal hernia is the reason why perineal hernia can become an emergency.

92. **d** This tends to be a chronic disease that is diagnosed by finding the organism in circulating white blood cells or in muscle biopsies. Thrombocytopenia is found in many rickettsial infections and some viral infections, but not generally in hepatozoonosis. Bone changes are not consistent, especially in the early stages.

93. **c** Ascites is commonly found in cirrhotic dogs with acquired portosystemic shunting. Though ascites may be found in dogs with congenital portosystemic shunt (due to severe hypoalbuminemia), it is rare in these dogs.

94. **d** Mucosal hypertrophy rarely causes ulceration. Gastric malignancy can easily cause upper gastrointestinal bleeding. Metoclopramide, intravenous fluids and antibiotics are inadequate therapy for gastrointestinal ulceration, though fluids may reasonably be incorporated into a therapeutic regimen with H-2 blockers or sucralfate.

95. **e** The most common necropsy finding is petechiation in the kidneys and liver. You cannot find the virus in white blood cells. Antibiotics are ineffective.

96. **c** Acepromazine is a central-acting antiemetic and is the most effective antiemetic of the drugs listed as answer choices. Misoprostol and cimetidine are used for gastric ulceration but are not antiemetics. Kaopectate is a poor antiemetic. Atropine is a parasympatholytic with only mediocre antiemetic efficacy.

97. **d** Serologic tests are not very sensitive for histoplasmosis. Osseous lesions are rare in this disease. *Cryptococcus* organisms have a capsule, while *Histoplasma* organisms do not. Most dogs with disseminated disease are presented because of weight loss and/or large bowel diarrhea.

98. **d** Inflammatory and neoplastic infiltrates usually produce a thickened gastric mucosa and/or firm wall. Mucosal hypertrophy is usually found in older, small-breed dogs. *Physaloptera* is a grossly visible nematode parasite.

99. **e** The prostate gland is ventral to the colon in the pelvic canal. If it is enlarged, it displaces the colon dorsally. Prostatomegaly is a common cause of constipation in dogs.

100. **b** Blastomycosis often affects the eyes. Histoplasmosis and coccidioidomycosis may affect the eyes but are uncommon. Sporotrichosis almost never affects the eyes. Coccidioidomycosis and cryptococcosis rarely cause marked peripheral lymphadenopathy.

101. **a** Chlorpromazine is an effective antiemetic but is not effective in treating ulceration.

102. **e** The acute fever, lymphadenopathy and especially the pitting edema are very suggestive of Rocky Mountain spotted fever, which is characterized by vasculitis. This is especially likely in an outdoor dog in summer. Borreliosis usually causes pain, not edema or lymphadenopathy.

103. **b** Hematochezia originates from infarcted gut mucosa, while vomiting is due to obstruction and pain. Hypoproteinemia and profuse diarrhea are sometimes seen in

animals with chronic intussusception. Abdominal distention is very rare in this condition, as is prolapse of the intussusception from the anus.

104. **a** Microhepatia is characteristic of hepatic atrophy (seen with portosystemic shunts). Decreased serum albumin and urea nitrogen levels also suggest hepatic insufficiency. Changes in serum alanine aminotransferase and alkaline phosphatase activities and/or bilirubin levels are possible but uncommon in these animals. Decreases in serum gamma glutamyltransferase and alanine aminotransferase activities and bilirubin levels are meaningless.

105. **b** Though it is relatively uncommon, reversible hepatic disease may occur and cause anorexia, vomiting and/or icterus.

106. **a** Contrast radiographs are notoriously insensitive for detecting gastric ulcers. Many affected animals can be treated successfully. Peripheral white blood cell counts are usually normal to modestly increased, unless perforation has occurred. Serum iron levels are low if intestinal bleeding is chronic.

107. **d** A large amount of intraabdominal fat would cause distention and provide excellent serosal detail on radiographs. Fat causes the intestines (which have a water density) to have excellent contrast. Effusion would obscure serosal contrast in the abdomen. Lymphadenopathy would probably decrease serosal contrast. Hepatic failure would cause weight loss and/or ascites, both of which would decrease contrast.

108. **e** Renal failure is more often seen in subacute or chronic leptospirosis. Renal biopsy may reveal the organisms in chronically affected kidneys. It is difficult to culture the organism and special media are needed if the attempt is to be made. Most leptospiral infections in dogs are chronic or subclinical.

109. **a** The described topical therapy is usually effective in animals with anal sacculitis.

110. **b** Keratoconjunctivitis sicca may occur after use of any sulfa drug. Azulfidine is salicylazosulfapyridine and has caused keratoconjunctivitis sicca. The salicylate moiety is thought to be the effective portion of the drug. The drug's main indication is for chronic or nonresolving large bowel diarrhea. Though it may cause salicylate toxicity in cats, it is used in selected patients, albeit carefully.

111. **d** H_2 blockers are not totally effective in protecting against ulceration induced by nonsteroidal antiinflammatories. Sucralfate is effective in allowing ulcers to heal. Affected animals are not helped by kaolin-pectin or milk diets.

112. **a** The history suggests a portosystemic shunt. Serum bile acid concentrations would be most useful in identifying this disorder.

113. **d** Flunixin meglumine is a nonsteroidal antiinflammatory drug that can readily produce gastrointestinal ulceration. Chlorpromazine does not facilitate ulcer healing but may lessen vomiting secondary to an ulcer.

114. **d** Of the diseases listed, leptospirosis is the most likely to cause icterus and fever. Blastomycosis could cause both, but this is very unlikely.

115. **c** This dog probably has extrahepatic biliary tract obstruction associated with acute pancreatitis. The history of vomiting and abdominal pain is consistent with pancreatitis. Schnauzers seem particularly prone to pancreatitis.

116. **e** The dog has an anal sac abscess, which should be lanced once it develops a discernable "head" or soft spot. Systemic antibiotics are indicated in animals with abscesses, as opposed to those with uncomplicated anal sacculitis.

117. **e** This is a progressive central nervous system disease that is usually fatal. Diagnosis requires histopathologic or serologic examination.

118. **a** Correction of the vascular ring does not ensure that the regurgitation will resolve. Some treated animals continue to vomit. Other congenital cardiac abnormalities, while possible, are not widely recognized. Likewise, congenital esophageal weakness is not recognized as a common problem in these animals. German Shepherds appear to have a predisposition for this disease.

119. **a** This question determines if you know the clinicopathologic effects of chronic inflammatory hepatic disease. Serum alanine aminotransferase activity is usually increased due to cell damage. Serum alkaline phosphatase activity is increased because of liver scarring. The serum albumin level is decreased because of hepatic insufficiency.

120. **a** Loss of gastric acid depletes body acid (hence, metabolic alkalosis) and chloride stores (hence, hypochloremia). Vomiting due to almost any reason may produce hypokalemia.

121. **c** *Nocardia* grows aerobically and may require long incubation before growth is evident. Sulfonamides are the drugs of choice. Quinolones are not effective. These patients are not human health risks.

122. **d** Of the organs listed, the urinary bladder is the most caudal organ in the abdominal cavity and can become greatly distended if the animal cannot urinate.

123. **d** This dog probably has acute pancreatitis, not pancreatic insufficiency. The latter is not commonly associated with acute pancreatitis. Radiographs (to rule out other diseases), nothing per os and intravenous fluids are indicated in dogs with suspected pancreatitis.

124. **c** Standard fecal flotation is often diagnostic. Fenbendazole or praziquantel is the treatment of choice. The life cycle requires an intermediate host. Coughing is the most common presenting complaint.

125. **b** Aspiration pneumonia is probably the most common cause of death, aside from euthanasia. Esophagitis is an uncommon cause of symptomatic esophageal disease in dogs. Surgery is usually contraindicated. H-2 blockers are used to diminish gastric acid production.

126. **d** Corticosteroids are useful for reducing the hepatic inflammatory response in dogs with chronic active hepatitis. Lactulose and neomycin are used for hepatic encephalopathy. Trientine is used for copper storage disorder.

127. **e** Despite the fact that many recognized cases of parvoviral enteritis are very severe, it is believed that most infections are relatively mild. The severity of the disease depends upon the size and virulence of the inoculum, presence or absence of other intestinal disease (*eg*, parasites) and the pup's maternal immunity.

128. **c** There appears to be an association between hepatic failure and gastrointestinal ulceration. Cirrhotic dogs that suddenly become worse may have a bleeding duodenal ulcer, which in turn causes hepatic encephalopathy due to the large amount of protein passing into the intestines.

129. **c** Metronidazole and clindamycin are the only drugs listed with good anaerobic efficacy. Metronidazole only kills anaerobic bacteria. Clindamycin is not very effective against Gram-negative bacteria, which would be expected in peritonitis due to intestinal leakage. Ampicillin plus amikacin has excellent aerobic efficacy.

130. **d** There is no effective medical therapy. Serologic testing is essentially useless. The gastrointestinal tract is commonly affected. Distal appendicular lesions are principally found in horses.

131. **d** Cardiac arrhythmias and gastric motility disturbances are common. Disseminated intravascular coagulation occurs in animals with severe, advanced gastric dilatation/volvulus. Recurrence is possible, especially if a gastropexy has not been performed.

132. **a** Loperamide is an opiate that increases segmental contraction and decreases intestinal secretion. Parasympatholytics are much less effective. Kaopectate is of dubious value.

133. **a** Though uncommon, there are reports of dogs living relatively long periods (weeks or months) despite rabies. Purulent or suppurative meningoencephalitis does not occur in rabies. Phenolic disinfectants are not needed to cleanse wounds.

134. **e** Copper storage disease is a very common cause of hepatic disease in Bedlington Terriers.

135. **e** Both Rocky Mountain spotted fever and ehrlichiosis can cause thrombocytopenia. Chloramphenicol is very effective in treatment of Rocky Mountain spotted fever. Many animals with acute Rocky Mountain spotted fever have a negative titer. *Rhipicephalus sanguineus* is the principal vector in the United States for ehrlichiosis, not Rocky Mountain spotted fever.

136. **c** Lipemia in a vomiting Miniature Schnauzer strongly suggests acute pancreatitis. The laboratory results are consistent with this diagnosis. Serum lipase activity is an inaccurate indicator of pancreatitis and affected dogs may have normal values.

137. **e** Oral antacids must be given frequently (4-6 times/day) to maintain a high gastric pH. Even then they may be vomited back up. H₂ blockers are usually more effective and for longer periods.

138. **b** Most affected dogs die if they are not treated. Diagnosis is principally by finding the organism in fine-needle aspirates of swollen lymph nodes. Finding fluke ova in the feces is suggestive but not diagnostic.

139. **e** The description of the feces is suggestive of whipworms. The parasites are often missed by fecal examination because they shed eggs periodically and the eggs are relatively heavy (they sink if the flotation solution is not made properly). Salmonellosis and prototheocosis are rare. Most rectal adenocarcinomas are easily found by rectal examination.

140. **c** A barium enema should reveal an obvious filling defect in a dog or cat with an ileocolic intussusception.

141. **c** Serologic testing has not been well evaluated in dogs. Dogs often have very few organisms in cutaneous lesions (as opposed to cats, which often have numerous organisms). The recommended therapy is with potassium iodide or possibly itraconazole.

142. **b** The dog obviously has chronic small intestinal diarrhea, meaning that it has malabsorption or maldigestion. Maldigestion is particularly common in German Shepherds. Serum trypsin-like immunoreactivity is the best test for maldigestion in dogs. Abdominal radiographs are rarely useful in dogs with either malabsorption or maldigestion. Because 5 fecal examinations have been negative, it is doubtful that another would be useful. Biopsy should be postponed until maldigestion has been ruled out.

143. **a** Dogs are relatively resistant to tetanus. Antitoxin is not effective once the toxin has bound to nerves. Phenobarbital and acepromazine are sometimes very helpful in management of these patients.

144. **a** This dog appears to be regurgitating because of esophageal disease, not vomiting due to gastrointestinal disease. Thoracic radiographs are needed to evaluate the esophagus.

145. **a** Cats usually are infected by *Mycobacterium bovis* and show gastrointestinal signs. Dogs usually are infected by *Mycobacterium tuberculosis* and show respiratory signs. Histopathologic and cytologic examinations are better means of diagnosis. Affected dogs should probably be euthanized because of the human health risk.

146. **e** Nonsteroidal antiinflammatory drugs are a major cause of gastrointestinal ulceration in dogs. Corticosteroids have comparatively low ulcerogenic potential.

147. **d** The latex agglutination test for cryptococcosis detects circulating antigen. It is one of the few sensitive, specific serologic tests for fungal infection. Aspergillosis is more common than cryptococcosis in the nose of dogs. *Cryptococcus* has a capsule, which makes cytologic diagnosis relatively easy. Ketoconazole is generally ineffective against central nervous system cryptococcosis.

148. **e** Endoscopy is not as good as fluoroscopy in demonstrating esophageal dysfunction. Surgery is almost never useful in these animals. Metoclopramide does not improve esophageal function. While some affected animals can be managed well with dietary therapy, the prognosis is guarded, as many die from aspiration pneumonia.

149. **a** Hypocalcemia is occasionally associated with pancreatitis. Hypercalcemia is not caused by pancreatitis, though it theoretically could cause pancreatitis. However, this is not thought to be clinically significant in dogs and cats.

150. **d** Chlorpromazine is a very effective central-acting antiemetic. Cimetidine is not an antiemetic. Atropine and aminopentamide are parasympatholytics and are not nearly as effective as chlorpromazine.

151. **a** Abdominal palpation may fail to detect an intestinal obstruction. Oral iodine contrast agents result in poor-quality gastrointestinal radiographs. Endoscopy is not useful if the foreign object is farther into the intestines than the endoscope can reach. Contrast radiographs are only needed if plain radiographs are not diagnostic. Dilated air- or fluid-filled intestinal loops are the most common finding on plain radiographs.

152. **c** The description of these protozoa suggests giardiasis. Metronidazole is an accepted therapy for these parasites.

153. **a** The dog is regurgitating and has aspiration pneumonia. Therefore, abdominal radiographs would be of dubious value. It is doubtful that a complete blood count or serum chemistry profile would be helpful. The dog's old age means that this is an acquired esophageal disease. Neuromuscular disease causes acquired esophageal weakness in dogs.

154. **d** Immunoproliferative enteropathy is a common cause of protein-losing enteropathy in Basenjis. These dogs often have increased serum globulin levels despite intestinal protein loss.

155. **a** *Coccidioides immitis* is a large organism containing small internal structures. An encapsulated yeast is likely *Cryptococcus*. Pleomorphic cigar-shaped organisms are likely *Sporothrix*. Nonseptate hyphae may be those of various other fungi.

156. **c** Boston Terriers are suspected to be at increased risk.

157. **b** Prednisolone may kill the dog if it has histoplasmosis (a reasonable differential diagnosis in this dog). Pyrantel would not kill whipworms, the parasite most likely to cause large bowel diarrhea. Azulfidine and azathioprine have many side effects. Dietary intolerance and/or fiber-reponsive disease are common causes of diarrhea and are safe to treat.

158. **e** The oocysts indicate coccidiosis. These protozoa are occasionally problematic in young dogs but rarely in older animals. This infection need not be treated. Also, none of the drugs listed is effective in coccidiosis.

159. **d** Corticosteroids commonly produce vacuolar hepatopathy, which characteristically increases serum alkaline phosphatase activity, but they have few other effects on the liver. The lymphopenia also suggests a corticosteroid effect. Portosystemic shunts often do not affect serum alanine aminotransferase or alkaline phosphatase activities.

160. **c** Portosystemic shunts are sometimes first considered in animals that do not recover from anesthesia as expected (due to hepatic insufficiency and slowed drug metabolism). Yorkshire Terriers seem predisposed to portosystemic shunts.

161. **b** In right lateral recumbency, the pylorus is the most dependent part of the stomach; thus, barium is most likely to pool there.

162. **b** Bismuth subsalicylate is an effective antisecretory agent (due to the salicylate moiety). Sucralfate and cimetidine are used for gastrointestinal ulceration. Atropine is a parasympatholytic and is much less effective than an opiate.

163. **b** Acute nosocomial diarrhea caused by *Clostridium* has been reported in dogs, especially those hospitalized in veterinary clinics.

164. **a** Many dogs with ulcers do not vomit blood. Ulcers would be a reason the barium is retained in 2 discrete areas of the stomach. Metoclopramide and chlorpromazine, while good antiemetic agents, are not useful for healing ulcers. Most affected dogs do not die from gastrointestinal ulceration.

165. **b** Approximately 70% of affected dogs have bacterial overgrowth in the small intestine. Fecal film digestion tests are worthless. Many animals do not respond to supplementation of pancreatic enzymes because the product used is inferior or is used with a high-fat diet. Hypoproteinemia is rare in affected animals. The most common cause is pancreatic atrophy.

166. **a** Xylazine is a satisfactory emetic in cats but not in dogs. Syrup of ipecac and salt water are very unreliable antiemetics. Apomorphine is the most consistently effective emetic in dogs.

167. **a** These puppies almost certainly became infected with hookworms from the dam. Pyrantel pamoate is safe and effective for such an infection.

168. **c** The mucus, absence of weight loss, and softness of the last portion of the fecal mass strongly suggest large bowel disease.

169. **e** Affected animals are often clinically normal. It is rare to find inclusions in platelets due to the periodicity of their appearance and the diminished number of platelets present at these times. Pancytopenia is not expected in this infection. Ticks carry both rickettsiae, and concurrent infections are probably common.

170. **d** Bones are common foreign bodies and are usually seen with plain radiographs. Even if the foreign object is radiolucent, there is often gas around it, which makes it visible radiographically. Barium is only contraindicated if a perforation is suspected. It is common for contrast esophagograms not to reveal an esophageal perforation.

171. **e** This description is classic for a congenital hepatic portosystemic shunt causing hepatic encephalopathy with polyuria and polydipsia.

172. **c** This is a common history for acute parvoviral enteritis. Coronaviral enteritis is usually relatively mild. Salmonellosis is very uncommon. The dog's age makes garbage ingestion unlikely. Foreign bodies usually do not produce severe diarrhea.

173. **d** Marked hemoconcentration is the hallmark of hemorrhagic gastroenteritis.

174. **e** Gastric dilatation/volvulus is a major cause of unproductive retching and abdominal pain in giant-breed dogs. Plain abdominal radiographs are usually diagnostic if physical examination is not.

175. **e** Histiocytic ulcerative colitis is almost only found in young to middle-aged Boxers. Some clinicians refer to the disease as "Boxer colitis."

176. **b** Ascites is possible but very unlikely in a dog with a congenital portosystemic shunt, unless very severe hypoalbuminemia is present.

177. **e** *Dipylidium caninum* is the most common tapeworm of dogs and cats. Its intermediate hosts are the flea and louse. Most affected animals do not show clinical evidence of infection.

178. **b** Parvovirus does not destroy villi directly, but destruction of crypts leads to subsequent loss of villi.

179. **d** The black, tarry stools suggest upper gastrointestinal bleeding, such as from an ulcer. Pancreatitis rarely causes gastric or duodenal ulceration.

180. **a** Xylazine paralyzes esophageal musculature and allows the organ to dilate with air. Thus, the patient appears to have megaesophagus on esophagograms. Acepromazine is the chemical restraint of choice in such studies.

181. **c**

182. **c** You must determine if the protruding mucosa is associated with rectal prolapse (the most common cause) or with an ileocolic intussusception that is so long that it protrudes from the rectum. A rectal prolapse forms a cul-de-sac near the rectum, but an ileocolic intussusception does not. Repelling the end of an ileocolic intussusception back into the descending colon would not benefit the patient.

183. **a** Bacterial metabolism of malabsorbed carbohydrates is probably the most common cause of flatulence. For example, beans often cause flatulence in people because raffinose in the beans is not absorbed and colonic bacteria metabolize it, producing gas.

184. **e** Hypoadrenocorticism commonly causes vomiting, but not hyperadrenocorticism.

185. **d** This is a likely case of parvoviral enteritis. Many affected patients do not show leukopenia if tested only once, early in the course of the disease. The severity, fever and acute onset suggest viral enteritis.

186. **d** Though tetracycline or doxycycline are usually used for ehrlichiosis, chloramphenicol is also effective. The diagnostic tests listed would probably not aid in diagnosis or change your therapy.

187. **a** Acute pancreatitis often obstructs the pancreatic duct but not the duodenum. Chronic pancreatitis may rarely cause duodenal obstruction because of scarring around the duodenum.

188. **e** Sudden gagging up of food or mucus, without prodromal nausea or retching, suggests regurgitation due to esophageal disease.

189. **c** Icterus is often not seen in significant hepatic disease in dogs. Pancreatitis (not exocrine pancreatic insufficiency) may cause icterus. Gallstones are rarely symptomatic in dogs. Vacuolar hepatopathy generally does not cause problems in dogs.

190. **a**

191. **d**

192. **c** The history is classic for congenital portosystemic shunt. This therapy is appropriate to symptomatically treat hepatic encephalopathy. High-protein meals and anticonvulsants are contraindicated because of the likely diagnosis. There is no reason to use aluminum hydroxide or prednisolone.

193. **c** Only intravenous fluids and preventing oral intake have been agreed upon as important in treating pancreatitis. Antibiotics are of dubious value, as septic pancreatitis is very rare in dogs and cats.

194. **c**

195. **d** Acute febrile gastroenteritis in a young dog is suggestive of parvoviral infection. Intussusception, gastrointestinal parasitism and dietary intolerance typically do not cause fever. Gastric ulceration is very unlikely in a 5-month-old dog.

196. **d** A hepatoma arising from the right side of the liver would displace the pylorus caudo-medially as described. Lymphosarcoma is a possibility, but it is often multicentric and unlikely to cause a solitary large mass in the cranial right abdominal quadrant. Hemangio-sarcoma is possible, but it is more likely to affect the spleen on the other side of the abdomen. A linear foreign body may displace the intestines, but it is doubtful that it would displace the pylorus as described.

197. **e** The dog probably has acute gastritis or perhaps a foreign body. Endoscopy (which requires anesthesia) is not indicated unless the dog's condition worsens. Also, you would not perform endoscopy without first ascertaining if the patient was a good anesthetic risk.

198. **a**

199. **d** There may be some inflammatory effusion around the pancreatitis, which is why the cranial right quadrant is hazy on a ventrodorsal abdominal radiograph. Ascites is rare.

200. **e** Most congenital hepatic portosystemic shunts are single vessels that anastomose with the azygos vein or the caudal vena cava.

201. **c** The clinical signs are referrable to neuromuscular weakness and muscular pain.

202. **d** Serum creatine phosphokinase activity increases as a result of leakage of the enzyme from damaged muscle.

203. **b** Beta-blockers cause bronchoconstriction and, as such, are contraindicated for use in asthmatic cats.

204. **a**

205. **c**

206. **e** Lymphosarcoma is the most common renal tumor of cats and is typically associated with a negative FeLV status. Renomegaly may be unilateral or bilateral.

207. **a** Hyperglobulinemia frequently occurs secondary to FIP and is usually classified as a polyclonal gammopathy.

208. **d** Though cats demonstrate hypersensitivity reactions, IgE has not yet been identified in this species.

209. **e** In comparison, the blood volume of dogs is about 7-8% of body weight.

210. **b** Historically, thiamin deficiency was always considered the first differential diagnosis for cervical ventroflexion in cats. Potassium deficiency should now also be given strong consideration.

211. **d** Affected cats have a better prognosis for long-term survival than do dogs.

212. **a** Bile acid concentrations are very useful for detecting liver disease in cats.

213. **b** Meningioma is the most common primary brain tumor of cats.

214. **c** Aortic thromboembolism is a frequent complication of hypertrophic cardiomyopathy.

215. **c** Horner's syndrome results from loss of sympathetic innervation.

216. **a** Diaphragmatic hernia muffles the heart and lung sounds.

217. **b** Hyperkalemic myocardiotoxicity and metabolic acidosis are classic findings with prolonged lower urinary tract obstruction.

218. **e** Deficiency of Factor XII is commonly recognized in cats.

219. **b** Respiration may cease with an incompatible transfusion; vomiting may occur when the rate of blood administration is excessively rapid.

220. **d** Arginine is an essential amino acid for cats. It is needed to "drive" the urea cycle, as it transforms ammonia to urea. Therefore, a deficiency of arginine may potentiate hepatic encephalopathy.

221. **c** Digoxin is contraindicated because it is a positive inotrope.

222. **b** The recognized blood groups of cats are A, B and AB. Severe transfusion reactions occur most frequently in type-B cats receiving type-A blood; type-B cats carry alloantibodies to type A. Of interest is the apparently higher incidence of type-B blood in purebred cats.

223. **e**

224. **a**

225. **d** Visceral mast-cell tumors are much more common in cats than in dogs. They should always be included in the differential diagnoses for splenomegaly. Cutaneous mast-cell tumors are less aggressive in cats than in dogs.

226. **c** Growth hormone is a powerful insulin antagonist and, therefore, exerts a diabetogenic effect.

227. **b** Cryptococcosis is distributed on a worldwide basis and is, therefore, most common; however, some geographic areas have another predominant mycosis, such as histoplasmosis.

228. **d** Latent infection is virtually impossible to demonstrate in everyday clinical practice. Bone marrow cultures must be submitted to special laboratories.

229. **c** The normal heart rate in cats is approximately 160-240 beats per minute.

230. **b** Methemoglobinemia reduces the oxygen-carrying capacity of blood.

231. **d** Acetylcysteine helps replenish hepatocellular supplies of glutathione.

232. **d** All of the aminoglycosides may cause neuromuscular blockade. This danger is potentiated with anesthesia.

233. **b**

234. **d** Amitraz is inappropriate for treatment of dermatophytosis. It is used to treat demodicosis in dogs.

235. **d** In cats, acromegaly is caused by pituitary tumors. In dogs, it is usually related to progestagens, either endogenous (intact bitch) or exogenous. Progestagens stimulate release of growth hormone. Insulin resistance occurs because of the antagonism of growth hormone to insulin.

236. **e** Cats have a higher renal threshold for glucose than dogs. Dogs have a threshold of about 180 mg/dl. Interestingly, diabetic cats appear to have a lower threshold (about 200 mg/dl) for glucose spillage than nondiabetic cats.

237. **d** "Walking dandruff" is *Cheyletiella* infestation.

238. **c** Cerebellar hypoplasia may be caused by panleukopenia virus, a parvovirus of cats.

239. **c** This is a classic presentation for food allergy in cats.

240. **b** It is important to change to a truly hypoallergenic diet and not just another commercial brand of diet. The diet should be tried for a minimum of 3 weeks.

241. **a** Some argue that cats are not infected by whipworms, yet the literature (and most current texts) indicate that it occurs sporadically.

242. **d** Digitoxin has a half-life of over 100 hours in cats. It undergoes extensive hepatic metabolism. It should not be used in cats.

243. **e** Phosphate-containing enemas are extremely dangerous in cats and small dogs. They can cause severe electrolyte disturbances, such as hypocalcemia and hypernatremia. Their use frequently results in death of the animal.

244. **e** Cats with hepatic lipidosis are notorious for their refusal to eat.

245. **c** This is a classic presentation for squamous-cell carcinoma on the head.

246. **d** This presentation is more representative of autoimmune skin disease.

247. **e** Basophilic stippling is not diagnostic of any particular disease. In cats, however, it can be supportive evidence of regenerative anemia.

248. **d** The kidneys, liver, spleen and mesenteric lymph nodes often provide diagnostic samples. The noneffusive form of FIP, usually more difficult to diagnose than the effusive form, shows pyogranulomas and vasculitis on tissue sections.

249. **a** Benzyl alcohol is a preservative frequently added to intravenous fluid products and sterile water (for drug reconstitution) intended for human use. The neurologic disturbance may ultimately be fatal, dictating that the veterinarian should use caution when purchasing fluids for use in cats.

250. **e** FIP produces a high-protein exudate that is nonseptic and contains relatively few cells. The relative cellularity may vary with the stage of the disease, however.

251. **b**

252. **c** Electrical alternans is an occasional electrocardiographic finding in cats with pericardial effusion.

253. **a** The mitral valve is usually the most commonly affected valve. The aortic valve is probably the second most commonly affected valve.

254. **c** In dogs, pleural effusion is generally recognized on radiographs after accumulation of about 100 ml of fluid in the pleural space.

255. **a** Chemotherapy is typically disappointing with this tumor.

256. **a** Canine insulin is identical to porcine insulin. Feline insulin, while not identical, is most similar to bovine insulin.

257. **c** Because many cats have occult infections, microfilariae are seldom identified. The occult test may be negative because fewer adults develop in cats than in dogs, and thus less antigen is present. The occult (antigen) test is becoming more reliable, however, as the sensitivity of this test increases. The antibody test is unreliable.

258. **d** Lymphoma is the most common gastrointestinal tumor of cats.

259. **e** Hemorrhage, thrombosis, petechiae and large numbers of parasites characterize cytauxzoonosis.

260. **e**

261. **a**

262. **d** Lymphoid hyperplasia, or reactive hyperplasia, is the most common cause of lymphadenomegaly in cats.

263. **e** Hyperglycemia and/or glucosuria are relatively common in stressed cats. One should never institute insulin therapy based on a single finding of either. If in doubt about diabetes mellitus, hospitalize the cat (allow time to acclimate) and continue to recheck glucose levels. A stressed cat can have a serum glucose level of 300 mg/dl.

264. **b** This antigen stimulates the immune system but does not elicit a virus-neutralizing response.

265. **b**

266. **e** The upper third premolar is the carnassial tooth.

267. **d** This test must be done by a diagnostic laboratory. Several stool samples are submitted.

268. **d** Aminoglycosides are relatively ototoxic in cats.

269. **d** Depletion of vitamin K-dependent factors prolongs prothrombin time and partial thromboplastin time.

270. **a** Anticoagulant rodenticide intoxication depletes the body of vitamin K-dependent factors.

271. **d** Latex agglutination is particularly useful because it is an antigen test. It can be helpful in monitoring therapy.

272. **d** A positive FIP titer may be generated in response to coronaviruses other than FIP virus. A positive titer is only evidence of exposure to a coronavirus, not specifically FIP virus.

273. **a** The adult cat has 30 teeth.

274. **b** An animal in diastolic failure should not receive intravenous fluids.

275. **d** Multicentric (generalized) lymphadenopathy is an uncommon presentation for feline lymphoma.

276. **a** Metronidazole is used most commonly.

277. **c** Vomiting during blood transfusion frequently indicates an excessive rate of administration.

278. **a** Acute onset of blindness with ocular hemorrhage in a geriatric cat should initiate an investigation into renal disease and its attendant hypertension.

279. **d** Sinus tachycardia is a common finding in stressed cats. It is also the most common arrhythmia in dogs. Ventricular tachycardia is the second most common arrhythmia of cats and dogs.

280. **d** Excessive chordae tendinae/papillary muscle cardiomyopathy is not a recognized form of cardiomyopathy in cats or dogs.

281. **d**

282. **c** This is a frequent finding in orange cats, and owners commonly ask the significance of the pigmentation. It is a benign lesion.

283. **e**

284. **e** Once the fluid is drained, antibiotics given intravenously reach adequate levels in the pleural space. Infusing antibiotic solutions into the chest exacerbates pleuritis.

285. **a** Metronidazole has good activity against most anaerobes, particularly *Bacteroides*. Penicillins may also be good choices. The cephalosporins have variable activity against anaerobes and may not be effective against *Bacteroides*. Aminoglycosides do not work in anaerobic environments. Base treatment on culture and sensitivity results.

286. **d** Brain tumors are among the more common causes of forebrain dysfunction. Meningioma is the most common primary brain tumor of cats.

287. **d** T₃ suppression is a relatively new test for diagnosing hyperthyroidism in cats with normal basal T₄ values.

288. **b**

289. **e** Electric heating pads may cause thermal burns. These are particularly dangerous for the unconscious or immobile patient. These have no place in clinical practice and their use only invites a lawsuit.

290. **c** Non-enveloped (hydrophilic) viruses, such as calicivirus and parvovirus, are difficult to kill with routine disinfection. Household bleach (sodium hypochlorite, Clorox) at 1:32 dilution is probably best.

291. **b**

292. **b**

293. **c** Clindamycin has been used more commonly recently.

294. **b** Oocysts do not sporulate for at least 24 hours after excretion. Ideally, someone other than the pregnant woman should clean the litterbox. The pregnant woman may be at greater risk for contracting toxoplasmosis from eating undercooked meat than from contact with cats.

295. **c**

296. **d** Aromatic amino acids worsen the signs of hepatic encephalopathy; branched-chain amino acids do not.

297. **c** Dilative cardiomyopathy has become increasingly rare because of taurine supplementation in most cat foods.

298. **a**

299. **c**

300. **b**

301. **d** Chloramphenicol is not used today as much as it has been in the past because of the concern for bone marrow suppression, both in the cat and the person administering the drug. The client should always be told to wear latex gloves when handling the drug. It may cause aplastic anemia in people.

302. **b** The same maximal rate of administration of 0.5 mEq/kg/hour should be used for dogs.

303. **d**

304. **d**

305. **c**

306. **c**

307. **e** The normal flora in a cat's mouth is a "mixed bag" of bacterial types.

308. **a** Amoxicillin or perhaps amoxicillin-clavulanic acid would be a good first choice to treat a bite abscess. A cephalosporin may not be indicated unless the less expensive beta-lactams are ineffective. Drainage of the abscess is as important as the antibiotic used.

309. **d** Lymphoma is the most common hepatic tumor in cats. It is usually metastatic from a distant site.

310. **a** Persian and Himalayan breeds are particularly sensitive to the effects of griseofulvin.

311. **d** This is a classic "nonobstructive feline urologic syndrome." The more currently accepted terminology is "feline lower urinary tract disorder."

312. **e** Both the obstructive and nonobstructive lower urinary tract syndromes are invariably associated with sterile urine.

313. **a** Stomatitis and gingivitis are "markers" for immunosuppression. They are frequently found in cats with retroviral immunosuppression.

314. **a** These are classic signs of dysautonomia.

315. **d** Steatitis is an inflammatory condition of adipose tissue. Diets high in polyunsaturated fats, such as fish and fish oils, require large amounts of vitamin E to prevent oxidation of fat. Vitamin E, the body's main defense against lipid peroxidation, is scant in many types of fish.

316. **b**

317. **d**

318. **c** Propranolol may be used for hypertrophic cardiomyopathy but is not recommended if the cat has embolism.

319. **d**

320. **b** Thyroid tumors are typically benign adenomas in cats. They are usually malignant in dogs.

321. **e**

322. **d** Mast cells produce histamine, an agonist for parietal cells.

323. **c** Dextrose-containing solutions should be avoided because of deranged glucose metabolism. Saline at 7% is hypertonic. Saline at 0.45% is hypotonic. Saline at 0.9% is the fluid of choice.

324. **b** Ptyalism is a prominent sign of hepatic encephalopathy in cats.

325. **e** 5-fluorouracil is a potent neurotoxin in cats and its use is likely to result in death of the patient.

326. **a** Deficiency of glucuronyl transferase limits the cat's ability to conjugate compounds to glucuronic acid and increase the water solubility of a compound.

327. **b** Cats do not have a glucocorticoid-induced isoenzyme of alkaline phosphatase.

328. **a**

329. **e**

330. **b**

331. **e**

332. **e**

333. **d**

334. **c** The higher osmolality is less favorable for bacterial growth.

335. **b** Thiacetarsamide has been recommended in the older literature. However, recent research suggests that it may be less effective than once thought and, in higher dosages such as those used to treat heartworms, it may be toxic. Arsenical compounds have an affinity for capillary beds.

336. **c** Cyanosis occurs as a result of life-threatening methemoglobinemia.

337. **b**

338. **b** Hyperthyroidism has not been reported as a sequel to use of megestrol acetate. This is a progestational agent.

339. **d** Cardiomyopathy caused by hyperthyroidism is sometimes called "thyrotoxic" heart disease.

340. **b** While the clinical signs of heart failure vary with the form of cardiomyopathy, ascites is a rarely recognized sign of heart failure in cats.

341. **b** About half of infected cats have nasal cavity involvement.

342. **c**

343. **c** Notoedric mange is intensely pruritic.

344. **d**

345. **e**

346. **a**

347. **d** 5% dextrose in water is an unacceptable choice. The dextrose is metabolized to free water and leaves the vascular compartment for the intracellular and interstitial tissues. Any of the others would be reasonable choices, depending on the electrolytes they contain.

348. **a** In reality, any of the signs listed may be seen. It is interesting, however, that vomiting is the most common clinical sign.

349. **c**

350. **b** Cats have a very high threshold for bilirubin elimination by the kidney (approximately 9 times higher than that of dogs). It is always an abnormal finding. The stressed cat may occasionally spill glucose into the urine because of "stress hyperglycemia."

351. **c** Cisplatin causes fulminant pulmonary edema in cats.

352. **b** Hypocalcemia will occur if the parathyroid glands cannot be preserved. In some cats, calcium homeostasis is transiently disrupted postoperatively, even if the parathyroids are preserved.

353. **c**

354. **c**

355. **b** Steatitis is associated with vitamin E deficiency.

356. **b**

357. **a** Rabid cats have a pronounced "furious" stage. "Dumb" rabies is less common in cats.

358. **a**

359. **b** Blood that autoagglutinates on a slide or in the blood tube is diagnostic of one type of autoimmune hemolytic anemia (AIHA). For this particular type, no further testing is necessary. Autoagglutination is pathognomonic for AIHA.

360. **e** Failure of autoagglutinated cells to disperse with an equal volume of saline is diagnostic of immune-mediated hemolytic anemia. Treatment consists of immunosuppressive doses of corticosteroids. Tetracycline may be added to the protocol in the event that *Hemobartonella felis* organisms are present but not identified.

361. **c**

362. **d**

363. **e** A brain tumor would be less likely because of this cat's age.

364. **d**

365. **b** These are classic signs of cerebellar hypoplasia.

366. **b**

367. **d** There appears to be little relation between hormones and mammary tumor development in cats. This is not the case in dogs.

368. **c** Normal cats suppress serum T$_4$ levels with the T$_3$ suppression test.

369. **c**

370. **b** Methimazole is associated with severe bone marrow suppression in some cats. Monitor the CBC closely.

371. **d**

372. **e**

373. **c** Heartworms live about 5 years in dogs.

374. **a**

375. **c**

376. **a**

377. **d**

378. **d** The response to prednisone is poor; these cats have a guarded prognosis.

379. **e**

380. **c** The lateral saphenous vein is frequently used in dogs. The medial saphenous vein is used in cats.

381. **c** Griseofulvin is extremely teratogenic.

382. **d**

383. **a**

384. **b** Caution is warranted when administering most drugs to cats with liver disease.

385. **b**

386. **e** A urine specific gravity above 1.035 should be attainable in cats with normal renal function.

387. **d** The plantigrade stance associated with diabetes mellitus is probably the major metabolic neuropathy of cats.

388. **c**

389. **a**

390. **d**

391. **a** Large doses of trimethoprim-sulfa are a good first choice to treat nocardiosis.

392. **c** The feline red blood cell is too small to detect spherocytosis. If immune-mediated hemolytic anemia is suspected, the erythrocyte fragility test may be useful.

393. **c**

394. **a**

395. **a**

396. **a**

397. **c**

398. **d** Calcium ions oppose the cardiotoxic effects of hyperkalemia but do not lower serum potassium levels.

399. **b** This is a classic description of Chediak-Higashi syndrome.

400. **d** Cats with Chediak-Higashi syndrome have a defect in neutrophil function, which renders them more susceptible to recurrent infections.

401. **c** Cytoplasmic inclusions are characteristic of chlamydial conjunctivitis. The other agents listed do not produce inclusions.

402. **a** Feline herpesvirus has a predilection for corneal epithelium. Keratitis is a common manifestation of feline herpesviral infection.

403. **c** Feline calicivirus has a predilection for oral epithelium. Vesicles that develop into ulcers are common on the tongue of infected cats.

404. **d** Calicivirus has a predilection for the lower respiratory tract. Virulent strains cause pulmonary lesions in young kittens.

405. **c** These signs are typical of upper respiratory infections caused by herpesvirus.

406. **d** Once infected, cats remain latent carriers of herpesvirus for life. Stress can cause recrudescence of the infection.

407. **d** Tetracycline is the drug of choice for treatment of *Chlamydia* infection.

408. **a** Idoxuridine is the only drug listed with efficacy against herpesvirus.

409. **a** Generalized peripheral lymph node lymphoma is the most common form in dogs, but it is relatively rare as compared with other forms in cats.

410. **e** Latent FeLV is nonreplicating by definition and therefore is undetectable by ELISA or the IFA test.

411. **d** Typically, erthrocytes in FeLV-infected cats are macrocytic, not microcytic.

412. **e** FeLV ELISAs are accurate if performed properly, but they often yield false positives due to technical error. Answers b and d improve accuracy.

413. **c** FeLV is excreted in massive amounts in saliva. Normal feline grooming behavior promotes transmission of the virus.

414. **b** Over 50% of cats with alimentary lymphoma are FeLV negative.

415. **a** Saliva testing is subject to a greater rate of false-positive and false-negative results. The other choices listed enhance test accuracy.

416. **d** Latent FeLV infection is not detected by conventional testing, only by *in-vitro* isolation from cultured bone marrow cells.

417. **b** ELISAs are more sensitive, detect earlier stages of infection, and are more prone to yield false-positive results.

418. **e** The result of ELISA becomes positive earlier than the result of the IFA test.

419. **b** Intestinal lymphoma occurs in aged cats; the other forms occur in young cats.

420. **c** FIV is commonly transmitted via cat bites.

421. **d** FIV antibody indicates exposure and infection. FIV infection is for life.

422. **b** Though the other listed signs occur, oral cavity lesions are present in well over 50% of cats with clinical disease related to FIV.

423. **d** Pyogranulomatous exudate is typical of effusive FIP.

424. **a** Immune-complex vasculitis is the key event in FIP coronavirus infection.

425. **b** Exudative anterior uveitis due to vasculitis is a common manifestation of FIP.

426. **d** This is a very nonspecific test and not a confirmatory diagnostic test of FIP.

427. **a** Feline enteric coronavirus is very prevalent in cats. It elicits antibodies indistinguishable from antibodies directed against FIP coronavirus.

428. **a** Cats ingest *Toxoplasma* cysts in muscles (raw meat) of rodents and meat-producing animals.

429. **e** An IgG antibody titer can indicate previous infection from years earlier; an IgM titer indicates recent or active infection.

430. **d** Of the drugs listed, only tetracycline is effective against hemobartonellosis.

431. **a** The capsule is characteristic of *Cryptococcus*.

432. **d** *Chlamydia* causes conjunctivitis but no internal ocular involvement.

433. **a** Panleukopenia virus can interfere with cerebellar development in the fetus.

434. **c** Serologic testing cannot distinguish between FIP and enteric coronaviral antibodies.

435. **e** Ketoconazole is the oral drug of choice for treatment of histoplasmosis.

436. **e** Hyperglobulinemia is a common finding in FIP but not in the other listed infections.

437. **a** Injection pain and systemic side effects are caused by vaccine adjuvants.

438. **c** In groups of cats, viruses are most likely to be transmitted by contact or aerosol.

439. **b** Asthma causes prominence of bronchial structures on radiographs. Air bronchograms indicate an alveolar fluid density, as occurs in pneumonia or edema.

440. **b** Terbutaline is an oral beta-2 adrenergic agent used as a bronchodilator.

441. **a** A bronchodilator is indicated; the only one listed is aminophylline.

442. **c** Nasopharyngeal polyps are common in cats.

443. **d** This lesion is typical of chronic lipidoid aspiration pneumonia.

444. **a** Eosinophils are typical in airway aspirates from asthmatic cats.

445. **e** Anaerobes are the most common type of bacteria found in pyothorax of cats.

446. **d** The twisted lung lobe and its air spaces become engorged with blood, producing a radiopaque lobe.

447. **d** Drainage and lavage of the pleural space are used in treatment of pyothorax.

448. **d** The fibrosing, walling-off process in pyothorax may encapsulate fluid into one hemithorax.

449. **d** A space-occupying cranial mediastinal mass, such as lymphoma, reduces compliance of the feline thorax.

450. **e** Air in the pleural space (pneumothorax) is resonant and tympanic on percussion.

451. **c** This is the definition of orthopnea.

452. **b** Aspiration pneumonia is a frequent complication of esophageal regurgitation.

453. **b** Fluid therapy promotes fluidity and enhances expectoration of respiratory secretions.

454. **d** *Cryptococcus* has a predilection for the nasal cavity of cats.

455. **d** Failure of the laryngeal orifice to open and close properly during respiration indicates laryngeal neuromuscular dysfunction.

456. **b** This treatment is for the pulmonary edema that results from electrocution.

457. **a** In asthma, bronchoconstriction is a major contributor to the signs of airway obstruction.

458. **c** With extensive thoracic wall injury, the flail or floating segment of chest wall collapses (rather than expands) on inspiration (negative intrapleural pressure).

459. **d** Stridor is a high-pitched inspiratory sound associated with upper airway (laryngeal) obstruction.

460. **a** Mediastinal and subcutaneous free air originates from an airway leak.

461. **d** Foreign bodies abruptly cause unilateral signs. The other choices are chronic or bilateral.

462. **b** *Campylobacter* infects many animal species and is of public health concern due to the potential for animal-to-human transmission.

463. **b** Metronidazole is not effective against *Salmonella.*

464. **d** Sulfasalazine is specifically indicated for treatment of colonic inflammation.

465. **b** Melena indicates upper gastrointestinal tract bleeding.

466. **a** Histamine from neoplastic mast cells stimulates gastric acid hypersecretion.

467. **c** Inflammatory bowel disease is usually lymphocytic or lymphocytic-plasmacytic.

468. **a** Intestinal adenocarcinomas often appear as circumferential stenosing intramural masses in older cats.

469. **a** Hypovolemia and shock are serious complications of viral gastroenteritis.

470. **e** These drugs enhance rhythmic segmentation contractions, delay transit and reduce mucosal fluid loss in diarrhea.

471. **d** Some cats respond to dietary management, such as hypoallergenic diets.

472. **d** This disease is characterized by a mucosal inflammatory process detected by histopathologic examination but not by radiography.

473. **e** Lactulose is a poorly absorbed disaccharide that induces osmotic catharsis.

474. **b** Mucus is secreted from the abundant goblet cells in the colon in response to local irritation or inflammation.

475. **e** Medical therapy is not effective and the nonfunctional colon must be removed.

476. **c** Serum bile acid determinations are the most sensitive screening test for shunts. The results of other tests of liver function (such as enzymes) are often normal.

477. **e** Cats are inherently resistant to corticosteroid hepatopathy, and it is unlikely to cause jaundice.

478. **e** Cats do not develop a corticosteroid-induced isoenzyme of alkaline phosphatase.

479. **b** Phenytoin is dangerous to cats. Phenobarbital is the preferred anticonvulsant.

480. **c** Acidosis and progressive hyperkalemia are typical of urethral obstruction.

481. **a** *Microsporum canis* is common in cats. The others listed are rare.

482. **c** Even standard human dosages of acetaminophen can be fatally toxic in cats.

483. **a** Azotemia with concentrated urine suggests prerenal azotemia due to dehydration.

484. **d** Cirrhosis is not an effect of taurine deficiency, but the other signs listed do occur.

485. **c** There are many causes, but chronic renal failure is the most common clinical setting for chronic hypokalemia.

486. **c** Each of these 3 is effective in restoring euthyroidism.

487. **a** Excessive thyroxine causes secondary cardiac hypertrophy and cardiomyopathy.

488. **e** Encephalopathy is not a manifestation of hyperthyroidism, whereas the other signs listed are very typical.

489. **c** A corticosteroid-induced isoenzyme of alkaline phosphatase does not occur in cats.

490. **e** Unlike dogs, cats do not develop diabetic cataracts because of a difference in their lens metabolic pathway.

491. **d** Megestrol is a progestational drug used for dermatologic and behavior therapy. It can cause diabetes mellitus in some cats.

492. **d** In this cat, the peak insulin effect (glucose nadir) occurs early and then wanes, as indicated by the afternoon and evening rise in glucose levels. This indicates a short duration of action of the insulin and the need for a longer-acting insulin or twice-daily insulin administration.

493. **b** Ultralente is the longest-acting insulin available.

494. **c** Methimazole can be used to maintain euthyroidism in hyperthyroid cats.

495. **a** Salicylates are very slowly metabolized in the feline species.

496. **d** Acetaminophen toxicity in cats causes methemoglobinemia and Heinz-body anemia.

497. **a** Over 70% of hyperthyroid cats have bilateral adenomas of the thyroid glands.

498. **b**

499. **a** Bilirubinuria is abnormal in any cat and is an important indicator of liver disease.

500. **d** Portosystemic shunts typically have minimal effect on serum bilirubin levels or enzyme activities.

501. **b**

502. **c**

503. **b**

504. **e**

505. **a**

506. **d**

507. **b**

508. **d**

509. **d**

510. **d**

511. **c**

512. **b**

513. **a**

514. **e**

515. **a**

516. **b**

517. **b**

518. **d**

519. **a**

520. **d**

521. **b**

522. **c**

523. **c**

524. **e**

525. **e**

526. **d**

527. **a**

528. **b**

529. **d**

530. **b**

531. **a**

532. **b**

533. **d**

534. **b**

535. **e**

536. **a**

537. **a**

538. **d**

539. **c**

540. **c**

541. **b**

542. **c**

543. **c**

544. **b**

545. **b**

546. **a**

547. **c**

548. **c**

549. **d**

550. **b**

551. **a**

552. **a**

553. **a**

554. **b**

555. **b**

556. **e**

557. **c**

558. **b**

559. **c**

560. **c**

561. **c**

562. **a**

563. **d**

564. **e**

565. **c**

566. **b**

567. **b**

568. **b**

569. **e**

570. **b**

571. **c**

572. **a**

573. **d**

574. **d**

575. **d**

576. **c** Prolonged use of dexamethasone, a relatively long-acting glucocorticoid, may produce Cushingoid signs.

577. **a**

578. **a**

579. **e**

580. **e**

581. **b**

582. **e**

583. **c**

584. **d**

585. **e**

586. **c** Cats contract toxoplasmosis by eating infected mice. Cats usually begin to hunt at 2-12 months of age. Once infected, cats only shed oocysts for 1-2 weeks. Even if reinfected, they do not again shed oocysts.

587. **d**

588. **c**

589. **c**

590. **d**

591. **b**

592. **d**

593. **c**

594. **a**

595. **d**

596. **a** The dog's age and the chronic clinical course strongly suggest a nasal tumor.

597. **a**

598. **d**

599. **e**

600. **e**

601. **b**

602. **a** The key is reduction in virulence while still maintaining viability.

603. **a** gp70 is present in feline leukemia virus, not parvovirus. Parvoviruses have no glycoprotein because they are non-enveloped.

604. **d** FOCMA is a cell membrane antigen and not a viral antigen.

605. **c**

606. **c**

607. **d** The general recommendation is to wait 2 weeks after vaccination, even though immunity may be generated before this time.

608. **c** A 4-fold increase in titer is the general standard for a rising titer.

609. **c** This is the only choice showing a 4-fold increase in titer between samples.

610. **a** CAV-1 (infectious canine hepatitis) vaccines may induce an antigen-antibody reaction in the cornea, producing the "blue eye" reaction.

611. **b** ICH, CHV and CPV are all DNA viruses.

612. **d** FCV, FIP and FeLV are all RNA viruses.

613. **e** Histopathologic examination is the only test that is "diagnostic" for FIP. Lesions are in the kidney.

614. **c** gp70 glycoprotein of the peplomer or spike of the virus is the key immunogen to stimulate neutralizing antibodies against FeLV.

615. **b** All viruses within one serotype are antigenically very similar, and thus stimulate similar antibody titers.

616. **d**

617. **e** ELISA is the most common test for antibodies to FIP virus.

618. **c**

619. **b** Both drugs are commercially available as eye ointments for antiherpes therapy.

620. **a**

621. **b** Antiserum can provide rapid although temporary protection, while MLV vaccines stimulate protection faster than inactivated vaccines.

622. **c** Both measles virus and canine distemper virus are morbilliviruses that stimulate cross-reactive protection.

623. **a**

624. **b** Like herpes simplex of people, local infection results in transport of virus via peripheral nerves to the nerve ganglia, where latent infection is established.

625. **c** FIP antibody titers are not diagnostic, but only indicate previous infection with a coronavirus, possibly FIP virus.

626. **c** Persistent viremia is only rarely reversible (less than 5% of infected cats).

627. **b**

628. **e** Panleukopenia virus may persist for years without a decrease in infectivity.

629. **b** Chlorhexidine is effective against herpesviruses, such as feline herpesvirus, but has no effect on nonenveloped viruses, such as feline calicivirus and parvovirus.

630. **c** Gentamicin and kanamycin remain on the mucosa of the respiratory system much longer than penicillins and other antibiotics, and hence are more effective in aerosols.

631. **d** Aerosol therapy can greatly reduce the number of bacteria and reduce clinical signs.

632. **b** Feline parvovirus requires an actively dividing cell for replication; hence, the clinical signs produced in panleukopenia are related to lysis of replicating cells.

633. **e**

634. **b** While FIP virus was once thought to be labile, studies have shown that the virus can persist up to 7 weeks at room temperature.

635. **b** Transfer only occurs within the first few hours after nursing, until the gut "closes" to antibody uptake.

636. **e** An anamnestic response to rhinotracheitis virus occurs at 21 days, but not if the vaccine is given earlier. Hence, one should not give 2 rhinotracheitis vaccines sooner than 3 weeks apart.

637. **e** They may be given by various routes, depending on the specific vaccine.

638. **b** Feline herpesvirus-1 is the most common cause of ulcers on the cornea of cats.

639. **c** Some strains of calicivirus commonly cause tongue ulcers.

640. **a**

641. **b**

642. **c** *Salmonella* may cause subclinical infections, but also may produce fatal infections.

643. **c** Because cats are frequently exposed to panleukopenia virus almost immediately upon entering some shelters, the efficacy of vaccines and antiserum (though rarely used now) are directly related to the speed of antibody induction.

644. **d**

645. **a** It is caused by *Mycobacterium lepraemurium*.

646. **c** Feline herpesvirus is quite labile and rapidly inactivated, but it may take a few days to completely inactivate the virus.

647. **d** Rabies virus excretion in infected cats and dogs begins shortly before clinical signs appear.

648. **b** FeLV infection of the crypt cells of the small intestine produces a chronic panleukopenia-like syndrome, in that the same cells are destroyed as in panleukopenia.

649. **a** Particles $<5\,\mu$ in diameter remain in aerosols until they reach the lung.

650. **e**

651. **d**

652. **b**

653. **d** Multivalent vaccines are commonly used. Each multivalent vaccine must be tested for possible interference between multiple components before licensure.

654. **b** Inactivated vaccines are safer for use in pregnant cats than modified-live-virus vaccines.

655. **e** Arbitrarily, 12 weeks has been selected as the cut-off for persistent viremia.

656. **c** Rabies virus, herpesvirus and morbilliviruses are enveloped and thus very susceptible to disinfectants.

657. **b**

658. **c**

659. **e** The serum neutralization test is very sensitive and specific.

660. **c**

661. **c** ELISAs can be set up to detect antibody and/or antigen.

662. **c** Canine parvovirus is very resistant to most disinfectants.

663. **e**

664. **b**

665. **c** While Negri bodies do occur in neurons of cats with rabies, histopathologic examination is no longer used routinely to diagnose rabies.

666. **e** The virus is single-stranded, non-enveloped, and resistant to most disinfectants.

667. **c** One cannot determine the time of infection from a single IgG antibody titer.

668. **e**

669. **c** Indirect fluorescent antibody testing detects virus or antigen within cells but not in fluid samples.

670. **c** The initial FIV test detected anti-FIV antibodies.

671. **e**

672. **c** All cats with clinical panleukopenia have leukopenia during the early acute phase.

673. **a**

674. **c** Clorox is highly effective against parvovirus.

675. **c**

676. **b** Modified-live-virus vaccines produce faster protection. One could use an approved intranasal modified-live-virus vaccine as well.

677. **e** Vaccinate as soon as possible. Time is critical.

678. **a**

679. **e**

680. **b**

681. **c**

682. **e**

683. **d**

684. **c**

685. **d**

686. **b**

687. **b**

688. **d** Dental disease is not directly related to diseases causing polyuria and polydipsia.

689. **b**

690. **d**

691. **a**

692. **c**

693. **e** The test for parvovirus infection is used on sick dogs, not as a screening test.

694. **c** Appetite is not necessarily a good indicator of small bowel versus large bowel disease.

695. **c**

696. **c**

697. **b**

698. **a**

699. **d**

700. **f**

701. **e**

702. **c**

703. **e**

704. **e** This cat is at least 8% dehydrated.

705. **d** A head tilt could be due to damage to the vestibular system, not the spinal cord.

706. **d** Lameness is not pertinent to this case.

707. **c** The vast majority of gastroenteritis is self-limiting.

708. **c** Ability to regulate body temperature takes several weeks to develop.

709. **d**

710. **c**

711. **c**

712. **b**

713. **a** Thoracic radiographs are useful to assess the degree of disease. Serum chemistry assays are useful to assess liver and kidney function before starting treatment.

714. **d**

715. **c**

716. **e**

717. **d**

718. **c** Shock causes a marked sympathetic response.

719. **e**

720. **d**

721. **a**

722. **b**

723. **c**

724. **c**

725. **d** The other tumors listed are relatively common skin tumors.

726. **d**

727. **d** Culture and sensitivity tests are the best way to determine which antibiotic is appropriate for treatment.

728. **c** This 8-week-old puppy is not old enough to develop problems from whipworm infection, as the prepatent period is 3 months.

729. **d**

730. **c**

731. **b**

732. **a**

733. **c** Parainfluenza virus, adenovirus or herpesvirus may act in concert with the bacterium *Bordetella bronchiseptica.*

734. **a**

735. **c** It takes approximately 6 months after infection for microfilariae to appear in the blood.

736. **c**

737. **d** Feline leukemia virus infection may indirectly cause upper respiratory disease through immunosuppression, allowing secondary bacterial infection.

738. **a** 55 lb = 25 kg. A dosage of 2 mg/kg = 2 x 25 = 50 mg. A 5% solution contains 5000 mg/dl, or 50 mg/ml. Therefore, the dog should receive 1 ml of the 5% furosemide solution.

739. **b** 28 lb = approximately 12.5 kg. 0.08 x 12.5 = approximately 1 kg, which, in fluid weight, is equivalent to 1 L (1000 ml). Not mentioned in the question, but also necessary to consider when treating with fluids, are maintenance needs and continuity losses (vomiting, diarrhea).

740. **d** Weight gain in the face of rehydration indicates overhydration. This is the earliest clinical sign. By the time other signs develop, life-threatening overhydration may be occurring.

741. **a** 360 ml ÷ 24 hours = 15 ml/hour. 60 drops = 1 ml. 60 drops x 15 ml = 900 drops. 900 drops ÷ 60 minutes = 15 drops/minute.

742. **c**

743. **b** The solution contains very small amounts of B vitamins, but a major percentage will be dextrose. Dextrose solutions of greater than 10% are too hyperosmolar for safe infusion into peripheral veins. The catheter should be a dedicated line and *never* used for intravenous medication. Frequent monitoring, particularly of blood glucose, PCV, total protein and electrolytes, is vital to successful total parenteral nutrition. Strict asepsis must be used; ideally a vented hood should be used to mix solutions in sterile containers not exposed to room air.

744. **c** This dog may have gastric dilatation-volvulus, an emergency situation that frequently requires surgery.

745. **c**

746. **c**

747. **b** Though less readily available than whole blood, packed red blood cells provide a higher concentration of red blood cells. They are useful for treatment of animals with acute blood loss, after fluid volume has already been replaced.

748. **c**

Notes

Notes

Notes

Section

8

Neurology

J.N. Kornegay

Recommended Reading

de Lahunta A: *Veterinary Neuroanatomy and Clinical Neurology.* 2nd ed. Saunders, Philadelphia, 1983.

Fraser CM: *The Merck Veterinary Manual.* 7th ed. Merck, Rahway, NJ, 1991. pp 564-626.

Kornegay JN: Neurologic disorders. *Contemp Issues Sm Anim Pract* 5:1992.

Kornegay JN: Feline neurology. *Prob Vet Med* 3:1991.

Oliver JE and Lorenz MD: *Handbook of Veterinary Neurologic Diagnosis.* Saunders, Philadelphia, 1983.

Practice answer sheet is on page 345.

Questions

1. *What are the principal muscle, peripheral nerve and spinal cord segments involved in the patellar reflex?*

   a. quadriceps femoris, femoral nerve, spinal cord segments L6-S1

   b. biceps femoris, femoral nerve, spinal cord segments L4-L6

   c. quadriceps femoris, sciatic nerve, spinal cord segments L4-L6

   d. biceps femoris, sciatic nerve, spinal cord segments L6-S1

   e. quadriceps femoris, femoral nerve, spinal cord segments L4-L6

2. *Which group of clinical signs is typical of lower motor neuron paralysis?*

   a. paralysis, hyperreflexia, hypotonus, severe muscle atrophy

   b. paralysis, hyporeflexia, hypertonus, mild muscle atrophy

   c. paralysis, hyporeflexia, hypotonus, severe muscle atrophy

   d. paralysis, hyperreflexia, hypertonus, mild muscle atrophy

   e. paralysis, hyporeflexia, hypotonus, mild muscle atrophy

---

Correct answers are on page 190.

3. The sensory distribution of the median nerve is to the:

   a. medial aspect of the palmar (caudal) aspect of the paw, distal to the carpus
   b. lateral aspect of the palmar (caudal) aspect of the paw, distal to the carpus
   c. medial aspect of the dorsal aspect of the paw, distal to the carpus
   d. lateral aspect of the dorsal antebrachium, proximal to the carpus
   e. medial aspect of the palmar (caudal) antebrachium, proximal to the carpus

4. On examination of a dog with progressive difficulty in using the right pelvic limb, you note that the dog drags this limb while walking. The right biceps femoris, cranial tibialis and gastrocnemius muscles are markedly atrophied. Postural reactions are absent in this limb but normal in the other 3 limbs. The patellar reflex in the affected limb is normal; however, the flexion and cranial tibialis reflexes are absent. Pain sensation is present in the medial digit but absent in the lateral digits. You find no hyperesthesia when the limb is examined. Based on these findings, you conclude that the most likely site of the lesion is in the:

   a. right femoral nerve
   b. L6-S1 spinal cord segments on midline
   c. bones of the right pelvic limb
   d. right sciatic nerve
   e. L4-L6 spinal cord segments on the right side

5. A dog is admitted to your hospital because of acute inability to use its pelvic limbs. You determine that conscious proprioception and the hopping reaction are absent in the pelvic limbs but normal in the thoracic limbs. The patellar and flexion reflexes are normal to slightly accentuated in the pelvic limbs. Pain sensation is absent in the pelvic limbs, and panniculus reflex is absent caudal to approximately the thoracolumbar junction. Based on these findings, you conclude that the most likely site of the lesion is the:

   a. L4-L6 spinal cord segments
   b. T2-L3 spinal cord segments
   c. C1-C5 spinal cord segments

   d. L6-S3 spinal cord segments
   e. coxofemoral joint on both sides

6. A cat is admitted to your hospital because of recent onset of head tilt to the right and horizontal jerk nystagmus, with the fast phase directed to the left. The cat is disoriented and seems slightly depressed. On evaluation of gait, the cat is ataxic and occasionally falls to the right. Conscious proprioception and the hopping reaction are normal on the left side but depressed on the right. The cat does not close its right eye when threatening gestures are made, and the right palpebral reflex is absent. All other cranial nerve functions are normal. Which area of the nervous system is affected?

   a. right peripheral vestibular system
   b. left brainstem
   c. right brainstem
   d. left peripheral vestibular system
   e. left and right peripheral vestibular system

7. In dogs, sacral spinal cord segments overlie which vertebral body?

   a. sacrum
   b. L7
   c. L6
   d. L5
   e. L4

8. Which clinical feature may be present in brachial plexus avulsion but is **not** present with radial nerve paralysis?

   a. loss of pain sensation over the dorsal aspect of the paw
   b. loss of the extensor carpi radialis reflex
   c. loss of the panniculus reflex on the side of the lesion
   d. abrasion of the dorsal aspect of the paw
   e. severe atrophy of the triceps brachii muscle

9. A 7-year-old male Labrador Retriever is admitted to your hospital with a history of progressive difficulty in walking with its pelvic limbs during the past 2 months. Your neurologic examination reveals depressed hopping

and conscious proprioception in the pelvic limbs, but these are normal in the thoracic limbs. The patellar reflexes are depressed bilaterally; pelvic limb flexion and the perineal reflex are normal. Pain sensation in the pelvic limbs is present. The panniculus reflex is normal. You note no hyperesthesia on spinal palpation, but the dog is stoic and does not readily respond to pain. No other abnormalities are identified on physical examination. The dog spends a lot of time outside without supervision, but the owners know of no trauma. Your differential diagnoses should include which group of diseases?

a. degenerative myelopathy, diskospondylitis, type-2 disk disease, lumbosacral malformation-malarticulation (cauda equina syndrome)

b. diskospondylitis, degenerative myelopathy, vertebral neoplasia, fibrocartilaginous embolism

c. degenerative myelopathy, fibrocartilaginous embolism, lumbosacral malformation-malarticulation (cauda equina syndrome), type-2 disk disease

d. diskospondylitis, vertebral neoplasia, vertebral fracture, type-2 disk disease

e. degenerative myelopathy, diskospondylitis, type-2 disk disease, vertebral neoplasia

10. *A 6-year-old female Great Dane is admitted to your hospital with a history of acute difficulty in walking. The dog was in a fenced yard when the owners left for work and could not stand when they returned. On neurologic examination, you find that hopping and conscious proprioception are normal on the left side in the thoracic and pelvic limbs but markedly depressed on the right. The dog is alert and cranial nerve reflexes are normal. All spinal reflexes are normal except for those of the right thoracic limb, which are depressed. There is no hyperesthesia on palpation of the cervical spine. The dog's condition gradually improves without treatment but the dog is left with paresis involving the right thoracic limb. The most likely cause of these signs is:*

a. fibrocartilaginous embolism

b. caudal cervical vertebral malformation-malarticulation

c. spinal trauma

d. vertebral neoplasia

e. type-1 disk disease

11. *A 5-year-old male Doberman Pinscher is admitted to your hospital with a history of progressive difficulty in walking during the past 5 days. On neurologic examination, you find that hopping is depressed in all 4 limbs. When you knuckle the dog's paws, it attempts to replace them but cannot. Attitude is normal but you suspect that the palpebral reflex is slightly depressed bilaterally, and jaw tone also seems weak. The dog has no evidence of hyperesthesia and is otherwise normal. You refer the dog to a local specialist, who finds no evidence of denervation on an electromyogram. You find several ticks on the dog and dip the animal twice, but signs do not improve. The dog remains in your hospital for 3 weeks, during which time it gradually returns to normal. The most likely cause of these signs is:*

a. polymyositis

b. botulism

c. myasthenia gravis

d. coonhound paralysis

e. tick paralysis

12. *Which segment of the lower motor neuron is affected by coonhound paralysis?*

a. dorsal spinal nerve roots and sensory axons of peripheral nerves

b. neuromuscular junctions

c. skeletal muscles

d. ventral spinal nerve roots and motor axons of peripheral nerves

e. ventral horn cells of the spinal cord

13. *Concerning degenerative myelopathy of German Shepherds and other large-breed dogs, which statement is most accurate?*

a. It affects middle-aged or older dogs.

b. It causes slowly progressive tetraparesis.

c. Most affected dogs have urinary and fecal incontinence.

d. Pain sensation is frequently lost due to dorsal root involvement.

e. Hyperesthesia is a frequent finding.

Correct answers are on page 190.

14. *Concerning the pathogenesis of diskospondylitis in dogs, organisms usually gain access to the vertebral column:*

 a. through direct extension from dermal lesions overlying or adjacent to the spine
 b. through hematogenous spread from infections elsewhere in the body
 c. by following fistulous tracts extending to and from the spine because of foreign body migration
 d. following contamination of surgical wounds after spinal surgery
 e. after initially localizing in epidural hematomas resulting from intervertebral disk herniation

15. *Which group of clinical signs is most compatible with a diagnosis of lumbosacral malformation-malarticulation?*

 a. paraparesis, depressed patellar reflexes, hyperesthesia on palpation of the caudal lumbar spine, urinary-fecal incontinence
 b. paraparesis, depressed pelvic limb flexor and perineal reflexes, no evidence of hyper-esthesia, normal urinary-fecal continence
 c. paraparesis, depressed patellar reflexes, no evidence of hyperesthesia, urinary-fecal incontinence
 d. paraparesis, normal spinal reflexes, hyperesthesia on palpation of the caudal lumbar spine, normal urinary-fecal continence
 e. paraparesis, depressed pelvic limb flexor and perineal reflexes, hyperesthesia on palpation of the caudal lumbar spine, urinary-fecal incontinence

16. *The breed most likely to have type-2 disk disease is the:*

 a. Beagle
 b. Pekingese
 c. Miniature Poodle
 d. Labrador Retriever
 e. Dachshund

17. *Concerning caudal cervical vertebral malformation-malarticulation (wobbler syndrome) in dogs, which statement is most accurate?*

 a. It is typically seen in 5- to 8-year-old Great Danes.
 b. It usually affects either the C3-C4 or C4-C5 vertebrae.
 c. Lower motor neuron signs in the thoracic limbs usually are restricted to atrophy of the infraspinatus and supraspinatus muscles.
 d. Because of the inherent risks of myelography, the decision to perform surgery should be based strictly on characteristic radiographic changes seen on survey radiographs.
 e. Surgical procedures used to treat the syndrome are relatively benign and rarely cause clinical deterioration.

18. *Concerning the pathogenesis of tick paralysis in dogs, toxin produced by the tick:*

 a. causes segmental demyelination
 b. inhibits presynaptic release of acetylcholine at the neuromuscular junctions
 c. affects muscle antigenicity, resulting in polymyositis
 d. causes degeneration of receptors on the muscle side of the neuromuscular junctions
 e. binds calcium, thereby preventing muscle relaxation

19. *Which dog breeds are affected with congenital myasthenia gravis?*

 a. Tibetan Mountain Dogs, Brittany Spaniels, Labrador Retrievers
 b. English Setters, Basset Hounds, Samoyeds
 c. Lhasa Apsos, Pekingese, German Shepherds
 d. English Bulldogs, Boston Terriers, Poulies
 e. Jack Russell Terriers, Smooth-Haired Fox Terriers, Springer Spaniels

20. *The clinical sign **least** likely to be observed in an animal with hydrocephalus is:*

 a. blindness
 b. intention tremor
 c. circling

d. altered mental attitude

e. compulsive walking

21. *Concerning neurologic signs associated with feline infectious peritonitis, which statement is most accurate?*

    a. Neurologic signs are usually associated with the dry (noneffusive) form of the disease.

    b. A positive fluorescent antibody test always indicates infection with the coronavirus causing feline infectious peritonitis.

    c. Neurologic signs usually improve dramatically following administration of glucocorticoids, and generally do not recur.

    d. Results of cerebrospinal fluid evaluation are usually normal.

    e. Only cats older than 3 years of age have shown neurologic signs with feline infectious peritonitis.

22. *Which clinical findings are most typical of cerebellar hypoplasia or dysplasia?*

    a. dysmetria and intention tremor that gradually improve, with the animal becoming normal by 1 year of age

    b. head tilt and nystagmus that do not resolve or worsen

    c. dysmetria and intention tremor that gradually worsen

    d. head tilt and nystagmus that gradually improve, with the animal becoming normal by 1 year of age

    e. dysmetria and intention tremor that do not resolve or worsen

23. *Concerning granulomatous meningoencephalitis (reticulosis) in dogs, which statement is most accurate?*

    a. Glucocorticoids are of no benefit in treatment.

    b. Neurologic deficits usually are not progressive.

    c. Poodles seem to be predisposed, and females are affected more commonly than males.

    d. Results of cerebrospinal fluid evaluation are normal in most affected dogs.

e. Lesions are most common in the gray matter of the cerebrum.

24. *Concerning the breed incidence of spinal cord diseases, which statement is most accurate?*

    a. Degenerative myelopathy occurs most commonly in Dachshunds.

    b. Caudal cervical vertebral malformation-malarticulation (wobbler syndrome) occurs most commonly in Dalmatians and Golden Retrievers.

    c. Spina bifida and associated dysraphic spinal cord lesions occur most commonly in English Bulldogs and Manx cats.

    d. Type-1 intervertebral disk disease occurs most commonly in Cocker Spaniels.

    e. Diskospondylitis occurs most commonly in miniature breeds of dogs.

25. *Which clinical sign is typical of foramen magnum brain herniation but is **not** a feature of caudal transtentorial brain herniation occurring alone?*

    a. apnea

    b. tetraplegia

    c. pupillary dilatation

    d. coma

    e. all of the above are features of both forms of brain herniation

26. *Concerning otitis media-interna in dogs and cats, which statement is most accurate?*

    a. The most common cause is extension of infection from the oral cavity through the auditory tube.

    b. Though some animals have concomitant otitis externa, signs rarely suggest external ear involvement.

    c. Nystagmus and ataxia usually are permanent, despite resolution of the infection.

    d. There may be fluid within the middle ear, as indicated radiographically by increased density of the tympanic bulla.

    e. Systemic antibiotics must be used in combination with topical therapy.

Correct answers are on page 190.

27. *Concerning idiopathic peripheral vestibular disease in cats, which statement is most accurate?*

   a. Occasionally it occurs after urinary tract infections, suggesting a possible bacterial cause.
   b. It occurs most commonly in late winter and early spring.
   c. Clinical signs usually do not resolve, but affected cats accommodate so that they are functional.
   d. Clinical involvement is always bilateral.
   e. One characteristic feature of bilateral involvement is loss of oculovestibular eye movements.

28. *Concerning distemper encephalitis in dogs, which statement is most accurate?*

   a. The different strains of canine distemper virus have remarkably similar virulence and tissue predilection.
   b. Demyelination generally develops in immunocompetent pups, as opposed to neuronal necrosis, which is seen more typically in immunodeficient pups.
   c. Dogs with neurologic involvement always have signs of systemic disease (fever, anorexia, etc) before manifesting neurologic dysfunction.
   d. Marked lymphocytosis is often seen, at times leading to a misdiagnosis of leukemia.
   e. All dogs with the neurologic form of canine distemper die, regardless of treatment.

29. *Concerning cranial trauma in dogs and cats, which statement is most accurate?*

   a. Brain injury with cranial trauma is more common in dogs than in cats.
   b. Affected animals almost always have hematomas that require surgical drainage.
   c. Shock should be treated only after specific steps have been taken to manage the effects of cranial trauma, so as to avoid brain herniation.
   d. Focal subpial brain hemorrhage with minimal malacia is termed contusion.
   e. Use of osmotic diuretics is always contraindicated in animals with cranial trauma because of the potential for induction of shock.

30. *The anticonvulsant preferred for long-term seizure control in dogs is:*

   a. primidone
   b. diphenylhydantoin (phenytoin)
   c. phenobarbital
   d. diazepam
   e. valproic acid

31. *Concerning seizures in dogs and cats, which statement is most accurate?*

   a. The most common form is the petit mal seizure.
   b. Partial seizures begin and usually remain relatively confined to a focal area of the brain.
   c. The process whereby exposure of normal neurons to spontaneous discharges increases their own inherent excitability is termed epileptogenesis.
   d. Animals with even a single seizure should be treated with long-term anticonvulsant medication to lessen the likelihood of subsequent seizures.
   e. Absorption and metabolism of anticonvulsants in dogs is consistent from dog to dog, so that there is no need to measure actual serum levels of the drug.

32. *Which drugs should be used in treatment of status epilepticus in dogs and cats?*

   a. phenobarbital, primidone
   b. diazepam, diphenylhydantoin (phenytoin)
   c. phenobarbital, diazepam
   d. primidone, diphenylhydantoin
   e. halothane, primidone

33. *Concerning cerebellar hypoplasia due to in-utero panleukopenia virus infection in cats, which statement is most accurate?*

   a. Though the cerebellum of affected cats is hypoplastic, clinical dysfunction is principally related to cerebrocortical dysfunction because of additional involvement there.
   b. The virus apparently has a direct cytopathic effect on neurons within the molecular and granule cell layers.

c. Signs of cerebellar hypoplasia are nonprogressive, which helps distinguish this condition from cerebellar abiotrophies.

d. The virus causes vasculitis, which may lead to *in-utero* thrombosis and infarction of the cerebellum and other areas of the nervous system.

e. Cerebellar hypoplasia is a minomer because, though microscopic lesions can be appreciated, the cerebellum usually is grossly normal.

34. *Concerning vasogenic brain edema, which statement is most accurate?*

a. The principal cause is hypoxia.

b. It primarily affects gray matter.

c. Fluid accumulates extracellularly.

d. It occurs subsequent to hydrocephalus.

e. It does not result in actual enlargement of the cerebrum.

35. *Concerning epidural and subdural hematomas in dogs and cats, which statement is most accurate?*

a. They are most commonly associated with inflammatory diseases causing vasculitis, with subsequent rupture of meningeal vessels.

b. They are commonly associated with cranial trauma.

c. They generally form soon after trauma but may not be manifested clinically for hours to days.

d. Epidural hematomas usually form after exteriorization of intracerebral hemorrhage.

e. Subdural hematomas have little clinical significance because they are usually of small volume.

36. *Neuronophagia is defined as a:*

a. process whereby neurons may themselves actively phagocytize cell debris, especially in instances of ischemic injury

b. process whereby neurons dedifferentiate to become glial cells, such as astrocytes

c. preneoplastic phase of neurons before development of neuroblastoma

d. process whereby necrotic neurons are removed by phagocytes

e. process whereby neurons contribute actively to resolution of vasogenic edema by imbibing fluid

37. *Concerning oligodendrogliomas in dogs, which statement is most accurate?*

a. They are most common is dolichocephalic breeds.

b. They usually affect young to middle-aged dogs.

c. They are generally gray and well demarcated grossly.

d. They most commonly involve the cerebrum.

e. They do not affect the ventricular system.

38. *Polymyositis in dogs is:*

a. a heritable degenerative myopathy especially prevalent in German Short-Haired Pointers

b. an inflammatory, immune-mediated myopathy potentially induced by certain viruses, *Toxoplasma gondii,* neoplasia or certain drugs

c. a myopathy of old dogs, typically causing a high erythrocyte sedimentation rate

d. usually associated with saddle embolism of the caudal aorta, with infarction and muscle necrosis

e. associated with antibodies to acetylcholine receptors at the neuromuscular junction

39. *Gliosis is a:*

a. process whereby astrocytes, oligodendroglia and microglial cells proliferate in response to neuronal injury

b. process whereby endothelial cells become hyperplastic subsequent to hypoxia

c. process whereby astrocytes become hyperplastic and hypertrophied due to a variety of diseases

d. process whereby neurons and astrocytes "communicate" through membranal attachments

e. process whereby microglia remove necrotic neurons

Correct answers are on page 190.

40. *Which of the following statements correctly distinguishes pseudolaminar cerebrocortical necrosis from laminar cerebrocortical necrosis?*

   a. Laminar cerebrocortical necrosis refers to necrosis of neurons in a single layer, while pseudolaminar cerebrocortical necrosis refers to an artifactual neuronal change associated with poor fixation.

   b. Laminar cerebrocortical necrosis refers to necrosis of a single layer of neurons, while pseudolaminar cerebrocortical necrosis refers to necrosis of multiple layers of neurons.

   c. Laminar cerebrocortical necrosis refers to necrosis of alternate layers of neurons, while pseudolaminar cerebrocortical necrosis refers to vacuoles occurring around neurons due to cytotoxic edema.

   d. Laminar cerebrocortical necrosis refers to necrosis of multiple layers of neurons, while pseudolaminar cerebrocortical necrosis refers to necrosis of a single layer.

   e. Laminar cerebrocortical necrosis refers to necrosis of layers 3 and 5 of the cerebral cortex, while pseudolaminar cerebrocortical necrosis refers to the changes in cerebrocortical neurons induced by injury to brainstem neurons.

41. *Hypoxic hypoxia is related to:*

   a. reduced PaO_2
   b. depleted blood hemoglobin
   c. impaired blood flow in certain areas of the cerebrum
   d. reduced cardiac output
   e. impaired tissue utilization of oxygen

42. *Which types of diseases typically cause lesions that are insidious in onset, gradually progress, and diffusely involve the nervous system?*

   a. vascular, neoplastic, inflammatory
   b. degenerative, inflammatory, metabolic
   c. inflammatory, toxic, traumatic
   d. neoplastic, degenerative, metabolic
   e. metabolic, traumatic, vascular

43. *Which one of the following is **not** a site at which lesions may cause obstructive (noncommunicating) hydrocephalus?*

   a. interventricular foramina between the lateral and 3rd ventricles
   b. 3rd ventricle
   c. mesencephalic aqueduct
   d. lateral aperture of 4th ventricle
   e. arachnoid villi

44. *Leptomeningitis is characterized by inflammation of the:*

   a. arachnoid and pia mater
   b. dura mater
   c. pia mater and dura mater
   d. arachnoid, dura mater and pia mater
   e. dura mater and arachnoid

45. *Which of the following is **not** a typical histologic feature of most forms of viral encephalitis?*

   a. perivascular cuffs of lymphocytes
   b. central chromatolysis
   c. microglial nodules
   d. gliosis
   e. nonsuppurative encephalitis

46. *Concerning meningiomas in dogs, which statement is most accurate?*

   a. They are friable, red and poorly demarcated on gross examination.
   b. They usually have features of malignancy.
   c. They occur most commonly at the cerebellopontine angle.
   d. They are most common in young to middle-aged dogs.
   e. They are most common in dolichocephalic breeds.

47. *What is the most detrimental potential danger of subfalcial brain herniation?*

   a. Infarction of the cingulate gyrus may lead to significant motor deficits.
   b. Infarction of the cingulate gyrus may lead to edema and hemorrhage, which could lead to other forms of brain herniation.
   c. Infarction of the cingulate gyrus often causes collapse of the interventricular foramen,

with resulting unilateral obstructive hydrocephalus.

d. Infarction of the cingulate gyrus often leads to loss of memory, such that the dog may no longer recognize its owners and is no longer housetrained.

e. Infarction of the cingulate gyrus creates a potential focus in which organisms may settle, leading to abscess formation.

48. *Concerning caudal transtentorial and foramen magnum brain herniation, which statement is most accurate?*

  a. Both usually do not cause significant paresis because brainstem compression occurs gradually.

  b. Both usually are self-limiting.

  c. Both typically cause compression of the mesencephalic aqueduct, which may lead to obstructive hydrocephalus.

  d. Both never occur concomitantly in an animal because of autoregulation of blood supply.

  e. Both often cause stupor because of involvement of the reticular activating system or its ascending input to the cerebrum.

49. *Concerning malignant hyperthermia, which statement is most accurate?*

  a. It is associated with accumulation of excessive chloride in the sarcoplasm of muscle.

  b. It is often induced by anesthetic agents, especially methoxyflurane.

  c. Muscles of affected animals become extremely hard and swollen.

  d. Serum creatine kinase activity is not elevated in affected animals because of the disease's rapidly progressive nature.

  e. It is strictly a biochemical lesion, with no histologic lesions seen.

50. *Which microscopic feature is **not** typical of myopathies?*

  a. variation of fiber size

  b. increased numbers of central nuclei

  c. proliferation of fibrous connective tissue

  d. hyalinized fibers

  e. numerous small, angulated fibers

51. *Concerning polymyositis in dogs, which statement is most accurate?*

  a. It is usually manifested as muscle weakness without evidence of muscle pain.

  b. On histologic examination of muscle, neutrophils usually predominate in the lesion.

  c. Muscle biopsies from some affected dogs may be histologically normal.

  d. Organisms that may induce immune-mediated destruction of muscle include *Trichinella spiralis* and *Leptospira*.

  e. Unlike degenerative myopathies, in which megaesophagus may develop, the esophagus is not affected in polymyositis.

52. *Which microscopic feature is **not** typical of normal neurons?*

  a. have a prominent nucleolus

  b. contain Nissl substance

  c. larger than glial cells

  d. have faintly eosinophilic cytoplasm

  e. arranged in layers in the cortex

53. *Which histologic changes are seen with muscle regeneration?*

  a. hyalinized fibers, variation in myofiber size

  b. basophilic myofibers, proliferating muscle nuclei

  c. basophilic myofibers, hyalinized myofibers

  d. proliferating muscle nuclei, fibrosis

  e. fibrosis, variation in myofiber size

54. *Which features characterize type-1 muscle myofibers?*

  a. "red" muscle, fast twitch, oxidative

  b. "white" muscle, slow twitch, nonoxidative

  c. "red" muscle, slow twitch, oxidative

  d. "white" muscle, fast twitch, oxidative

  e. "white" muscle, slow twitch, oxidative

Correct answers are on page 190.

Answers

1. **e**		28. **b**
2. **c**		29. **d**
3. **a**		30. **c**
4. **d**		31. **b**
5. **b**		32. **c**
6. **c**		33. **c**
7. **d**		34. **c**
8. **c**		35. **c**
9. **e**		36. **d**
10. **a**		37. **d**
11. **b**		38. **b**
12. **d**		39. **c**
13. **a**		40. **b**
14. **b**		41. **a**
15. **e**		42. **b**
16. **d**		43. **e**
17. **c**		44. **a**
18. **b**		45. **a**
19. **e**		46. **e**
20. **b**		47. **b**
21. **a**		48. **e**
22. **e**		49. **c**
23. **c**		50. **e**
24. **c**		51. **c**
25. **a**		52. **d**
26. **d**		53. **b**
27. **e**		54. **c**

Oncology

S.M. Cotter, E.T. Keller

Recommended Reading

Duncan JR and Prasse KW: *Veterinary Laboratory Medicine.* 2nd ed. Iowa State University Press, Ames, 1986.
Ettinger S: *Textbook of Veterinary Internal Medicine.* 3rd ed. Saunders, Philadelphia, 1990.
Kirk RW and Bonagura JD: *Current Veterinary Therapy XI.* Saunders, Philadelphia, 1992.
Theilen GH and Madewell BR: *Veterinary Cancer Medicine.* 2nd ed. Lea & Febiger, Philadelphia, 1987.
Withrow SJ and MacEwen EG: *Clinical Veterinary Oncology.* Lippincott, Philadelphia, 1989.

Practice answer sheet is on page 347.

Questions

1. Which of the following drugs is **least** nephrotoxic?

   a. amphotericin B
   b. vincristine
   c. amikacin
   d. cisplatin
   e. gentamicin

2. Chemotherapy with cyclophosphamide most commonly induces:

   a. cardiotoxicity
   b. pancreatitis
   c. hemorrhagic cystitis
   d. pulmonary fibrosis
   e. peripheral neuropathy

3. Which metabolic abnormality is **not** commonly associated with tumor lysis syndrome?

   a. hyperkalemia
   b. hyperuricemia
   c. hyperphosphatemia
   d. hyponatremia
   e. hypocalcemia

4. Which of the following is **not** a valid reason for radiation therapy of a spinal cord tumor?

   a. the patient is unable to tolerate surgery
   b. the tumor is grossly inoperable
   c. the lesions are widely separated along the spine
   d. the tumor is radiosensitive
   e. previous radiotherapy for this spinal tumor has failed

Correct answers are on pages 200-202.

5. *For long-term control of hypercalcemia in an animal with neoplasia, the most effective therapy is:*

    a. intravenous fluids
    b. diuretics
    c. corticosteroids
    d. antineoplastic therapy
    e. calcitonin

6. *Which drug is indicated for a dog that has received an adrenalectomy for adrenal carcinoma?*

    a. potassium chloride
    b. amikacin
    c. dexamethasone
    d. piperazine
    e. lysodren

7. *The tumor most likely to be associated with hypoglycemia is:*

    a. insulinoma
    b. lymphosarcoma
    c. osteosarcoma
    d. melanoma
    e. lipoma

8. *Which tumor is most likely to be associated with hypertension?*

    a. Sertoli-cell tumor
    b. pheochromocytoma
    c. lymphoma
    d. hemangiosarcoma
    e. adenocarcinoma

9. *A dog is presented for weakness. Physical examination demonstrates pale mucous membranes. A complete blood count shows anemia, schistocytes and nucleated red blood cells. The tumor most compatible with these findings is:*

    a. splenic hemangiosarcoma
    b. lymphoma
    c. multiple myeloma

    d. hepatic adenocarcinoma
    e. interstitial-cell tumor of the testicle

10. *An owner presents her dog because of exercise intolerance. You test the dog and observe that it collapses upon exercise. This collapse is immediately reversed by edrophonium hydrochloride, suggesting a diagnosis of myasthenia gravis. The tumor most likely to cause these signs is:*

    a. pancreatic islet-cell carcinoma
    b. lymphoma
    c. thymoma
    d. prostatic adenocarcinoma
    e. malignant melanoma

11. *Initial treatment of multiple metastases is best performed using:*

    a. any well-known chemotherapeutic agent
    b. a combination of doxorubicin, cyclophosphamide and vincristine
    c. a chemotherapeutic agent effective against the primary tumor
    d. L-asparaginase
    e. resection, followed by whole-body irradiation

12. *Metastasis:*

    a. is more common via hematogenous vs lymphatic routes
    b. is a random-chance event
    c. is a complex series of biologic steps
    d. is most likely to affect the first organ contacted by the primary tumor
    e. always involves the regional lymph node first

13. *Spirocerca lupi infection is associated with osteosarcoma and fibrosarcoma in the:*

    a. liver
    b. lungs
    c. brain
    d. esophagus
    e. ear

14. In dogs, the biologic behavior of hemangio-pericytoma is commonly characterized by:

a. pulmonary metastases
b. regional lymph node metastases
c. local recurrence after resection
d. moderate recurrence of hypercalcemia
e. a well-encapsulated, readily excisable mass

15. The most common syndrome associated with hemangiosarcoma is:

a. disseminated intravascular coagulation
b. hypercalcemia
c. myasthenia gravis
d. polyuria and polydipsia
e. hyponatremia

16. Which of the following is **least** likely to cause neutropenia and leukopenia in dogs with cancer?

a. chemotherapy
b. immune-mediated mechanisms
c. myelophthisis (infiltration of bone marrow with cancer cells)
d. disseminated intravascular coagulation
e. hypersplenism

17. Pancytopenia (absence of all 3 cell lines in the peripheral blood) is most likely to be associated with:

a. hemolytic disease
b. disseminated intravascular coagulation
c. myelophthisis (infiltration of bone marrow with cancer cells)
d. gastrointestinal ulcer
e. initiation of chemotherapy

18. Which of the following is **not** associated with diminished platelet production?

a. myelophthisis
b. estrogen-secreting Sertoli-cell tumor
c. chemotherapy
d. disseminated intravascular coagulation
e. myelodysplasia

19. Mycosis fungoides is best described as a lesion of abnormal lymphocytes arising in the:

a. spleen
b. skin
c. liver
d. lung
e. kidney

20. Which of the following is most likely to be observed in a dog with mast-cell tumors?

a. monoclonal gammopathy
b. elevated serum creatine phosphokinase activity
c. occult blood in feces
d. leukocytosis
e. low urine specific gravity

21. The primary differential diagnosis to consider in a feline leukemia virus-negative 9-year-old cat with a cranial mediastinal mass is:

a. lymphoma
b. thymoma
c. sarcoma
d. feline infectious peritonitis granuloma
e. hemangiosarcoma

22. What approximate percentage of mammary masses in cats are typically malignant?

a. 10%
b. 25%
c. 50%
d. 65%
e. 90%

23. What is the most important prognostic factor for survival of cats with mammary tumors?

a. cat's age
b. cat's breed
c. location of affected gland
d. tumor size
e. multiple sites of tumors

Correct answers are on pages 200-202.

24. *Multiple myeloma is a neoplastic disorder of:*

    a. liver cells
    b. granulocytes
    c. splenocytes
    d. plasma cells
    e. osteocytes

25. *Monoclonal gammopathy is most often seen in animals with:*

    a. hemangiosarcoma
    b. osteosarcoma
    c. malignant melanoma
    d. multiple myeloma
    e. acute lymphocytic leukemia

26. *For a 10-year-old female dog with a 3-cm nodule of the fourth left mammary gland, which treatment is most appropriate?*

    a. observation with periodic reexamination
    b. cytologic examination of fine-needle aspirates, with observation if it is a benign neoplasm
    c. excisional biopsy, followed by histopathologic examination and further surgery if the surgical margins are not free of tumor cells
    d. chemotherapy, regardless of the tumor type
    e. unilateral radical mastectomy

27. *Ovariohysterectomy can help reduce the frequency of mammary neoplasia if performed before the:*

    a. first estrous cycle
    b. second estrous cycle
    c. third estrous cycle
    d. fourth estrous cycle
    e. fifth estrous cycle

28. *In dogs, hemangiosarcoma is most likely to be definitively diagnosed by:*

    a. cytologic evaluation of fine-needle aspirates
    b. the history and clinical signs
    c. cytologic evaluation of abdominocentesis fluid
    d. histologic examination of a wedge biopsy of the spleen
    e. histologic evaluation of multiple sections of the spleen

29. *Which 2 drugs should **not** be used in cats because of potentially life-threatening toxic reactions?*

    a. doxorubicin and vincristine
    b. 5-fluorouracil and cisplatin
    c. L-asparaginase and cytosine arabinoside
    d. methotrexate and cyclophosphamide
    e. chlorambucil and prednisone

30. *In dogs, which endocrine disorder is **not** usually associated with a neoplastic syndrome?*

    a. hyperparathyroidism
    b. hypothyroidism
    c. hyperadrenocorticism
    d. hyperinsulinism
    e. hypergastrinemia

31. *Feline immunodeficiency virus is most likely to be transmitted by:*

    a. shared food bowls
    b. the queen's milk or colostrum
    c. bite of an infected cat
    d. reciprocal grooming behavior of cats
    e. fomites

32. *Which of the following does **not** characterize lentiviral infections?*

    a. prolonged incubation before onset of clinical signs
    b. persistent viremia and a weak neutralizing antibody response
    c. neural lesions
    d. transmission to multiple species
    e. tendency to undergo genetic mutation and genetic drift

33. A client brings in her white cat to your practice in the Arizona Sun Belt. She believes her cat was injured in a cat fight, as it has a sore on its nose that has not healed for several months. On examination of the cat, you notice an eroded area on the nasal planum and several crusts on the ear tips. The history and clinical findings are most compatible with:

a. mycosis fungoides
b. malignant melanoma
c. mast-cell tumors
d. squamous-cell carcinoma
e. basal-cell tumor

34. A dog is presented to you because of multicentric lymphadenopathy. The **least** likely cause of this problem is:

a. lymphoma
b. systemic lupus erythematosus
c. blastomycosis
d. gastrointestinal foreign body
e. generalized pyoderma

35. A dog has persistent hematuria that has not responded to antibacterials selected by urinary culture results. The diagnostic test that would provide the most useful information in determining the cause of persistent hematuria is:

a. urinalysis
b. repeat urine culture
c. double-contrast cystogram
d. trial of therapy with another antibacterial
e. serum chemistry panel

36. Which diagnostic test is **least** helpful in diagnosis of multiple myeloma?

a. quantitation of urinary protein by dipstick
b. skeletal survey radiographs
c. cytologic examination of bone marrow aspirates
d. serum protein electrophoresis
e. urine protein electrophoresis

37. Primary bone tumors commonly metastasize to the:

a. regional lymph node and liver
b. kidney and spleen
c. lungs and bone
d. brain and regional lymph node
e. lung and spleen

38. Which radiographic finding is most likely to differentiate a primary bone tumor (eg, osteosarcoma) from osteomyelitis?

a. osteolytic and osteoproductive lesion within the medullary cavity
b. radiographic lesion crossing the joint space
c. marked progressive osteolytic response
d. osteocortical erosion
e. lesion located primarily in the metaphysis

39. A client presents his 7-year-old Irish Setter for evaluation of intermittent epistaxis from the left nostril for the past 4 weeks. Physical examination reveals loosening of the third and fourth premolars and first and second molars. The most appropriate course of action is to:

a. administer antibiotics for a tooth root abscess
b. administer anesthesia for tooth extraction and antibiotics for a tooth root abscess
c. obtain a serum chemistry profile to evaluate for renal secondary hyperpara- thyroidism ("rubber jaw")
d. administer anesthesia and make nasal radiographs to evaluate for a nasal tumor
e. obtain aerobic bacterial cultures of the nasal cavity to identify rhinitis

40. The best treatment for nasal adenocarcinoma is:

a. immunostimulation
b. radiation therapy
c. chemotherapy
d. resection
e. immunosuppression

Correct answers are on pages 200-202.

41. You submit a bone biopsy from a dog with suspected osteosarcoma. The pathologist reports that the sample consists of reactive bone. What is the most appropriate course of action?

 a. send a sample to another pathologist for another opinion
 b. biopsy another portion of the opposite leg for comparison
 c. diagnose a healing fracture based on the pathology report
 d. rebiopsy the site for a suspected tumor
 e. inform the owner that there is no cancer present

42. Which test is most likely to support the diagnosis of a brain tumor?

 a. serum chemistry profile
 b. computed tomography
 c. skull radiographs
 d. cerebrospinal fluid analysis
 e. complete blood count

43. You diagnose a brain tumor in a dog with a 2-year history of seizures. The owners decline definitive treatment, such as radiation therapy or surgery; however, they do not want to euthanize their dog, if possible. What is the most appropriate course of action?

 a. the tumor is progressive and there is no way to provide a good quality of life for this dog, so euthanasia is the best option
 b. chemotherapy is very helpful for brain tumors and, therefore, should be administered
 c. administer corticosteroids, as they often help decrease neurologic signs associated with brain tumors
 d. administer antibiotics for associated secondary infection
 e. hospitalize the dog and administer mannitol to decrease peritumoral edema

44. The 2 most common oral tumors of cats are:

 a. lymphoma and osteosarcoma
 b. epulis and plasmacytoma
 c. melanoma and fibrosarcoma
 d. squamous-cell carcinoma and fibrosarcoma
 e. melanoma and plasmacytoma

45. An owner presents his 12-year-old Labrador Retriever because he noticed a small mass on the gums. You resect the mass down to the level of the gum line. Histopathologic examination identifies the mass as an acanthomatous epulis. The most appropriate course of action is to:

 a. refer the patient for radiation therapy, as these tend to recur
 b. advise the owner to observe the dog, as these often do not recur
 c. recommend chemotherapy, as these tumors typically cause metastatic disease
 d. recommend dental prophylaxis every 6 months so that new masses will not form
 e. recommend euthanasia, as these tumors spread rapidly

46. An owner presents her dog to you because of a cutaneous mass. Cytologic examination of a fine-needle aspirate reveals individualized round cells. Which type of tumor is **least** likely to be associated with these findings?

 a. hemangiosarcoma
 b. mast-cell tumor
 c. plasmacytoma
 d. histiocytoma
 e. transmissible venereal tumor

47. A dog with seizures has neurologic signs compatible with a lesion compressing the dorsal cerebral cortex, strongly suggestive of meningioma. The most appropriate prognosis to give the owner is:

 a. very poor due to irreversible brain damage from compression by the tumor
 b. very poor due to the high metastatic rate of meningiomas
 c. excellent due to the remarkable response to radiation therapy
 d. good due to the ability to resect these meningiomas in this location
 e. good due to the efficacy of chemotherapy for meningiomas

48. A 3-year-old cat is presented because of weakness. Physical examination reveals pallor of the mucous membranes. A complete blood count reveals anemia and thrombocytopenia. A reticulocyte count reveals nonregenerative anemia. The most appropriate diagnostic test to obtain more definitive information is:

a. serum chemistry profile
b. abdominal radiographs
c. thoracic radiographs
d. bone marrow aspirates
e. Coombs' test

49. Bone marrow aspiration:

a. requires costly equipment and cannot be done in private practice
b. is a relatively easy and inexpensive procedure, and can be performed in private practice
c. is a very difficult procedure and should be done at a referral institution
d. is fraught with high risks and should be done at a referral institution
e. is usually not diagnostic and should not be performed

50. The cachexia associated with neoplasia is related to:

a. decreased caloric intake
b. improper caloric intake due to pica
c. decreased nutrient absorption
d. aberrant nutrient metabolism
e. decreased nutrient digestion

51. Concerning mammary tumors in dogs, which statement is most accurate?

a. About 80% are benign.
b. The most common metastatic site is bone.
c. Postoperative chemotherapy significantly decreases the rate of recurrence.
d. Ovariohysterectomy at the time of tumor removal significantly decreases the rate of recurrence.
e. Ovariohysterectomy before the first heat period significantly lowers the risk of mammary tumors.

52. A 12-year-old male German Shepherd has had weakness and epistaxis for 2 days. A large splenic mass is palpable in the abdomen. Nonclotting bloody fluid is aspirated from the abdominal cavity. The prothrombin time and partial thromboplastin times are slightly prolonged. The packed cell volume is 28%, total protein level is 7.2 g/dl, and platelet count is 80,000/μl. The most likely cause of the bleeding is:

a. immune-mediated thrombocytopenic purpura
b. von Willebrand's disease
c. disseminated intravascular coagulation
d. hypersplenism
e. myeloma

53. All of the following may be associated with an elevated packed cell volume **except**:

a. renal tumor
b. right-to-left cardiac shunt
c. dehydration
d. hemorrhagic gastroenteritis
e. erythroleukemia

54. A 12-year-old dog is presented for regurgitation of undigested food. Thoracic radiographs show a dilated esophagus and a 5-cm-diameter cranial mediastinal mass. The most likely diagnosis is:

a. esophageal carcinoma
b. lymphoma
c. thyroid carcinoma
d. thymoma
e. systemic mast-cell tumor

55. Of the following diseases, which 2 have the best prognosis?

a. acute lymphoblastic leukemia, erythroleukemia
b. acute granulocytic leukemia, skin lymphoma
c. erythroleukemia, mycosis fungoides
d. acute granulocytic leukemia, megakaryocytic leukemia
e. well-differentiated lymphocytic leukemia, polycythemia vera

---

Correct answers are on pages 200-202.

56. Which side effect is most likely to occur after use of the following drugs?

    a. cystitis from chlorambucil
    b. myelosuppression from l-asparaginase
    c. urticaria from doxorubicin
    d. hepatic necrosis from cyclophosphamide
    e. pancreatitis from vincristine

57. A dog is being treated for lymphoma with l-asparaginase, vincristine and cyclophospha-mide. Immediately after the drugs are given IV simultaneously, the dog collapses with pale mucous membranes and vomiting. After 10-15 minutes the dog's condition improves. The schedule calls for all 3 drugs to be repeated 3 weeks later. Considering the immediate reaction after the previous treatment, the safest approach for the next treatment would be to:

    a. omit vincristine
    b. omit l-asparaginase
    c. omit cyclophosphamide
    d. give all of the drugs again, but with a 25% reduction in dose for each
    e. give all of the drugs at the same dose, but as an intravenous drip over 1 hour

58. In addition to corticosteroids, what drug should be given to a dog with multiple inoperable mast-cell tumors?

    a. aspirin
    b. cimetidine
    c. propranolol
    d. cyclophosphamide
    e. doxorubicin

59. A 14-year-old Norwegian Elkhound is presented because of lethargy. Physical findings are negative except for moderate splenomegaly. A hemogram shows packed cell volume 32%, WBC count 95,000/μl, 10% neutrophils, 89% small lymphocytes and 1% monocytes. The platelet count is 120,000/μl. A bone marrow aspirate shows about 40% small lymphocytes, 20% myeloid cells and 30% erythroid cells. The most likely diagnosis is:

    a. hypersplenism
    b. hypoadrenocorticism

    c. reactive lymphocytosis
    d. chronic lymphocytic leukemia
    e. acute lymphoblastic leukemia

Questions 60 and 61

60. A young adult female Shepherd-cross was found as a stray by a veterinary student on externship in Africa. The student noticed vulvar bleeding and palpated an irregular friable mass just inside of the vaginal opening. What is the most likely diagnosis?

    a. granulomatous vaginitis
    b. vaginal hyperplasia
    c. leiomyosarcoma
    d. squamous-cell carcinoma
    e. transmissible venereal tumor

61. What treatment is most likely to benefit this dog?

    a. testosterone
    b. ovariohysterectomy
    c. vincristine
    d. cisplatin
    e. ivermectin

62. A 4-year-old cat that has been lethargic for 2 weeks has splenomegaly and a rectal temperature of 99 F. The packed cell volume is 9% and WBC count is 10,000/μl, with 150 nucleated RBCs/100 WBCs and a normal differential WBC count. The reticulocyte count is less than 1%. Concerning this case, which statement is most accurate?

    a. The findings often occur with immune-mediated hemolytic anemia.
    b. The findings often occur with a red cell malignancy.
    c. A bone marrow aspirate is not indicated in this case.
    d. The anemia is regenerative, as indicated by the nucleated red blood cells.
    e. The corrected WBC count is 5000/μl.

63. Which combination of paraneoplastic syndrome and tumor is **least** likely to occur?

    a. myasthenia gravis with thymoma

b. bleeding tendencies with myeloma
c. peptic ulceration with pancreatic tumor
d. ACTH secretion with fibrosarcoma
e. hypercalcemia with anal-sac carcinoma

64. *Which of the following is **least** likely to be present in a patient with acute leukemia?*

a. neutrophilia
b. anemia
c. thrombocytopenia
d. eosinopenia
e. lymphopenia

65. *A cat is **unlikely** to develop lymphoma if it has antibodies against:*

a. feline leukemia virus (FeLV) core antigen
b. FeLV envelope antigen
c. FeLV reverse transcriptase
d. feline oncornavirus cell membrane antigen (FOCMA)
e. any FeLV antigen

66. *Feline leukemia virus (FeLV) differs from other retroviruses, such as bovine leukemia virus or human immunodeficiency virus, in that a major route of FeLV transmission is via:*

a. blood
b. semen
c. urine
d. arthropod vectors
e. saliva

67. *The term myeloproliferative disease usually refers to all of the following **except**:*

a. acute granulocytic leukemia
b. acute lymphoblastic leukemia
c. erythroleukemia
d. thrombocythemia
e. myelofibrosis

68. *Which of the following is more characteristic of polycythemia rubra vera than of polycythemia secondary to a renal tumor?*

a. elevated packed cell volume, red blood cell count and hemoglobin concentration

b. erythroid hyperplasia in bone marrow
c. abnormal red blood cell morphology
d. low serum erythropoietin level
e. secondary heart failure

69. *Lymphoma in dogs, as compared with lymphoma in cats, is more likely to be manifested as:*

a. a mediastinal mass
b. renal masses
c. intestinal thickening
d. generalized lymphadenopathy
e. lymphoblastic proliferation in several organs

70. *What complication is most likely to occur in a dog with an estrogen-secreting Sertoli-cell tumor of the testicle?*

a. hypercalcemia
b. polycythemia
c. aplastic anemia
d. disseminated intravascular coagulation
e. hemolysis

71. *Which of the following is most likely to occur with myeloma?*

a. duodenal ulcers
b. hepatic failure
c. microangiopathic hemolysis
d. lytic bone lesions in the vertebrae
e. splenomegaly

72. *Concerning radiation therapy, which statement is most accurate?*

a. Sensitivity of cells to radiation increases in the G1 phase of the cell cycle.
b. Hypothermia combined with irradiation enhances tumor cell kill while minimizing damage to normal tissues.
c. Hypoxic tumor cells are especially sensitive to radiation.
d. Adenocarcinomas, osteosarcomas and fibrosarcomas in dogs and cats are most likely to respond to radiation.
e. Megavoltage radiation is less likely to cause skin damage than is orthovoltage radiation.

Correct answers are on pages 200-202.

73. *An owner says that her only cat died a month ago from feline leukemia virus (FeLV) infection, and she now would like to get a new kitten. The most appropriate advice for her is:*

    a. to wait at least 6 months before obtaining a new kitten

    b. to adopt an adult cat rather than a kitten because kittens are more susceptible to FeLV infection

    c. it is safe to adopt a new kitten with no special precautions

    d. it is safe to adopt a kitten now if it is first vaccinated against FeLV infection

    e. to first clean the floors with sodium hypochlorite solution (Clorox) and destroy any dishes used by the previous cat

74. *A form of lymphoma affecting the skin is:*

    a. reticuloendotheliosis

    b. mycosis fungoides

    c. Marek's disease

    d. myelofibrosis

    e. B-cell lymphoma

75. *Which of the following syndromes is most often associated with polycythemia?*

    a. renal carcinoma

    b. erythroleukemia

    c. iron overload

    d. testosterone-secreting tumors

    e. mitral insufficiency with early left heart failure

Answers

1. **b** Vincristine rarely causes nephrotoxicity in veterinary patients.

2. **c** Hemorrhagic cystitis is usually sterile and may be induced by use of this drug.

3. **d** Hyponatremia is not a common component of the tumor lysis syndrome, whereas the other elements are released from blood cells and the increased phosphorus causes decreased calcium levels.

4. **e** If the primary tumor has not responded to radiation therapy, metastatic lesions are unlikely to be responsive to radiation therapy.

5. **d** Antineoplastic therapy is most important to control the cause of hypercalcemia.

6. **c** Function of the remaining adrenal gland is suppressed, so supplementation with dexamethasone is important.

7. **a** Insulinomas produce excessive insulin, which causes hypoglycemia. It should be noted that any tumor can cause hypoglycemia.

8. **b** Pheochromocytomas produce epinephrine and norepinephrine, which induce hypertension.

9. **a** Hemangiosarcoma often causes microangiopathic hemolytic anemia, which results in schistocyte production. Splenic malfunction allows circulation of nucleated red blood cells.

10. **c** Myasthenia gravis most commonly has been associated with thymoma as a paraneoplastic syndrome.

11. **c** The metastatic tumor is most likely, but not always, to respond similarly to the primary tumor.

12. **c** It is a complex series of steps.

13. **d** *Spirocerca lupi* causes granulomatous lesions in the thoracic esophagus that undergo neoplastic transformation.

14. **c** The metastatic rate of hemangiopericytomas is very low; however, they tend to be fairly aggressive locally and recur readily after surgery.

15. **a** A large percentage of dogs have some form of disseminated intravascular coagulation or coagulopathy associated with hemangiosarcoma.

16. **d** Disseminated intravascular coagulation causes coagulopathy, platelet disorders and

anemia, but the white blood cell count is typically normal.

17. **c** The fact that all 3 cell lines are affected indicates that the bone marrow is involved. Recent initiation of chemotherapy would not cause anemia, as the red blood cell life span is very long. Disseminated intravascualr coagulation involves platelets and red blood cells only.

18. **d** Disseminated intravascular coagulation causes increased consumption of platelets, but does not actually cause decreased production of platelets.

19. **b** Mycosis fungoides is a T-cell lymphoma that is epidermotropic.

20. **c** Mast-cell tumors may release histamine, which activates histamine receptors of parietal cells in the gastric mucosa. This causes increased gastric acidity and gastric ulceration, which leads to bleeding and positive fecal occult blood.

21. **b** Thymoma is the most likely diagnosis, as it is observed in older cats. Lymphoma should be a secondary consideration; however, cranial mediastinal lymphoma is typically seen in cats that average 3 years old and are FeLV positive.

22. **e** Most mammary masses in cats are adenocarcinomas.

23. **d** The size of the tumor appears to be the most important prognostic factor. Tumors less than 2 cm in diameter are associated with longer survival times than tumors larger than 2 cm in diameter.

24. **d** Multiple myeloma is a proliferative disorder of plasma cells.

25. **d** Multiple myeloma is a disease of plasma cells, which produce immunoglobulins that result in monoclonal gammopathy.

26. **c** Approximately 50% of mammary masses are benign. Excisional biopsy may be curative, but if the histologic examination indicates a malignancy, further excision may be required. Fine-needle aspiration may miss the malignant part of the tumor.

27. **d** Studies have shown that before the fourth estrous cycle, the risk of mammary tumors is reduced significantly by ovariohysterectomy.

28. **e** The entire spleen should be evaluated, as histologic diagnosis of hemangiosarcoma may be missed otherwise.

29. **b** 5-fluorouracil causes neurologic signs and death. Cisplatin causes pulmonary edema and death.

30. **b** Hypothyroidism is typically due to immune-mediated thyroid destruction, whereas the other endocrine disorders typically involve a gland secreting a hormonal substance or a hormonal stimulatory substance.

31. **c** Casual contact does not cause transmission of this disease. Bite wounds have been experimentally demonstrated to cause infection.

32. **d** Typically, the lentiviruses are very species specific.

33. **d** Squamous-cell carcinoma typically occurs on the eyelids, nasal planum, and ears of white cats exposed to excessive sunlight. The lesions often appear as nonhealing wounds.

34. **d** The other diseases are associated with lymphadenopathy.

35. **c** Double-contrast cystography is indicated in chronic hematuria.

36. **a** Light protein chains (Bence Jones proteins) are typically secreted in the urine and are not detected by urinary dipstick methods.

37. **c** The lungs and bones appear to be the most common sites for osteosarcoma metastases.

38. **b** Primary bone tumors typically do not cross the joint space, whereas osteomyelitis is not limited by the joint space.

39. **d** The most common cause of nasal epistaxis in older dogs is nasal tumor; therefore, evaluation for this disease is warranted.

40. **b** Radiation therapy can increase survival times for nasal adenocarcinomas. Chemotherapy and immunotherapy have not been evaluated thoroughly, but at this stage they are generally ineffective. Surgery alone does not appear to prolong survival times.

41. **d** It is not unusual to obtain a histopathologic diagnosis of reactive bone on a superficial biopsy of the primary bone tumor. Therefore, it is important to rebiopsy the bone.

42. **b** Computed tomography is most likely to aid detection of a brain tumor. CSF analysis is typically supportive by demonstrating increased total protein.

43. **c** Corticosteroids often help decrease peritumoral inflammation and provide or allow for a good quality of life for several weeks.

44. **d** Squamous-cell carcinoma is the most common oral tumor, accounting for over 90% of oral tumors in cats. Fibrosarcoma is the next most common tumor.

45. **a** These tumors are typically very responsive to radiation therapy; however, surgery is also a good option. They generally recur if not excised completely.

46. **a** Cytologic examination of hemangiosarcoma reveals spindle-shaped cells, indicating its mesenchymal origin.

47. **d** Meningioma in the cerebral cortical area is highly accessible to surgery. These tumors can be readily removed, with a good quality of life following resection. Radiation therapy is moderately effective. Chemotherapy is not very effective for these tumors.

48. **d** The involvement of 2 separate blood lines usually indicates a bone marrow disorder.

49. **b** Bone marrow aspiration is an inexpensive procedure that can yield excellent diagnostic information.

50. **d** Cancer cachexia is due to increased energy consumption by the tumor, which causes aberrant nutrient metabolism.

51. **e** The beneficial effect is lost partially after the first few estrous cycles and lost totally after 2 1/2 years of age.

52. **c** Disseminated intravascular coagulation frequently occurs in dogs with splenic hemangiosarcoma.

53. **e** All forms of acute leukemia cause myelophthisic anemia.

54. **d** Thymomas are associated with esophageal dilatation secondary to myasthenia gravis.

55. **e** Lymphocytic leukemia usually responds to an alkylating agent and corticosteroids. Polycythemia vera responds to phlebotomy and hydroxyurea.

56. **e** The risk of urticaria is lessened by giving the drug slowly intravenously.

57. **b** Intravenous or intraperitoneal l-asparaginase may cause anaphylaxis. The reaction is likely to recur if the drug is given again.

58. **b** This is used to inhibit duodenal ulcers, which are likely to form because histamine from the tumor stimulates HCl secretion by the stomach.

59. **d** This disease is characterized by a high count of normal lymphocytes.

60. **e** Transmissible venereal tumor is enzootic in Africa, often in young adults.

61. **c** The cure rate is high after 3-4 injections given once a week.

62. **b** In cats, anemia that is nonregenerative, with many circulating nucleated red blood cells, may be caused by erythroid malignancy.

63. **d** This combination has not been reported.

64. **a** In acute leukemia, production of normal neutrophils, red blood cells and platelets is decreased.

65. **d** FOCMA is on the surface of tumor cells transformed by FeLV.

66. **e** FeLV is more contagious than bovine leukemia virus or human immunodeficiency virus.

67. **b** The term refers to nonlymphoid hematopoietic neoplasia.

68. **d** The high packed cell volume in polycythemia vera inhibits erythropoietin production. Some renal tumors secrete erythropoietin.

69. **d** The typical presentation in dogs with lymphoma is lymphadenopathy.

70. **c** Aplastic anemia occurs with estrogen toxicity.

71. **d** "Punched-out" lesions may be seen on radiographs.

72. **e** Megavoltage radiation penetrates skin better than orthovoltage radiation, allowing it to focus on deeper sites.

73. **c** The virus only lives a few hours to a few days in a household after an infected cat leaves the premises.

74. **b** This is a T-cell tumor with characteristic histopathologic changes.

75. **a** This tumor secretes erythropoietin.

Section

10

Ophthalmology

D.E. Brooks

Recommended Reading

Gelatt K: *Veterinary Ophthalmology*. Lea & Febiger, Philadelphia, 1991.

Slatter D: *Fundamentals of Veterinary Ophthalmology*. Saunders, Philadelphia, 1990.

Practice answer sheet is on page 349.

Questions

1. Accommodation of the canine lens for near vision occurs when the:

   a. ciliary muscle contracts and the zonules relax
   b. ciliary muscle contracts and the zonules are stretched
   c. iris muscles contract and squeeze the lens into a more spherical shape
   d. ciliary muscle relaxes to allow the cornea to alter its shape
   e. iris muscles contract to pull the lens rostrally

2. Which cranial nerves compose the afferent and efferent limbs of the pupillary light reflex?

   a. trigeminal and trochlear nerves
   b. optic and oculomotor nerves
   c. optic and abducent nerves
   d. trigeminal and facial nerves
   e. optic and facial nerves

3. Which enzyme is associated with formation of aqueous humor?

   a. collagenase
   b. protease
   c. carbonic anhydrase
   d. sorbitol dehydrogenase
   e. prostaglandin synthetase

4. What is the normal range of intraocular pressures in dogs and cats?

   a. 5-10 mm Hg
   b. 10-15 mm Hg
   c. 15-25 mm Hg
   d. 30-40 mm Hg
   e. 40-50 mm Hg

Correct answers are on pages 208-210.

5. Which parasympatholytic mydriatic drug has the shortest duration of effect?

    a. atropine
    b. tropicamide
    c. homatropine
    d. epinephrine
    e. cyclopentolate

6. Which drug is a beta-adrenergic antagonist useful for glaucoma therapy?

    a. epinephrine
    b. pilocarpine
    c. demecarium
    d. apraclonidine
    e. timolol maleate

7. Gonioscopy is a diagnostic technique used for examination of the:

    a. lens
    b. eyelids
    c. retina
    d. iridocorneal angle
    e. vitreous

8. Use of the Schiotz tonometer is generally contraindicated in the presence of:

    a. hyphema
    b. corneal laceration
    c. posterior lens luxation
    d. anterior uveitis
    e. cataract

9. Which drug is most effective for treatment of feline herpesviral infection involving the eye?

    a. trifluorothymidine
    b. flucytosine
    c. mitomycin
    d. apraclonidine
    e. nystatin

10. Topical corticosteroids are contraindicated for use in animals with:

    a. lens-induced uveitis
    b. episcleritis
    c. glaucoma
    d. corneal ulcers
    e. pannus

11. Mechanical debridement and use of topical antibiotic solutions are beneficial in treatment of persistent corneal erosions in Boxers. What other listed drug is also indicated?

    a. sodium chloride
    b. dexamethasone
    c. idoxuridine
    d. nystatin
    e. cromolyn sodium

12. Which topical medication is useful in treatment of keratoconjunctivitis sicca in dogs?

    a. timolol maleate
    b. atropine
    c. cyclosporine A
    d. 5% sodium chloride
    e. nystatin

13. What is the most common eyelid tumor in cats?

    a. melanoma
    b. squamous-cell carcinoma
    c. meibomian-gland adenoma
    d. mast-cell tumor
    e. fibrosarcoma

14. Cytologic examination of conjunctival scrapings from a cat with conjunctivitis reveals predominantly neutrophils, a few mononuclear cells, and basophilic cocci on the cell membranes. What type of conjunctivitis is present?

    a. herpesviral
    b. mycoplasmal
    c. chlamydial
    d. allergic
    e. bacterial

15. Removal of the gland of the third eyelid for "cherry eye" in dogs has been associated with subsequent development of:

a. retinal detachment
b. eversion of the cartilage of the third eyelid
c. keratoconjunctivitis sicca
d. squamous-cell carcinoma of the third eyelid
e. glaucoma

16. *Linear, dendritic areas of fluorescein dye retention in the cornea of a cat with a painful eye are associated with infection by:*

a. *Mycoplasma*
b. *Chlamydia*
c. *Streptococcus*
d. herpesvirus
e. *Cryptococcus*

17. *Which breed of dog is most sensitive to the ocular side effects of vaccination against infectious canine hepatitis?*

a. Poodle
b. Afghan
c. Labrador Retriever
d. German Shepherd
e. Rottweiler

18. *About 20% of naturally infected dogs and a smaller percentage of dogs vaccinated against infectious canine hepatitis develop:*

a. glaucoma
b. retinal detachment
c. corneal ulceration
d. anterior uveitis
e. cataracts

19. *You detect a brownish-black, focal, midstromal corneal lesion in a Persian cat. The lesion does not retain fluorescein dye, but stains with rose bengal. What is the most likely cause of this lesion?*

a. melanoma
b. foreign body
c. corneal sequestrum
d. corneal dermoid
e. iris prolapse

20. *What ocular condition is recessively inherited in Basenjis?*

a. persistent pupillary membranes
b. cataracts
c. retinal dysplasia
d. entropion
e. anterior uveitis

21. *The term "China eye" is a lay term for heterochromia iridis. What is the clinical appearance of the iris in this condition?*

a. albinotic
b. blue and white
c. heavily pigmented
d. blue
e. blue and yellow-brown

22. *Blindness in glaucoma ultimately results from damage to the:*

a. cornea
b. iris
c. retina
d. lens
e. optic nerve

23. *What term is used to describe the ophthalmoscopic appearance of caudal displacement of the optic nerve in glaucoma patients?*

a. cupping
b. atrophy
c. degeneration
d. dysplasia
e. hypoplasia

24. *The term for enlargement of the globe in response to chronic elevation of intraocular pressure is:*

a. exophthalmos
b. proptosis
c. buphthalmos
d. luxation
e. strabismus

Correct answers are on pages 208-210.

25. *A dilated, nonresponsive pupil is a clinical sign of:*

    a. iritis
    b. cataracts
    c. glaucoma
    d. episcleritis
    e. iridal cysts

26. *Which medication can be used in emergency situations by the owner to treat sudden acute attacks of glaucoma in dogs?*

    a. intravenous acetazolamide
    b. topical pilocarpine
    c. topical timolol maleate
    d. intravenous mannitol
    e. oral glycerine

27. *Controlled application of intense cold (cryotherapy) to what part of the eye is useful in managing chronic elevation of intraocular pressure in dogs and cats?*

    a. cornea
    b. ciliary body
    c. iris
    d. lens
    e. choroid

28. *What breed of cat is most at risk of developing primary glaucoma?*

    a. Persian
    b. Himalayan
    c. Scottish Fold
    d. Siamese
    e. Russian Blue

29. *What type of cataract is associated with anterior uveitis and is characterized by a wrinkled anterior capsule?*

    a. incipient
    b. immature
    c. mature
    d. hypermature
    e. intumescent

30. *Which condition is associated with sudden onset of cataracts in dogs?*

    a. Addison's disease
    b. Cushing's disease
    c. diabetes mellitus
    d. systemic hypertension
    e. malignant lymphoma

31. *Which of the following occurs as a result of normal aging of the lens?*

    a. lenticonus
    b. lenticular sclerosis
    c. microphakia
    d. cataracts
    e. persistent tunica vasculosa lentis

32. *In dogs, which type of cataract surgery involves aspiration of the cataract following ultrasonic disruption through a very small corneal or limbal incision?*

    a. discission-aspiration method
    b. extracapsular method
    c. intracapsular method
    d. photodisruption phacolysis method
    e. phacoemulsification method

33. *Persistent hyperplastic primary vitreous is a congenital defect of the vitreous that is most common in:*

    a. Doberman Pinschers
    b. German Shepherds
    c. Labrador Retrievers
    d. Toy Poodles
    e. Beagles

34. *The tapetum of dogs and cats is located in which layer of the eye?*

    a. sclera
    b. choroid
    c. retinal pigment epithelium
    d. inner nuclear layer of the retina
    e. outer nuclear layer of the retina

35. *Which retinal cell is adapted for night vision?*

    a. cone
    b. rod
    c. Müller cell

d. ganglion cell

e. amacrine cell

36. Which electrodiagnostic test is useful for evaluating mass retinal function?

   a. electroretinography
   b. early receptor potentials
   c. visual-evoked potentials
   d. electrooculography
   e. oscillatory potentials

37. On ophthalmoscopic examination, hyper-reflective tapetal regions indicate damage to the:

   a. choroid
   b. sclera
   c. retina
   d. vitreous
   e. lens

38. The axons of which retinal cells comprise the optic nerve?

   a. Muller cells
   b. rods
   c. cones
   d. ganglion cells
   e. retinal pigment epithelial cells

39. Nyctalopia or night blindness is a cardinal sign of:

   a. optic neuritis
   b. retinal detachment
   c. glaucoma
   d. cataracts
   e. progressive retinal atrophy

40. In cats, a deficiency of which nutrient can cause central retinal degeneration?

   a. tryptophan
   b. taurine
   c. vitamin A
   d. proline
   e. methionine

41. A syndrome of vision loss without associated fundic abnormalities has been observed in overweight female dogs. Many affected dogs are also polyuric and polydipsic. This syndrome is known as:

   a. progressive retinal atrophy
   b. hemealopia
   c. sudden acquired retinal degeneration
   d. Collie eye anomaly
   e. neuronal ceroid lipofuscinosis

42. Which form of Collie eye anomaly can progress to vision loss?

   a. blood vessel tortuosity
   b. choroidal hypoplasia
   c. retinal dysplasia
   d. persistent pupillary membranes
   e. optic nerve colobomas

43. Which clinical sign is **not** associated with Horner's syndrome?

   a. miosis
   b. ptosis
   c. enophthalmos
   d. nictitans prolapse
   e. exophthalmos

44. Feline dysautonomia is differentiated from Horner's syndrome by the presence of:

   a. miosis
   b. mydriasis
   c. nictitans prolapse
   d. enophthalmos
   e. cataracts

45. A 2-year-old Labrador Retriever is presented with acute onset of exophthalmos, pain on opening the mouth and unilateral nictitans protrusion. The dog has a slight fever and leukocytosis. What is the most likely cause of these signs?

   a. intraocular neoplasm
   b. glaucoma
   c. orbital neoplasm
   d. orbital cellulitis/abscess
   e. Horner's syndrome

Correct answers are on pages 208-210.

46. Corneal endothelial dystrophy in Boston
    Terriers is characterized initially by:

    a. corneal ulceration
    b. keratoconus
    c. corneal edema
    d. corneal pigmentation
    e. corneal vascularization

47. What is the most common primary
    intraocular tumor of dogs?

    a. lymphosarcoma
    b. melanoma
    c. mast-cell tumor
    d. adenocarcinoma
    e. astrocytoma

48. Topical anesthetics are used diagnostically
    rather than therapeutically because repeated
    short-term use can cause:

    a. corneal ulcers
    b. bradycardia

    c. iridal cysts
    d. glaucoma
    e. cataracts

49. The fundus of a dog demonstrates an optic
    nerve in focus at −6 diopters with the direct
    ophthalmoscope. The blood vessels appear
    slightly smaller than normal. What is the most
    likely cause of these findings?

    a. retinal detachment
    b. progressive retinal atrophy
    c. glaucoma
    d. normal variation
    e. prior chorioretinitis

50. What does the term "haws" refer to in cats?

    a. squamous-cell carcinoma
    b. heterochromia iridis
    c. iridal neovascularization
    d. iridal cysts
    e. bilateral nictitans protrusion

Answers

1. **a** When the ciliary muscle is in the contracted state, the lens zonules are relaxed and the eye is accommodated for near vision.

2. **b** The optic nerve is the afferent nerve and the oculomotor is the efferent nerve.

3. **c** Carbonic anhydrase catalyzes the formation of carbonic acid from carbon dioxide and water.

4. **c** Intraocular pressure ranges from 15 to 30 mm Hg in dogs and cats.

5. **b** Tropicamide has the shortest duration of action. Atropine and cyclopentolate have the longest and homatropine is intermediate. Epinephrine is an adrenergic drug.

6. **e** Timolol maleate is the only beta-antagonist in this list. It has varying results in lowering intraocular pressure in dogs and cats. Epinephrine is an alpha and beta agonist. Apraclonidine is an alpha agonist, while

pilocarpine and demecarium are parasympatholytic agents.

7. **d** Gonioscopy utilizes a special corneal lens to examine the iridocorneal angle in glaucoma patients.

8. **b** The weight of the Schiotz tonometer precludes its use in conditions of corneal weakness.

9. **a** Trifluorothymidine is the most effective agent against feline herpesvirus. The other drugs listed are not used for antiviral therapy.

10. **d** Patients with corneal ulcers should not receive corticosteroid medication. Corticosteroids have no benefit for glaucoma unless uveitis is also present.

11. **a** 5% NaCl is a hyperosmotic drug used to reduce corneal edema in this condition.

12. **c** Cyclosporine A is a T-lymphocyte inhibitor and is thought to relieve the immune-mediated attack on the lacrimal gland, a common cause of keratoconjunctivitis sicca.

13. **b** This is by far the most common feline eyelid tumor.

14. **b** Inclusions on the surface of inflammatory cells are characteristic of *Mycoplasma*.

15. **c** The third eyelid gland produces a large percentage of the tear film in dogs. Surgical removal may be associated with subsequent keratoconjunctivitis sicca.

16. **d** Dendritic ulcers are typical of feline herpetic keratitis.

17. **b** The Afghan and Greyhound are most susceptible to side effects of such vaccination.

18. **d** The "corneal blue-eye" reaction is due to anterior uveitis from infection with hepatitis virus.

19. **c** Corneal sequestra are associated with herpesvirus, entropion in Persians and previous corneal ulceration.

20. **a** These are common in this dog breed.

21. **d** The iris is blue in China eye.

22. **e** While all parts of the eye are affected by elevated intraocular pressure, blindness results from damage to the optic nerve.

23. **a** Cupping refers to caudal movement of the laminal cribosa in response to increased intraocular pressure. The other terms are histologic in nature.

24. **c** Buphthalmos means the eye has enlarged due to stretching of the cornea and sclera.

25. **a** Glaucoma causes damage to the iris sphincter muscle, resulting in a fixed and dilated pupil.

26. **e** Oral glycerine can be used by owners to reduce intraocular pressure while awaiting more aggressive therapy by the veterinarian.

27. **b** Freezing the ciliary body at multiple sites is beneficial in reducing production of aqueous humor.

28. **d** There are many reports of primary glaucoma in Siamese cats.

29. **d** Hypermature cataracts have a wrinkled anterior capsule due to loss of lens proteins into the anterior chamber. These lens proteins incite anterior uveitis.

30. **c** Saturation of the hexokinase enzyme in the lens results in accumulation of sorbitol in the lens. The sorbitol osmotically draws water into the lens, resulting in disruption of lens fibers and a cataract.

31. **b** Aging of the lens results in dehydration and hardening of the lens nucleus.

32. **e** Phacoemulsification is ultrasonic cataract surgery.

33. **a** This is a hereditary condition in Doberman Pinschers.

34. **b** The tapetum of carnivores is in the dorsal choroid.

35. **b** Rods are for night vision and cones for day vision.

36. **a** Electroretinograms are used for evaluating mass retinal responses.

37. **c** Damage that causes thinning to the overlying retina makes it easier to see the tapetal reflection, so it appears brighter than normal or hyperreflective.

38. **d** Ganglion cell axons form the optic nerve.

39. **e** Progressive retinal atrophy is characterized by loss of rod cells initially, which causes nyctalopia.

40. **b** Taurine deficiency is associated with development of retinal degeneration and blindness in cats.

41. **c** Dogs with progressive retinal atrophy are night blind. Hemeralopic dogs are day blind. There are no gender differences in Collie eye anomaly. Neuronal ceroid lipofuscinosis causes neurologic disturbances.

42. **e** Colobomas can progress to retinal detachment. The other choices are nonprogressive.

43. **e** Horner's syndrome is due to loss of sympathetic innervation to the eye. Enophthalmos is due to loss of adrenergically innervated orbital smooth muscle tone.

44. **b** Fixed and dilated pupils characterize this loss of parasympathetic innervation to the eye.

45. **d** Orbital abscesses arise suddenly and are very painful. These dogs may be febrile and have elevated WBC counts.

46. **c** Endothelial dystrophies result in edema initially. Chronic edema can cause all the other changes later.

47. **b** Melanomas are the most common primary intraocular tumor. Lymphosarcoma is more common, but is metastatic to the eye of dogs.

48. **a** Topical anesthetics are toxic to the corneal epithelium and cause ulcers.

49. **c** If the optic nerve is in focus at –6 diopters instead of 0 diopters, it is displaced caudally. Glaucoma is the only choice that could cause this. Progressive retinal atrophy, retinal detachment and retinitis would cause pallor of the nerve, not cupping. Normal variation would be an optic nerve in focus from 0 to –3 diopters.

50. **e** Haws refers to idiopathic bilateral nictitans protrusion in cats.

Notes

Pharmacology and Pharmacy Procedures

S. Hudson Duran

Recommended Reading

Bennett K: *Compendium of Veterinary Products.* 1st ed. North American Compendiums, Port Huron, MI, 1991.

Booth NH and McDonald LE: *Veterinary Pharmacology and Therapeutics.* 6th ed. Iowa State University Press, Ames, 1988.

Brumbaugh G and Davis LE: Clinical pharmacology. *Vet Clin No Am* (Equine Pract) 3:1-254, 1987.

Hinchcliff KW and Jernigan AD: Applied pharmacology and therapeutics I. *Vet Clin No Am* (Food Animal Pract) 7:633-814, 1991.

Hinchcliff KW and Jernigan AD: Applied pharmacology and therapeutics II. *Vet Clin No Am* (Food Animal Pract) 8:1-168, 1992.

Johnston D: *The Bristol Veterinary Handbook of Antimicrobial Therapy.* 2nd ed. Veterinary Learning Systems, Trenton, NJ, 1987.

Koterba A *et al: Equine Clinical Neonatology.* Lea & Febiger, Philadelphia, 1990.

Plumb D: *Veterinary Drug Handbook.* Pharma Vet Publishing, White Bear Lake, MN, 1991.

Short CE: *Principles and Practice of Veterinary Anesthesia.* Williams & Wilkins, Baltimore, 1987.

Veterinary Pharmaceuticals and Biologicals 91/92. 7th ed. Veterinary Medicine Publishing, Lenexa, KS, 1991.

Practice answer sheet is on page 351.

Questions

1. *Approved veterinary drugs are:*

   a. drugs whose use for certain diseases in certain species has been approved by the Food and Drug Administration

   b. drugs prescribed by veterinarians

   c. drugs that may be purchased at a retail pharmacy

   d. drugs that may be purchased at a feed store

   e. drugs used in human medicine

Correct answers are on pages 219-222.

2. *All of the following are examples of extra-label use of a veterinary drug* **except**:

   a. the drug is used as directly indicated on the label
   b. the drug is used for a species other than those indicated on the label
   c. the route of administration is different than that indicated on the label
   d. the disease treated is different than those indicated on the label
   e. the dosage interval is different than that indicated on the label

3. *Extra-label use of veterinary drugs is legal only if:*

   a. a client asks for at least a week's supply of medication
   b. a client insists on ordering the medication over the phone
   c. a cat breeder must treat all of her cats for a respiratory problem
   d. there is a cheaper human drug than the available veterinary product
   e. there is a valid veterinarian-client-patient relationship, with the animal's medical diagnosis established

4. *All dosages charted in an animal's medication records should be expressed in:*

   a. milliliters (ml)
   b. cubic centimeters (cc)
   c. milligrams (mg), grams (g) or units (U)
   d. number of capsules
   e. number of tablets

5. *A 7% solution of chloral hydrate contains:*

   a. 7 g in 10 ml
   b. 7 g in 100 ml
   c. 7 g in 1000 ml
   d. 7 mg in 100 ml
   e. 7 mg in 1000 ml

6. *A milliequivalent (mEq) is calculated by dividing the milligram (mg) molecular weight by the valence, which gives mg/mEq. If potassium chloride (KCl) has a molecular*

weight of 74.5, how many milliequivalents are in 1 gram of KCl?

   a. 74.5 mEq
   b. 7.45 mEq
   c. 13.4 mEq
   d. 20 mEq
   e. 134 mEq

7. *A vial of sodium penicillin G powder contains 5 million units. If you add 18 milliliters (ml) of sterile water to the vial, the concentration will be 250,000 units/ml. What volume of powder was originally in the vial?*

   a. 4 ml
   b. 2 ml
   c. 1 ml
   d. 20 ml
   e. 5 ml

8. *By law, veterinary technicians are permitted to dispense veterinary drugs to clients:*

   a. provided the client has been in the clinic for a prior visit
   b. only if the technician is familiar with the drug
   c. only if the veterinarian is away and has given general permission
   d. only if the technician is over 21 years of age
   e. only in the presence and under the direct supervision of a licensed veterinarian

9. *You plan to dispense an external parasiticide to a client. In what type of container should the insecticide be dispensed?*

   a. the original container, with a safety cap
   b. a clear glass bottle, appropriately labeled
   c. an amber glass bottle, appropriately labeled
   d. a plastic 1-gallon container
   e. a plastic container with a wide mouth

10. *What is the osmolarity of an isotonic solution?*

   a. 750 mOsm/L
   b. 300 mOsm/L
   c. 1000 mOsm/L

d. 200 mOsm/L
e. 150 mOsm/L

a. 4-6 hours
b. 6-8 hours
c. 8-10 hours
d. 1-2 hours
e. 12-18 hours

11. *United States Pharmacopeia (USP)
Standards state that drugs used in human
medicine must contain ±10% of the amount of
those ingredients indicated on the label. USP
standards for veterinary drugs are:*

a. ±10%
b. ±5%
c. ±15%
d. ±20%
e. ±25%

12. *Aminoglycoside antibiotics, such as
gentamicin and amikacin, are used in
veterinary medicine to treat infections caused
by Gram-negative bacteria. Types of toxicities
associated with these drugs are:*

a. nephrotoxicity, ototoxicity and neurotoxicity
b. nephrotoxicity, hepatotoxicity and
cardiotoxicity
c. cardiotoxicity, bone marrow suppression and
immunosuppression
d. neurotoxicity, cardiotoxicity and bone
marrow suppression
e. immunosuppression, hepatotoxicity and
neurotoxicity

13. *Gentamicin and amikacin are antibiotics
with a narrow therapeutic index, meaning the
dosage must be carefully controlled so as to
prevent toxicity. The safest way to monitor the
response to these antibiotics is to:*

a. measure levels in serum to make sure they
are within the safe range
b. give very low dosages
c. use these drugs for no more than 1 day
d. use these drugs for 3 days, withhold the
drugs for another 3 days, then resume
treatment for 3 more days
e. keep the animal well nourished while the
drugs are being given

14. *A dog has a serum creatinine level of 3 mg/dl.
You plan to begin ampicillin therapy at 25
mg/kg body weight. How often should you give
the drug?*

15. *What key words should you look for when
purchasing fluids for intravenous injection?*

a. sterile, distilled
b. distilled, bacteriostatic
c. sterile, pyrogen free
d. autoclaved, distilled
e. bacteriostatic

16. *Lactated Ringer's Injection USP is **not**
compatible with:*

a. calcium chloride
b. potassium chloride
c. sodium chloride
d. sodium bicarbonate
e. potassium acetate

17. *An animal has an allergic reaction to
xylazine. Another drug that should **not** be
administered to this animal is:*

a. ketamine
b. acepromazine
c. thiamylal sodium
d. guaifenesin
e. detomidine

18. *If you wish to prepare 1000 ml of a 5%
guaifenesin solution in 5% dextrose, how much
of each ingredient will the solution contain?*

a. 100 grams of dextrose and 100 grams of
guaifenesin
b. 5 grams of dextrose and 5 grams of
guaifenesin
c. 50 grams of dextrose and 50 grams of
guaifenesin
d. 10 grams of dextrose and 10 grams of
guaifenesin
e. 0.5 grams of dextrose and 0.5 grams of
guaifenesin

Correct answers are on pages 219-222.

19. *The half-life of a drug is the time it takes for:*

    a. the drug to be totally eliminated from the body
    b. the drug to kill half of the bacteria causing an infection
    c. drug concentrations in the body to be reduced by one-half
    d. half of a usual course of therapy
    e. half of the recommended dosage to resolve disease

20. *All of the following drugs have narrow therapeutic indexes (safety margins) **except**:*

    a. theophylline
    b. penicillin
    c. gentamicin
    d. digoxin
    e. phenobarbital

21. *Cimetidine and ranitidine are:*

    a. antacids used for reflux esophagitis
    b. anthelmintics used for hookworm infections
    c. antibiotics used against Gram-positive bacteria
    d. H2 antagonists used for gastrointestinal ulcers
    e. injectable laxatives

22. *The more water soluble a drug is, the higher its accumulation in:*

    a. fatty tissues
    b. the brain
    c. bone or teeth
    d. the liver and spleen
    e. serum or plasma

23. *In addition to its main use, cimetidine is also used to treat:*

    a. keratoconjunctivitis sicca (dry eye)
    b. congestive heart failure
    c. malignant melanoma
    d. endocrine alopecia
    e. lungworm infection

24. *A lipophilic (fat-loving) drug tends to accumulate in:*

    a. teeth
    b. serum
    c. urine
    d. plasma
    e. soft tissues

25. *In dogs, digoxin has an elimination half-life of:*

    a. 30-112 minutes
    b. 14-56 hours
    c. 7-15 days
    d. 72-96 hours
    e. 21-30 days

26. *When given by injection, oxytetracycline should be given:*

    a. with calcium products
    b. very slowly intravenously
    c. by any convenient route
    d. with blood products
    e. very rapidly as an intravenous bolus

27. *Atropine has all of the following clinical uses **except**:*

    a. antispasmodic
    b. inhibit salivation
    c. bronchoconstriction
    d. diagnosis of sinus node dysfunction
    e. treatment of sinus bradycardia

28. *Aminophylline, prednisone and terbutaline are used in combination to treat:*

    a. infections with Gram-positive bacteria
    b. intestinal malabsorption
    c. squamous-cell carcinoma
    d. chronic obstructive pulmonary disease
    e. diabetes insipidus

29. *The anticoagulant heparin can be added to saline to make a solution used to flush intravenous catheters, so as to prevent*

---

obstruction by blood clots. How much heparin should be added to each milliliter of saline to make such a flushing solution to be used in adult animals?

a. 1 unit per ml
b. 2 units per ml
c. 3 units per ml
d. 5 units per ml
e. 10 units per ml

30. *Whole blood, plasma, and blood substitutes should:*

a. be kept at room temperature for 24 hours before use
b. be given in the same intravenous line as other medications
c. not be used to dilute any drugs
d. be mixed with calcium products before use
e. be given with dextrose solutions

31. *Antineoplastic agents, such as vincristine and doxorubicin, should be:*

a. cautiously handled so as to avoid human and environmental contamination
b. mixed with calcium solutions and infused as a bolus intravenous injection
c. prepared at least 24 hours before intended use so as to allow precipitation of contaminants
d. used only when the prognosis for recovery is poor
e. used only in animals less than 3 years of age

32. *Amprolium is used to treat:*

a. heartworm infection
b. coccidiosis
c. congestive heart failure
d. paronychia
e. otitis externa

33. *When given orally once a month for heartworm prevention in dogs, the recommended dosage of ivermectin is:*

a. 200 μg/kg

b. 2 μg/kg
c. 300 μg/kg
d. 6 μg/kg
e. 50 mg/lb

34. *After administration of hetacillin potassium, the drug is metabolized and appears in tissue and blood as:*

a. ampicillin and amoxicillin
b. hetacillin and carbenicillin
c. ampicillin and hetacillin
d. amoxicillin and penicillin
e. penicillin and carbenicillin

35. *Strong tincture of iodine USP is comprised of:*

a. 2% iodine in water
b. 2% iodine in alcohol
c. 7% iodine in water
d. 7% iodine in alcohol
e. 15.6% iodine in water

36. *Xylazine hydrochloride is classified as:*

a. an alpha-1 adrenergic agonist
b. an alpha-2 adrenergic antagonist
c. an alpha-2 adrenergic agonist
d. a beta-1 adrenergic agonist
e. a beta-2 adrenergic agonist

37. *Yohimbine is classified as:*

a. an alpha-1 adrenergic agonist
b. an alpha-1 adrenergic antagonist
c. an alpha-2 adrenergic agonist
d. an alpha-2 adrenergic antagonist
e. a beta-1 adrenergic agonist

38. *Epinephrine should **not** be given with any of the following medications **except**:*

a. dextrose 5% injection USP
b. sodium bicarbonate
c. warfarin sodium
d. ascorbic acid
e. Hetastarch

Correct answers are on pages 219-222.

39. A dog is having a seizure. The drug of choice to immediately stop the seizure is:

a. phenytoin per os
b. acepromazine intramuscularly
c. xylazine intravenously
d. diazepam intravenously
e. ketamine intramuscularly

40. In dogs, primidone is metabolized to:

a. phenobarbital
b. diazepam
c. xylazine
d. ketamine
e. acepromazine

41. Records on use of controlled substances in a veterinary practice should be maintained by:

a. a veterinary technician with a license in that state
b. a clerk with experience in inventory control
c. a hospital administrator with a key to the controlled substances cabinet
d. an office manager
e. a veterinarian registered with the Drug Enforcement Administration

42. Concerning a veterinarian's dispensing of medication to hospital staff members for use in treating themselves, which statement is most accurate?

a. It is permitted if they present a prescription written by a physician.
b. It is permitted if the drugs are used on the premises.
c. It is permitted if they have been employed by the hospital for at least 3 years.
d. It is permitted if they are blood relatives.
e. It is not permitted under any circumstances.

43. Concerning the legality of dispensing outdated drugs (after the date of expiration indicated on the label), which statement is most accurate?

a. It is permitted within 1 month after the date of expiration.

b. It is permitted within 2 months after the date of expiration.
c. It is permitted within 3 months after the date of expiration.
d. It is permitted within 6 months after the date of expiration.
e. It is not permitted under any circumstances.

44. A drug that is a direct respiratory stimulant is:

a. epinephrine
b. norepinephrine
c. doxapram
d. ketamine
e. calcium

45. Magnesium hydroxide, an ingredient in some antacids, can be given orally in treatment of:

a. constipation
b. diarrhea
c. emesis
d. nausea
e. indigestion

46. Which drug is used in dogs and cats to treat gastric ulcers but is **not** absorbed?

a. cimetidine
b. ranitidine
c. neomycin
d. sucralfate
e. omeprazole

47. According to the Controlled Substances Act of 1970, anabolic steroids have some potential for abuse, and therefore are classified as:

a. Schedule I
b. Schedule II
c. Schedule III
d. Schedule IV
e. Schedule V

48. Oxfendazole is an anthelmintic in the same class of drugs as:

a. fenbendazole

b.   levamisole

c.   ivermectin

d.   pyrantel pamoate

e.   trichlorfon

49. *A client calls and says she left the container of diethylcarbamazine citrate oral liquid in her car for 3 weeks during the summer. Concerning the potency of the drug after such storage, which statement is most accurate?*

a.   It has probably lost potency.

b.   It has probably gained potency.

c.   It will regain any lost potency if placed in the refrigerator.

d.   It will lose any excessive potency if placed in the refrigerator.

e.   It is probably unaffected and can be used without concern.

50. *Veterinary prescription medications should be dispensed in:*

a.   white envelopes with a self-sealing adhesive flap

b.   brown envelopes with a gummed flap sealed by moistening

c.   child-proof amber vials and bottles

d.   transparent plastic cups with a pop-off top

e.   transparent plastic bags with a "zip-lock" closure

51. *All of the following are nonsteroidal anti-inflammatory drugs except:*

a.   phenylbutazone

b.   aspirin

c.   flunixin

d.   dexamethasone

e.   dipyrone

52. *Which of the following is the most potent glucocorticoid?*

a.   dexamethasone

b.   prednisone

c.   prednisolone

d.   methylprednisolone

e.   hydrocortisone

53. *Glucocorticoids are* **contraindicated** *in all of the following conditions* **except:**

a.   first trimester of gestation

b.   last trimester of gestation

c.   systemic fungal infections

d.   corneal ulcers

e.   trauma or shock

54. *What is the main adverse effect of phenylbutazone?*

a.   pulmonary edema

b.   crystals in the urine

c.   gastric ulcers

d.   cardiac decompensation

e.   dryness of the mouth

55. *Which glucocorticoid is metabolized to prednisolone?*

a.   dexamethasone

b.   prednisone

c.   betamethasone

d.   hydrocortisone

e.   cortisone

56. *You plan to give a dog sucralfate for treatment of a gastric ulcer. Which drug enhances healing of gastric ulcers, when given with sucralfate?*

a.   cimetidine

b.   ranitidine

c.   famotidine

d.   antacids

e.   no other drug

57. *Enrofloxacin should be used with caution when treating:*

a.   young dogs

b.   dogs with infections by Gram-negative bacteria

c.   dogs with marginal cardiopulmonary functions

d.   brachycephalic dogs

e.   dolichocephalic dogs

Correct answers are on pages 219-222.

58. In dogs, overdosage of ivermectin can produce all of the following **except**:

    a. tremors
    b. ataxia
    c. mydriasis
    d. weight loss
    e. degenerative joint disease

59. Cloxacillin sodium is an antibiotic that is effective against:

    a. lecithinase-producing micrococci
    b. E coli
    c. penicillinase-producing staphylococci
    d. Proteus
    e. collagenase-producing enterobacteria

60. The major toxicity associated with flunixin meglumine is:

    a. ototoxicity
    b. liver toxicity
    c. renal toxicity
    d. glaucoma
    e. gastrointestinal ulcers

61. Dobutamine, a drug used for treatment of heart failure, is classified as:

    a. a beta-1 adrenergic antagonist
    b. an alpha-1 adrenergic agonist
    c. an alpha-2 adrenergic agonist
    d. a beta-1 adrenergic agonist
    e. a histamine type-2 antagonist

62. A dehydrated animal is best treated by intravenous infusion of:

    a. dextrose 15% injection USP
    b. dextrose 10% injection USP
    c. dextrose 20% injection USP
    d. dextrose 50% injection USP
    e. acetated Ringer's injection USP

63. One gram of dextrose contains 3.4 calories. How many calories are contained in 1 liter of 5% dextrose?

    a. 170 calories
    b. 2000 calories
    c. 50 calories
    d. 500 calories
    e. 1000 calories

64. Because of the likelihood of adverse reaction, solutions of B vitamins should **never** be administered:

    a. intramuscularly
    b. orally
    c. subcutaneously
    d. as an intravenous bolus
    e. by slow intravenous infusion after dilution in 1-2 liters of fluid

65. The diuretic of choice to combat pulmonary edema in an animal with congestive heart failure is:

    a. thiazide
    b. chlorothiazide
    c. aldosterone
    d. furosemide
    e. ethacrynic acid

66. Tiletamine hydrochloride is an injectable anesthetic closely related to:

    a. acepromazine
    b. diazepam
    c. ketamine
    d. guaifenesin
    e. xylazine

67. Therapeutic drug monitoring involves:

    a. periodic physical examination of animals that have been treated with drugs.
    b. testing of animals for possible anaphylactic reaction before treatment with a drug
    c. measurement of serum or plasma levels of a drug to maintain levels in the optimal range
    d. close visual observation of animals in the first 8 hours after a drug is administered
    e. periodically obtaining tissue or exudate specimens for culture during a course of drug therapy

Answers

1. **a** Approved drugs are those for which experimental data document safety and efficacy for a particular disease in certain species.

2. **a** Extra-label use involves use of an approved drug in a manner not consistent with the drug's label.

3. **e** A veterinary drug may be used in an extra-label fashion only when a proper veterinarian-client-patient relationship exists, with a medical diagnosis established, and when there is no approved drug available to treat the disease properly. Animals so treated must be easily identified and/or kept separate from others on the premises.

4. **c** All records of the medication should be cited in metric units of the total dose given. For example, 500 mg of flunixin (not 10 ml).

5. **b** A 7% solution contains 7 g/dl. Remember, percent is parts (in this case, grams) per 100.

6. **c** There are 13.4 milliequivalents (mEq) in 1 gram (1000 mg) of potassium chloride. The equation is

$$mEq = \frac{mg}{molecular\ weight/valence}$$

7. **b** First divide the initial amount (5 million units) by the final amount (250,000 units/ml). 5,000,000 ÷ 250,000 = 20 ml. Then subtract the volume of diluent added (18 ml). 20 − 18 = 2 ml of powder originally in the vial.

8. **e** Veterinary technicians are permitted to dispense drugs only in the presence of a licensed veterinarian.

9. **a** All insecticides should be dispensed in the original container, with all EPA information on the label and in a safety-cap container or spray container.

10. **b** An isotonic solution has an osmolarity of 300 mOsm/L, which is the same osmotic pressure as for body fluids. A solution with an osmolarity less than 300 mOsm/L is hypotonic and could cause lysis of red blood cells. A solution with an osmolarity greater than 300 mOsm/L is hypertonic.

11. **d**

12. **a** Aminoglycosides can produce nephrotoxicity, ototoxicity and neurotoxicity.

13. **a** The safest way to monitor patients receiving aminoglycosides is to obtain serum samples and measure peak and trough levels to make sure drug levels are within the safe, therapeutic range.

14. **e** Ampicillin is eliminated primarily by the kidneys and normally administered every 6 hours for 7-10 days. If an animal has a serum creatinine value of 3 mg/dl (normal, 1-2 mg/dl), this indicates reduced renal function, so the drug should be given less frequently as it is not being eliminated at a normal rate. A good rule of thumb is: serum creatinine x normal dosage interval = adjusted dosage interval. 3 x 6 = 18 hours.

15. **c** Only fluids that are sterile and pyrogen free should be given intravenously.

16. **d** Lactated Ringer's USP contains calcium chloride. Mixing with sodium bicarbonate forms an insoluble precipitate, calcium carbonate.

17. **e** Detomidine and xylazine are chemically related. Animals that have an adverse reaction to xylazine may also react to detomidine.

18. **c** A 5% dextrose-5% guaifenesin solution contains 5 grams of dextrose and 5 grams of guaifenesin per 100 ml, which is equal to 50 grams of each per 1000 ml.

19. **c** The half-life of a drug is the time it takes for the drug concentration to decrease by one-half. Usually in animals, 99% of the drug is cleared from the animal's body in 10 half-lives.

20. **b** Theophylline, phenobarbital, digoxin, amikacin and gentamicin all have narrow safety ranges and could cause adverse reactions and toxicities if serum levels are not monitored. Penicillin has a larger margin of safety.

21. **d** Cimetidine and ranitidine are H2 antagonists that block gastric acid secretion, which
aids treatment of ulcers. Because there are no
H2 antagonists approved for veterinary use,
these drugs can only be used in accordance
with extra-label laws.

22. **e** Water-soluble drugs, such as gentamicin,
tend to remain in the serum or plasma and are
often used for Gram-negative septicemia.

23. **c** Cimetidine acts as an immunostimulant
and is sometimes used to treat melanomas in
horses and dogs.

24. **e** A lipophilic drug has an affinity for such
areas as soft tissue, the outer layers of the
lungs, and bone.

25. **b** Digoxin has a variable half-life in dogs,
ranging from 14 to 56 hours. Serum levels of
the drug should be monitored after initiation
of therapy and at least once a month during
therapy.

26. **b** Oxytetracycline chelates (binds) calcium.
The vehicles used in some oxytetracycline
products, such as propylene glycol, can cause
anaphylaxis if these drugs are given by rapid
intravenous injection. Because of their pH or
vehicles, some products cannot be given
intramuscularly.

27. **c** Atropine causes bronchodilation.

28. **d** Aminophylline (a bronchodilator), prednisone (an antiinflammatory glucocorticoid)
and terbutaline (a selective beta-2 adrenergic
agonist) can be given in combination to treat
chronic obstructive pulmonary disease.

29. **e** Heparinized saline is commonly prepared
at a concentration of 10 units/ml. A commercial preparation of heparin is available 1000
units/ml. To prepare a sterile solution, add 1
ml of heparin to 100 ml of sodium chloride
injection 0.9% USP. In neonates, a
concentration of 1 unit/ml is often used.

30. **c** Whole blood, plasma and blood substitutes
should not be used as diluents of any drugs,
and can be infused only by piggyback with
sodium chloride injection 0.9% USP.

31. **a** Antineoplastic agents can pose a threat to
human health if not handled properly. EPA
guidelines, including disposal of medical waste,
should be observed. This may require that you
attend a continuing education class on safe
preparation of drugs used in cancer therapy.

32. **b** Amprolium is used in prevention and
treatment of coccidiosis caused by *Eimeria
bovis* and *E zurnii* in calves.

33. **d** The ivermectin dosage for heartworm
prevention in dogs is very small (6 μg/kg).
There are 1000 μg in 1 mg. Certain breeds of
dogs, such as Collies, are more sensitive to
ivermectin, though the dosage used for
heartworm prevention should be safe, as it is
extremely low.

34. **c** Hetacillin potassium is chemically related
to ampicillin. Some of the drug is metabolized
to ampicillin, while some remains as hetacillin.

35. **d** Strong tincture of iodine USP is a 7%
tincture, which has an alcohol base. It is
commonly used to dip the umbilical cord of
newborn calves. Mild tincture of iodine is a 2%
solution and can be used to dip the umbilical
cord of foals.

36. **c** Xylazine is an alpha-2 adrenergic agonist.
It stimulates alpha-2 receptors and is a
sedative/analgesic with muscle relaxant
properties.

37. **d** Yohimbine is an alpha-2 adrenergic
antagonist and can be used to reverse xylazine.

38. **a** Epinephrine is usually given by
intravenous bolus injection. If it must be
diluted, it should be added to dextrose 5%
injection USP.

39. **d** Diazepam is the drug of choice for rapid
control of seizures. Other anticonvulsants can
be used for maintenance therapy, such as
primidone, phenobarbital and phenytoin. All of
these drugs require monthly monitoring of
serum levels to ensure accurate dosage.

40. **a** Primidone is converted to phenobarbital
and other active metabolites, and is monitored
in the serum as phenobarbital.

41. **e** A veterinarian registered with the DEA
and prescribing controlled substances should
keep accurate records.

42. **e** A veterinarian is not permitted to dispense
any drugs to people. Severe penalties are
associated with this offense.

43. **e** Only drugs that are in date (not expired)
and stored in proper containers at the proper
temperature may be legally dispensed by or on
prescription of a licensed veterinarian.

44. **c** Doxapram has a direct stimulatory effect
on the medullary respiratory center.

45. **a** Magnesium hydroxide is often found in antacids and is also used as a laxative. When added to magnesium hydroxide, the constipating antacid aluminum hydroxide seems to provide a balanced antacid.

46. **d** Sucralfate is an alkaline aluminum complex of sucrose sulfate that acts locally rather than systemically. It forms a barrier at the ulcer site and protects the ulcer from further damage caused by pepsin, acid or bile.

47. **c** Anabolic steroids, such as boldenone, stanozolol, nandrolone, testosterone, chorionic gonadotropin and any growth stimulants, are currently Schedule-III controlled substances due to their potential for abuse.

48. **a** Fenbendazole and oxfendazole are benzimidazole anthelmintics.

49. **a** Diethylcarbamazine citrate, used for heartworm prevention in dogs, decomposes when exposed to temperatures over 30 C (86 F) and when exposed to light. Always dispense this drug in an amber bottle.

50. **c** Any medication that could be ingested by a child should be dispensed in amber safety-cap vials or bottles.

51. **d** Dexamethasone is a glucocorticoid and not a nonsteroidal antiinflammatory; however, it does have antiinflammatory activity.

52. **a** Dexamethasone is a fluorinated prednisolone glucocorticoid. Fluorination of the drug molecule gives the greatest antiinflammatory effects.

53. **e** Glucocorticoids are contraindicated in all pregnant animals. Deformities may occur in the first trimester, and abortions may occur in the last trimester, particularly with the longer-acting glucocorticoids, such as methylprednisolone, dexamethasone, betamethasone and triamcinolone. Fungal infections and corneal ulcers may worsen with glucocorticoid treatment.

54. **c** The major toxicity associated with phenylbutazone is gastric ulcers. The dosage should be tapered to small amounts or the drug should be used for short periods only, as it accumulates.

55. **b** Prednisone is metabolized to prednisolone by the liver.

56. **e** Sucralfate requires an acidic environment to be effective. All of the other drugs listed increase the pH of the stomach and decrease the efficacy of sucralfate.

57. **a** Enrofloxacin is contraindicated in small and medium-sized dogs 2-8 months of age, and in large-breed dogs of all ages. Changes in articular cartilage have been noted when the drug was given at 2-5 times recommended doses for 30 days, though clinical signs have only been seen at 5 times the recommended dose.

58. **e** Excessive ivermectin dosages may produce tremors, ataxia, mydriasis and weight loss when administered to dogs. Collie breeds seem to be more sensitive to toxicities.

59. **c** Cloxacillin sodium is a penicillin that is effective against penicillinase-producing staphylococci. Other drugs in that category are oxacillin, dicloxacillin, and antibiotics combined with clavulanate sodium or clavulanic acid.

60. **e** Flunixin meglumine causes severe irritation of the gastrointestinal tract in dogs, and should be used with great caution in horses with gastrointestinal ulcers. The dosage and frequency of administration may also need to be adjusted in dehydrated horses. Prophylactic treatment with ranitidine or sucralfate may be helpful in preventing gastric ulcers.

61. **d** Dobutamine is a direct beta-1 adrenergic agonist that is used as a rapid-acting injectable positive inotropic agent for short-term treatment of heart failure. It must be diluted in sodium chloride or dextrose 5% injection and infused continuously intravenously because of its short half-life.

62. **e** Acetated Ringer's injection is the fluid of choice. Hypertonic dextrose solutions would act as an osmotic diuretic and further dehydrate the animal.

63. **a** Dextrose normally has 4 kilocalories per gram; however, hydrous dextrose is used to prepare 5% dextrose injection. It has 3.4 calories per gram. 3.4 calories x 50 grams per liter of dextrose equals 170 calories.

64. **d** B vitamins must never be administered by direct intravenous injection, as anaphylactic reactions can result in death due to massive release of histamine.

65. **d** Furosemide is the diuretic of choice for congestive heart failure. It is approved for use in dogs, cats, horses and cattle. The response is very rapid and the drug may be effective in animals nonresponsive to other diuretics.

66. **c** Tiletamine hydrochloride is an injectable anesthetic closely related to ketamine. It is commercially available in combination with zolazepam hydrochloride and is approved for use in dogs.

67. **c** Therapeutic drug monitoring involves measuring the amount of drug in the serum or plasma of the diseased animal to achieve the best therapeutic dosage, with the least toxicity.

Notes

12

Preventive Medicine

P.C. Bartlett, C.N. Carter,
J.D. Hoskins

Recommended Reading

August JR: *Consultations in Feline Internal Medicine.* Saunders, Philadelphia, 1991.

Brander GC *et al: Veterinary Applied Pharmacology and Therapeutics.* Bailliere Tindall, London, 1991.

Ettinger SJ: *Textbook of Veterinary Internal Medicine: Diseases of the Dog and Cat.* 3rd ed. Saunders, Philadelphia, 1989.

Georgi JR and Georgi ME: *Parasitology for Veterinarians.* 5th ed. Saunders, Philadelphia, 1990.

Greene CE: *Infectious Diseases of the Dog and Cat.* 2nd ed. Saunders, Philadelphia, 1990.

Morgan RV: *Handbook of Small Animal Practice.* 2nd ed. Churchill Livingstone, New York, 1992.

Panel Report on the Colloquium on Feline Leukemia Virus/Feline Immunodeficiency Virus: Tests and Vaccination. *JAVMA* 199:1271-1487, 1991.

Proceedings of the Heartworm Symposium, 1989. American Heartworm Society, Washington, DC.

Sherding RG: *The Cat: Diseases and Clinical Management.* Churchill Livingstone, New York, 1989.

Veterinary Pharmaceuticals and Biologicals. 7th ed. Veterinary Medicine Publishing, Lenexa, KS, 1991.

> *Practice answer sheet is on page 353.*

Questions

1. *According to the AVMA Compendium on Rabies Control, which of the following should be used by practicing veterinarians to record rabies vaccination of dogs and cats?*

   a. any self-designed form with complete information is adequate

   b. the National Association of State Public Health Veterinarians form #50 ("Rabies Vaccination Certificate") or a computer-generated form containing the same information

   c. an entry in the medical record, along with an appropriate rabies tag

   d. any computer-generated certificate

   e. no formal recording of rabies vaccinations is required

Correct answers are on pages 236-239.

2. *Concerning vaccination of wild animals against rabies, which statement is most accurate?*

   a. Rabies vaccines are now available and approved for use in pet raccoons and skunks.

   b. Any wild animal can be vaccinated against rabies, as long as it has been adequately domesticated by its owner.

   c. There are no licensed rabies vaccines approved for use in wild animals, with the exception of ferrets

   d. Rabies vaccines licensed for use in dogs can be used on pet coyotes, foxes and wolves.

   e. The AVMA does not consider rabies in wild animals to be a real threat in the United States and, therefore, vaccination is optional.

3. *The AVMA recommends that all dogs and cats be vaccinated against rabies, as per which preexposure guidelines?*

   a. vaccinate at 4 months of age using a vaccine effective for at least 1 year, with an annual booster

   b. vaccinate at 4 months of age using a vaccine effective for 3 years

   c. vaccinate at 2 months of age using any approved vaccine, with an annual booster

   d. vaccinate at 6 months of age using a vaccine effective for at least 1 year, with an annual booster

   e. vaccinate at 3 months of age and revaccinate according to National Association of Public Health Veterinarians recommendations for the specific vaccine used

4. *The AVMA Compendium on Rabies Control states that "Any animal bitten or scratched by a wild, carnivorous mammal (or a bat) that is not available for testing should be regarded as having been exposed to rabies." In this situation, how should pet dogs and cats be managed (postexposure management)?*

   a. the animal should be confined and observed for 10 days, and released upon examination by a licensed veterinarian

   b. the animal should be euthanized, regardless of vaccination status

   c. the animal should be vaccinated against rabies and placed in strict isolation for 90 days

   d. unvaccinated dogs and cats should be euthanized immediately; if the owner is unwilling to do this, the animal should be isolated for 6 months and vacccinated 1 month before release; currently vaccinated animals should be revaccinated and observed for 90 days

   e. vaccinated animals are likely to be adequately protected and require no further action; unvaccinated animals should be vaccinated and observed for 90 days

5. *What is the appropriate management of a dog or cat that bites a person?*

   a. the animal should be immediately euthanized, regardless of ownership status and the animal's head sent to the local state health department for rabies examination

   b. the animal should be confined and observed for 10 days; if any signs of illness arise, a veterinarian should evaluate the animal and report to the health department; if signs of rabies emerge, the animal should be humanely killed and the head sent to the local or state health department for rabies examination

   c. the animal should be immediately given a rabies booster, confined and observed for 30 days

   d. the animal should be simply observed for 10 days and released after examination by a licensed veterinarian

   e. a copy of the bite report must be given to the local or state health department

6. *Which of the following is **not** a characteristic of an ideal disinfectant?*

   a. broad spectrum of activity against bacteria, viruses and fungi

   b. does not promote development of resistant populations of organisms

   c. not inactivated by proteinaceous substances

   d. simple and inexpensive to use

   e. no residual action

7. *Dogs infected with parvovirus shed large numbers of virus particles and present a significant threat to susceptible animals. Which of the following describes appropriate management of such animals and the environment to protect other dogs from infection?*

   a. isolate infected dogs from other dogs until a week after full recovery and disinfect the premises with dilute (1:30) chlorine bleach solution

   b. dogs routinely shed virus for up to 6 months and should be isolated for at least that period, followed by a thorough detergent cleaning of the environment

   c. isolate infected dogs and disinfect the premises only if unvaccinated animals will be in the area

   d. isolate infected dogs until they recover and disinfect the premises with chloroxylenol

   e. isolate infected dogs until they are no longer febrile; no environmental disinfection is required, as parvovirus is extremely labile

8. *Concerning peroxides (eg, hydrogen peroxide), which statement is most accurate?*

   a. They are some of the most effective antiseptics.

   b. They are known for their long-term residual activity.

   c. They provide a mechanical cleansing action via release of oxygen but have only a mild antiseptic action.

   d. They have virtually no use in the medical environment.

   e. Most peroxides are virucidal.

9. *Concerning quaternary ammonium compounds (eg, benzalkonium chloride), which statement is most accurate?*

   a. They are very effective against a broad range of organisms.

   b. They are virucidal only.

   c. They are bactericidal only.

   d. They are relatively ineffective against bacterial spores, viruses and fungi, and are inactivated by organic matter.

   e. Their effects are not hampered by organic matter.

10. *Iodophor disinfectants (eg, povidone-iodine) are surgical scrubs. Concerning iodophors, which statement is **least** accurate?*

    a. Scrubbing of hands and surgical sites with an iodophor reduces bacterial populations for up to 8 hours.

    b. Iodophors are effective against a broad range of bacteria, viruses and fungi.

    c. Iodophors act as oxidizing agents, though they are less active than chlorine.

    d. Iodophors are known for their action against spores.

    e. Iodophors can irritate the skin.

11. *Which disinfectant has the best overall antimicrobial activity?*

    a. chlorine/iodine

    b. benzalkonium chloride

    c. chlorhexidine

    d. benzoyl peroxide

    e. hydrogen peroxide

12. *Oral use of the organophosphate cythioate every third day can help provide effective flea control. Concerning use of cythioate, which statement is most accurate?*

    a. Cythioate should not be given to Cocker Spaniels.

    b. Cythioate should not be given to Greyhounds or cats.

    c. Cythioate can be used in pregnant animals, sick animals or animals recovering from surgery.

    d. Cythioate can be used concomitantly with other anticholinesterase drugs.

    e. The primary sign of cythioate toxicity is blindness.

13. *Which of the following is a recognized method of preventing ascariasis in dogs?*

    a. no raw meat in the diet

    b. boiling of all drinking water

    c. treatment of newborn pups with niclosamide

    d. treatment of the postparturient bitch with metronidazole

    e. treatment of the preparturient bitch with fenbendazole

---

Correct answers are on pages 236-239.

14. Hookworm infections are a serious problem in catteries. Which of the following is **not** a method to prevent and control ancylostomiasis in cats?

   a. good general sanitation
   b. exposure to sunlight and drying of the environment
   c. cleaning litterboxes at least once a week
   d. cleaning surfaces with dilute chlorine bleach (1% solution)
   e. regular treatment of cats with an approved anthelmintic (*eg*, pyrantel pamoate, piperazine)

15. Heartworm infection in dogs can be prevented by all of the following **except**:

   a. diethylcarbamazine daily
   b. ivermectin monthly
   c. milbemycin oxime monthly
   d. standard adulticide dose of thiacetarsamide sodium twice a year
   e. metronidazole weekly

16. Concerning prevention and control of herpesvirus-1 and calicivirus respiratory infection in cats, which statement is most accurate?

   a. Intranasal vaccines offer rapid protection but may result in mild disease and possibly a carrier state.
   b. Parenteral vaccines take longer to act than intranasal products, and usually cause mild clinical disease and carrier states.
   c. Cats often develop oral ulcers after chewing at an intramuscular vaccination site when inactivated products are used.
   d. Vaccination may cause severe central nervous system signs.
   e. If administered properly, the vaccines are totally effective.

17. Concerning vaccination and immunity in dogs and cats, which statement is **least** accurate?

   a. Colostrum-deprived dogs and cats should be given the initial vaccination approximately 2-3 weeks earlier than normal.
   b. Maternal antibodies can provide 3-6 months of protection against most diseases but can also interfere with development of active immunity from vaccination.
   c. Live agents in vaccines should be attenuated so that they remain antigenic and replicate in the recipient but do not produce illness.
   d. The agents in killed (inactivated) vaccines are immunogenic but do not replicate in the host.
   e. Vaccine failures are most common in very young and very old animals.

18. Only modified-live vaccines have been shown to protect dogs against distemper. Which of the following best describes the most reasonable vaccination regimen against canine distemper in a puppy that received adequate colostrum?

   a. vaccinate at 3- to 4-week intervals, beginning at 5-8 weeks of age, until the animal is 12 weeks of age
   b. vaccinate at 3- to 4-week intervals, beginning at 12 weeks of age, until the animal is 20 weeks of age
   c. vaccinate at 4- to 5-week intervals, beginning at 4 weeks of age, until the animal is 16 weeks of age
   d. vaccinate at 4- to 5-week intervals, beginning at 6 weeks of age, until the animal is vaccinated for rabies
   e. vaccinate at 8-week intervals, beginning at 8 weeks of age, for a total of 3 vaccinations

19. A possible complication of immunization with canine adenovirus-1 vaccine is:

   a. acute retinitis
   b. subacute poliomyelitis
   c. thromboembolism
   d. anterior uveitis
   e. paralysis of cranial nerve V

20. Concerning vaccination of dogs against infectious tracheobronchitis (kennel cough), which statement is **least** accurate?

   a. Parenteral vaccinations probably provide little prolonged protection.

---

b. Intranasal vaccines are no more promising than parenterally administered products.

c. Vaccination is most recommended when animals will be at increased risk (*eg,* in kennels, at dog shows, etc).

d. Puppies can be given the intranasal vaccine as young as 2-3 weeks of age, as maternal antibodies do not interfere as much as with parenteral products.

e. Annual or more frequent boosters are indicated for animals with a high potential for exposure.

21. *Vaccination of dogs against parvoviral enteritis has become an essential preventive measure in practice. Concerning canine parvovirus, which statement is **least** accurate?*

a. Parvovirus is as contagious as distemper virus but is more resistant in the environment.

b. Because of the stable environmental properties of canine parvovirus, it is estimated that at least 90-95% of dogs must be immunized to prevent spread of the disease.

c. Killed parvovirus vaccines produce a shorter duration of immunity than modified-live-virus products.

d. Modified-live-virus products are not recommended for immunosuppressed animals, pregnant bitches, or puppies 5 weeks of age or younger.

e. Bitches should receive a booster with inactivated vaccine just after breeding or during the last trimester of gestation.

22. *One of your clients actively shows Dobermans and is concerned about exposure to viral diarrhea agents causing some recent outbreaks. Which of the following constitutes the best preventive medicine program?*

a. 2 weeks before each show, administer a vaccine against distemper, adenovirus-2, parvovirus and leptospriosis

b. 2 weeks before each show, administer a modified-live-virus parvovirus vaccine

c. 2 weeks before each show, administer a modified-live-virus parvovirus vaccine and an inactivated coronavirus vaccine

d. before shipment to each show, administer hyperimmune serum intravenously

e. regularly expose the dogs to animals that are known carriers of parvovirus and coronavirus

23. Leptospira *vaccines are usually comprised of inactivated bacterins of* L canicola *and* L icterohemorrhagiae. *Concerning these products, which statement is most accurate?*

a. Vaccination is recommended at 6 weeks of age to avoid problems with allergic reactions.

b. Most *Leptospira* bacterins do not protect against a carrier state, which may occur after exposure to virulent organisms.

c. Anaphylaxis is never a problem with *Leptospira* bacterins.

d. *Leptospira* bacterins produce extremely long-lasting immunity as compared with other agents in canine vaccines.

e. *Leptospira* bacterins are ideal in combination with inactivated adjuvanted vaccines, such as canine coronavirus.

24. *A new client with a kitten is asking questions about feline distemper (feline panleukopenia). Which of the following is **least** appropriate in advising this client?*

a. Two modified-live-virus or 3 inactivated vaccine doses should be given at 3- to 4-week intervals, beginning at 8-9 weeks of age.

b. Boosters should be given every 2 years if modified-live-virus products are used and annually if inactivated products are used.

c. Inactivated vaccines should be used in pregnant, immunosuppressed or diseased animals, and in kittens less than 4 weeks of age.

d. Modified-live-virus products must not be used in kittens less than 4 weeks of age because of the risk of cerebellar degeneration.

e. Immune serum can give some protection for unvaccinated kittens in the face of exposure.

Correct answers are on pages 236-239.

25. *Concerning vaccination of cats against feline leukemia virus (FeLV), which statement is* **least** *accurate?*

   a. Only healthy, afebrile cats should be vaccinated; FeLV-infected cats should not be vaccinated.
   b. All cats at risk of exposure should be vaccinated.
   c. Prevaccination testing for FeLV is unnecessary in cats that have been exposed to FeLV or whose exposure status is unknown.
   d. Transient viremia develops in many FeLV-vaccinated cats after subsequent virus exposure.
   e. Vaccines should be administered according to the manufacturer's recommendations.

26. *Concerning diagnostic testing for feline leukemia virus (FeLV) infection, which statement is* **least** *accurate?*

   a. Enzyme-linked immunosorbent assay detects the p27 core antigen in serum, plasma, tears or saliva.
   b. The indirect fluorescent antibody test detects the p27 core antigen in white blood cells.
   c. Enzyme-linked immunosorbent assays of saliva and tears may yield false-positive results.
   d. Vaccination interferes with FeLV testing procedures.
   e. After screening by enzyme-linked immunosorbent assay, a positive or equivocal result should be confirmed by an indirect fluorescent antibody test.

27. *Hemobartonellosis can cause severe anemia in both dogs and cats. Which of the following is the best preventive medicine program for this disease?*

   a. vaccination
   b. preventing exposure to infected animals
   c. establishing premunition via serial transfusions of infected blood
   d. vaccination and quarterly prophylaxis with oxytetracycline

   e. control of ectoparasites (fleas, ticks) and proper screening of blood donors for infection

28. Toxoplasma *is an intracellular coccidian parasite that infects virtually all warm-blooded species, including people. Cats are the definitive host. Prevention of this disease in all species is aimed at reducing the incidence in cats, thereby decreasing the number of infective oocysts in the environment. Concerning prevention and control of toxoplasmosis, which statement is most accurate?*

   a. Cats should be fed only dry or canned commercially processed food or thoroughly cooked meats, and should not be allowed to hunt or roam at large.
   b. Cats with *Toxoplasma* titers should be euthanized.
   c. All infected cats should be treated with clindamycin.
   d. A new commercially available subunit vaccine prevents clinical illness and shedding of the organism.
   e. Additions of sulfadiazine and pyrimethamine to the food is an effective prophylactic measure.

29. *Concerning prevention and control of borreliosis (Lyme disease), which statement is most accurate?*

   a. Many commercially available vaccines provide good protection.
   b. Immunomodulating drugs work well in preventing borreliosis and should be used when exposure to ticks is probable.
   c. Lifetime prophylactic administration of oxytetracycline to outdoor dogs and people in high-risk occupations provides excellent protection.
   d. It may take up to 24 hours of tick feeding before the *Borrelia* organism is secreted in the tick's saliva.
   e. No progress has been made in developing a borreliosis vaccine, as no species have been found to generate an active immune response.

30. *Concerning Rocky Mountain spotted fever, which statement is **least** accurate?*

    a. It can be prevented by preventing access of dogs to wooded areas, and quickly removing any attached ticks.
    b. It cannot be totally eliminated in an area by tick eradication, as the rickettsia life cycle is maintained by ticks feeding on rodents and other wild hosts.
    c. Infected dogs are immune to reinfection after they recover.
    d. Vaccination with an inactivated product provides long-lasting immunity.
    e. The causative rickettsia is inactivated in overwintering ticks but becomes reactivated by the tick's first blood meal in the spring.

31. *Prevention of salmonellosis in dogs and cats is difficult because:*

    a. the organism is very resistant to all known disinfectants and drugs
    b. dogs and cats have a propensity to develop a chronic carrier state or latent infection
    c. the organism is easily aerosolized
    d. salmonellae are a common contaminant in commercial pet foods
    e. disinfection of kennels, cages, food dishes and utensils is impossible

32. *Herpesvirus infection in a dog kennel is best controlled by:*

    a. testing incoming dogs for the carrier state and removing all infected dogs
    b. artificial insemination and cesarean delivery, with serologic testing of all neonates and removal of all infected pups
    c. vaccination of all dogs twice yearly
    d. maintaining warm environmental temperature for neonates, and administration of hyperimmune globulin to puppies at high risk during the first few days of life
    e. disinfection of the environment

33. *Concerning the prevention of feline immunodeficiency virus infection, which statement is most accurate?*

    a. Infected cats should be isolated from uninfected cats and overcrowding should be avoided.
    b. The newest vaccine available appears to confer adequate protection for up to 1 year.
    c. Routine disinfection of facilities provides adequate control.
    d. Annual prophylactic therapy with lymphokine modulators provides adequate control.
    e. Annual prophylactic therapy with interleukins yields excellent results.

34. *Which of the following is **least** effective in preventing pseudorabies in dogs and cats?*

    a. avoid contact with pigs
    b. do not feed raw pork to dogs or cats
    c. vaccinate with an inactivated product
    d. avoid contact with animals with suspected pseudorabies
    e. avoid contact with guinea pigs

35. *Salmon poisoning is a potentially fatal disease of domestic and wild canids, transmitted by a helminth. How is salmon poisoning best prevented?*

    a. allow dogs to eat only decomposed fish, as the metacercariae are only viable in fresh fish
    b. vaccinate with an attenuated product in enzootic areas (Washington, Oregon, northern California, British Columbia)
    c. freeze infected fish at -20 C for 24 hours or thoroughly cook fish before feeding to dogs
    d. give prophylactic doses of fenbendazole in enzootic areas
    e. give prophylactic doses of metronidazole in enzootic areas

---

Correct answers are on pages 236-239.

36. *Chlamydial infections can cause keratitis and possibly encephalitis in dogs, and ocular, nasal and lower respiratory problems in cats. What is the best way to prevent chlamydiosis in cats?*

    a. prevent contact with infected animals

    b. give prophylactic antibodies to animals at high risk of infection

    c. induce premunition by intramuscular injection of live chlamydial organisms

    d. vaccinate with an inactivated or modified-live vaccine

    e. test for infection and euthanize infected animals to limit exposure to uninfected animals

37. *Which drug is metabolized to form formaldehyde, is primarily excreted in the urine, and is used as a long-term prophylactic to help prevent recurring urinary tract infections?*

    a. ammonium chloride

    b. rifampin

    c. methenamine

    d. ethambutol

    e. mupirocin

38. *Concerning botulism, which statement is most accurate?*

    a. It has been experimentally reproduced in cats, but no natural infections have been confirmed.

    b. Botulinus toxin cannot be destroyed by heat.

    c. Raw meat or carrion is rarely implicated in cases of botulism.

    d. Commercially available vaccines lessen the clinical signs of botulism in dogs.

    e. The clinical signs of botulism directly reflect endothelial damage caused by the organism.

39. *An outbreak of tetanus in a veterinary hospital is most likely attributable to:*

    a. bites from an infected animal

    b. inhalation of aerosolized organisms from a convalescing patient

    c. improper sterilization of surgical instruments

    d. indirect transmission via a variety of insects

    e. contact with contaminated fomites

40. *Concerning control of dermatophytosis in a cattery, which statement is **least** accurate?*

    a. Infected animals should be segregated from all others during treatment.

    b. Sanitizing materials and grooming instruments used on infected cats must be kept separate from those used on uninfected cats so as to prevent cross contamination.

    c. Handlers must change clothes and first work with uninfected cats before working with infected cats.

    d. Treatment should include clipping, topical antifungal rinses and systemic griseofulvin or ketoconazole until cultures are negative.

    e. Large doses of corticosteroids can help prevent severe onychomycosis.

41. *Which of the following constitutes sound advice for cat owners wishing to prevent periodontal disease in their cat?*

    a. routine cleansing of the teeth with a soft toothbrush and swabbing of the teeth and gums with 0.1% chlorhexidine

    b. daily administration of prophylactic antibiotics for the life of the animal

    c. feeding of dry cat food with embedded "microbrushes"

    d. regular cleansing of the teeth with fine-grain sandpaper or steel wool

    e. routine culture of oral flora, with periodic antibiotic prophylaxis based on sensitivity tests

42. *Which of the following is most important in prevention of urolithiasis in cats?*

    a. decreasing the urine volume

    b. reducing urine concentration of calculogenic crystalloids

    c. decreasing the solubility of calculogenic crystalloids

d. alkalinizing the urine
e. limiting dietary intake of zinc

43. *Concerning risk factors for pancreatitis in dogs and cats, which statement is most accurate?*

a. Animals that exercise vigorously are at higher risk.
b. Animals that suffer from heat stroke are more likely to succumb to pancreatitis.
c. Hypolipoproteinemia can precipitate acute pancreatitis.
d. Pancreatitis is more prevalent in obese animals.
e. Specific drugs do not cause pancreatitis.

44. *Which of the following constitutes the most reasonable postoperative management for preventing recurrence of gastric dilatation-volvulus in dogs?*

a. do not feed dry dog food
b. give parasympatholytic drugs before each meal to help prevent gastrointestinal spasms
c. give multiple small feedings each day of moistened, softened foodstuffs, with restricted water intake and exercise before and after meals
d. feed special nonallergenic foods
e. avoid ectoparasite control programs because certain insecticides can precipitate gastric dilatation

45. *Trichobezoars (hairballs) are a common problem in cats. How are they best prevented in cats?*

a. give mineral oil directly per os or in the animal's food each day
b. train the cat not to groom
c. give enzymes that dissolve any hair material in the gastrointestinal tract
d. give petrolatum-based lubricants per os and encourage frequent grooming by the client

e. palpate the animal regularly to detect tricholbezoars and perform surgery before they cause problems

46. *How is tapeworm infection best prevented in dogs and cats?*

a. tick control
b. improved hygiene
c. adequate cooking of beef
d. louse control
e. flea control

47. *Cat scratch disease in people is thought to be caused by a small Gram-negative bacillus. What appropriate advice can you provide clients regarding prevention of this disease in family members?*

a. train children to be gentle with pets to avoid scratching and biting, and declaw cats that will be exposed to children
b. have cats tested serologically every year to identify carriers and remove them from the household
c. treat cats prophylactically with oxytetracycline to eliminate infection
d. wear protective clothing when around cats
e. euthanize cats that scratch people

48. *Trichuriasis (whipworm infection) is a common cause of large intestinal diarrhea in dogs. Which of the following constitutes a good management/prevention program for this disease?*

a. flea control
b. when worm segments are seen in the feces, treat with pyrantel pamoate
c. routine fecal examinations for characteristic double-operculated eggs and treatment with fenbendazole
d. keep the environment disinfected and counsel clients on the zoonotic potential of trichuriasis
e. avoid feeding raw meat and prevent access to infected rodents

49. *About 25-50% of Americans have antibodies to* Toxoplasma *organisms. Which of the following describes the most prudent means of preventing exposure of human beings to this disease?*

   a. cats should not be allowed to reside in the same building with children and pregnant women.

   b. people regularly exposed to cats should be serologically evaluated annually and treated if positive

   c. cat litter should be changed daily, and consumption and/or handling of raw meat avoided

   d. domestic cats should be given prophylactic therapy

   e. cats should be vaccinated annually against toxoplasmosis with an inactivated or modified-live product

50. *Coccidia are obligate intracellular parasites normally found in the intestinal tract of dogs and cats. Concerning the epizootiology of coccidiosis, which statement is **least** accurate?*

   a. Coccidiosis is usually seen in conjunction with poor sanitation of premises.

   b. Insect control is important, as cockroaches and flies can act as mechanical vectors of oocysts.

   c. Animals should not be fed uncooked meat.

   d. Coccidiostatic drugs can be given to infected bitches just before or after whelping to help control the spread of infection in puppies.

   e. Coccidial oocysts cannot survive freezing temperatures.

51. *Approximately how many people die from dog bites every year in the United States?*

   a. 2
   b. 20
   c. 200
   d. 2,000
   e. 20,000

52. *What United States agency regulates use of tick and flea sprays in veterinary practice?*

   a. Department of Agriculture
   b. Drug Enforcement Administration
   c. Environmental Protection Agency
   d. Centers for Disease Control
   e. Occupational Safety and Health Administration

53. *Use of a tick or flea dip in a manner **not** specified on the label is:*

   a. acceptable if the product is applied by a licensed veterinarian

   b. only legal if no licensed product is available for the species being treated

   c. only legal by special permit

   d. strictly prohibited

   e. legal but unethical

54. *In a state in which no rabies occurred in dogs during the past year, a dog bites a child. During the 10-day rabies observation period, the dog begins acting sick and agitated, and showing signs that could be those of rabies or other diseases. The most appropriate course of action is to:*

   a. euthanize the dog and send the head to the laboratory for rabies testing

   b. confirm the diagnosis before euthanizing the dog

   c. wait to see if the dog survives the full 10 days; if so, the bitten child will need not worry about rabies

   d. have a sample of the dog's blood tested for a rabies titer

   e. wait a few days for clinical signs to more fully develop

55. *In a state in which no rabies occurred during the past year, a currently vaccinated dog bites a person. The most appropriate course of action is to:*

   a. euthanize the dog and send the head to a laboratory for rabies testing

   b. revaccinate the dog and isolate it for 30 days

   c. observe the dog for 10 days; if the dog is healthy after 10 days, the bitten person need not worry about rabies

d. have a sample of the dog's blood tested for a rabies titer

e. revaccinate the dog but do not isolate or observe it

56. *How do children contract toxocariasis?*

   a. from ingestion of raw meat
   b. by direct contact with dogs infected with roundworms
   c. from ingestion of roundworm eggs in dog feces
   d. by inhaling aerosol from infected animals
   e. by ingestion of uncooked or undercooked chicken eggs

57. *Toxoplasmosis is often transmitted to people by:*

   a. bite wounds
   b. cat feces
   c. dog feces
   d. raw milk
   e. contamination of food with rodent feces

58. *In the United States, most cases of ringworm in people are caused by contact with:*

   a. dogs
   b. cats
   c. horses
   d. cattle
   e. other people

59. *Are cats susceptible to human immunodeficiency virus (HIV) infection, which causes acquired immunodeficiency syndrome (AIDS) in people?*

   a. yes, but they cannot transmit it to people
   b. no, but they are susceptible to a different feline immunodeficiency virus, which has similar manifestations
   c. yes, and they can transmit the disease to people
   d. no, but they can act as a carrier and transmit the disease to people

   e. yes, they can become infected and can act as a reservoir

60. *Visceral larva migrans in people is caused by:*

   a. *Toxoplasma*
   b. *Toxocara*
   c. *Ancylostoma*
   d. *Hypoderma*
   e. *Dermacentor*

61. *Dogs or cats being prepared for shipment or entering a boarding facility should be vaccinated how many weeks before the event?*

   a. 16-18 weeks
   b. 12-14 weeks
   c. 8-10 weeks
   d. 4-6 weeks
   e. 1-2 weeks

62. *Rabies vaccine is **not** recommended for dogs younger than what age?*

   a. 7 months
   b. 6 months
   c. 5 months
   d. 4 months
   e. 3 months

63. *What is the youngest age at which puppies and kittens can be safely treated with insecticides for fleas and ticks?*

   a. 1 week
   b. 1 month
   c. 2 months
   d. 3 months
   e. 4 months

64. *At what age should most kittens first be presented for initial immunizations?*

   a. 4-6 weeks
   b. 8-10 weeks
   c. 12-14 weeks
   d. 16-20 weeks
   e. 24-30 weeks

Correct answers are on pages 236-239.

65. At what age should most puppies first be presented for initial immunizations?

   a. 2-4 weeks
   b. 8-10 weeks
   c. 12-16 weeks
   d. 16-20 weeks
   e. 24-30 weeks

66. Feline leukemia virus vaccine can be safely administered to kittens as young as:

   a. 2 weeks of age
   b. 3 weeks of age
   c. 4 weeks of age
   d. 5 weeks of age
   e. 6 weeks of age

67. Cheyletiellosis most commonly affects what area on cats?

   a. chin
   b. legs
   c. ventral thorax
   d. back
   e. eyelids

68. The passive antibodies transferred from immune dams to the fetus during gestation may make puppies and kittens unresponsive to vaccination for what period at the beginning of life?

   a. 3-6 weeks
   b. 6-8 weeks
   c. 2-3 weeks
   d. 6-7 days
   e. 10-12 days

69. The most common cause of vaccination failure in young dogs and cats is:

   a. disease at the time of vaccination
   b. the presence of maternal antibodies
   c. ineffective vaccine
   d. human error in mixing or administering the vaccine

   e. congenital or acquired immunodeficiency

70. Which of the following is most likely to cause vaccination failure?

   a. attenuation of the vaccine components
   b. storage at refrigeration temperatures
   c. no disinfectant used on needles or syringes
   d. wrong strain or type of microbe used to make the vaccine
   e. mixing with a sterile diluent

71. Which of the following is **least** likely to contribute to vaccination failure?

   a. vaccination of an anesthetized patient
   b. fever or hypothermia
   c. general debilitation
   d. very young or very old age
   e. use of glucocorticoids or cytotoxic agents

72. Human errors that may cause vaccination failure include all of the following **except**:

   a. vaccinating during estrus
   b. improper mixing of vaccine
   c. incorrect route of administration
   d. storing vaccine at very warm temperatures
   e. vaccinating too frequently

73. Which genetic engineering technique is **not** used in production of vaccines?

   a. genetic manipulation to construct mutants of a virus, bacterium, parasite or cancer cell
   b. production of vaccines against the pathogen's vector
   c. removal of pathogenic genes that affect the pathogen's multiplication properties
   d. insertion of fragments of DNA material into immunogenic proteins of a virus, bacterium, parasite or cancer cell
   e. production of vaccines containing mutant strains of the pathogen

74. Concerning disease in cats, which statement is most accurate?

a. Feline infectious peritonitis occurs most commonly in middle-aged cats.

b. Temperature-sensitive feline infectious peritonitis vaccine provides protection against coronavirus challenge in healthy cats.

c. Male cats are affected more frequently with feline infectious peritonitis than are female cats.

d. Feline infectious peritonitis virus is resistant to most household detergents and disinfectants.

e. Natural infection with feline enteric coronaviruses results in production of antibody that can be serologically distinguished from that produced by infection with feline infectious peritonitis virus.

75. At what age should puppies be given canine distemper-measles vaccine?

a. 4-6 weeks
b. 6-12 weeks
c. 14-18 weeks
d. 20-24 weeks
e. 24-32 weeks

76. What approximate percentage of maternal antibodies is transferred from the dam to the fetus via the placenta and to puppies and kittens via colostrum?

a. 100% colostral and 0% transplacental
b. 95-99% colostral and 1-5% transplacental
c. 50% colostral and 50% transplacental
d. 1-5% colostral and 95-99% transplacental
e. 0% colostral and 100% transplacental

77. A 9-week-old kitten has a serous ocular discharge and mild sneezing. The kitten is still eating and, according to the owner, very active. In conjunctival scrapings stained with Giemsa stain, epithelial cells contain intracytoplasmic inclusions. The most likely cause of disease in this kitten is infection with:

a. feline leukemia virus
b. calicivirus
c. *Chlamydia*
d. rhinotracheitis virus
e. *Toxoplasma*

78. The intranasal vaccine against feline viral rhinotracheitis and feline calicivirus infection may cause adverse effects in young kittens. After vaccine administration, these adverse effects are usually observed within:

a. 36-48 hours
b. 4-7 days
c. 10-14 days
d. 14-21 days
e. 12-24 hours

79. Concerning canine adenovirus type 1 in dogs, which statement is **least** accurate?

a. It causes ocular lesions.
b. It causes renal lesions.
c. The vaccine protects susceptible dogs against infectious canine hepatitis and infectious tracheobronchitis.
d. It causes virus shedding in urine.
e. The vaccine is approved for intranasal use.

80. Concerning Bordetella infection in dogs, which statement is most accurate?

a. *Bordetella bronchiseptica* cannot reside within the trachea and bronchi of asymptomatic dogs.
b. *Bordetella bronchiseptica* vaccine administered by the parenteral route is not recommended for male and female dogs used for breeding.
c. *Bordetella bronchiseptica* vaccine given by the intranasal route is not recommended for puppies as young as 2-4 weeks of age.
d. *Bordetella bronchiseptica* is naturally spread from dog to dog by aerosol.
e. *Bordetella bronchiseptica* is naturally spread from dog to dog by contaminated feces.

Correct answers are on pages 236-239.

81. A 20-week-old puppy has a serous nasal discharge, depression, inappetence and diarrhea of 2 days' duration. The total white blood cell count is 10,500 cells/µl (normal range, 6000-17,000 cells/µl), with 7500 segmented neutrophils/µl (normal range, 3000-11,500 cells/µl). Which virus is most likely involved?

a. canine leukemia virus
b. canine parvovirus-2
c. canine coronavirus
d. canine herpesvirus
e. canine rotavirus

82. Canine coronavirus vaccine is labeled by the manufacturer for first recommended use in puppies as young as:

a. 7-10 days
b. 2-3 weeks
c. 10-12 weeks
d. 4-6 weeks
e. 14-20 weeks

83. The indirect fluorescent antibody test (IFA) and the enzyme-linked immunosorbent assay (ELISA) detect feline leukemia virus (FeLV) infection in affected cats of all ages. To confirm FeLV infection in a 12-week-old kitten before FeLV vaccination, what diagnostic test is most appropriate to conduct in a veterinary hospital?

a. virus isolation and identification
b. ELISA for gp70 antigen
c. IFA for feline oncornavirus cell membrane antigen
d. Western immunoblotting technique on serum
e. ELISA for p27 antigen

84. At what age can puppies safely begin receiving heartworm preventive?

a. 1-2 weeks
b. 24-30 weeks
c. 12-16 weeks
d. 6-8 weeks
e. 4-5 weeks

85. Hookworm infection in dogs can be prevented by regular administration of:

a. fenbendazole, piperazine or praziquantel
b. cythioate, pyrantel pamoate or clotrimazole
c. thiacetarsamide, ivermectin or dichlorvos
d. diethylcarbamazine, oxibendazole or milbemycin
e. amprolium sulfadimethoxine or fenthion

86. In the United States, which drug is approved for treatment of hookworm infection in cats?

a. fenbendazole
b. pyrantel pamoate
c. thenium closylate
d. ivermectin
e. no drug has been approved for treatment of hookworm infection in cats

87. Which drug is used for treating giardiasis in dogs and cats?

a. milbemycin oxime
b. metronidazole
c. fenbendazole
d. nitroscanate
e. febantel-praziquantel

Answers

1. **b** The NASPHV form #50 is recommended by the AVMA and is available from vaccine manufacturers. Computer-generated forms are acceptable, as long as all of the information on form #50 is present.

2. **c** Because there are no vaccines licensed for wild animals, the AVMA stongly encourages that states pass laws prohibiting ownership of wild animals and wild animals crossbred to domestic dogs and cats as pets.

3. **e** The NASPHV urges that only vaccines with a 3-year duration of immunity should be used to protect the largest fraction of dog and cat populations at any time.

4. **d** Euthanasia for exposed and unvaccinated animals is recommended because of the high probability for infection and shedding of the virus, which can lead to other exposures. The 6-month confinement period is justified, based on cases of rabies in domestic animals, for which the time of exposure to onset of clinical signs has been shown to be several months in duration.

5. **b** The 10-day observation period ensures that animals that may have exposed human beings to rabies virus are promptly indentified, as virus is shed in the saliva no more than a few days before the onset of clinical signs.

6. **e** Disinfectants should have some residual action to guard against recontamination of a surface.

7. **a** Chloroxylenol is not virucidal. Puppies nearing the end of maternal antibody protection (6-20 weeks) are at particular risk, as passive antibodies still interfere with vaccination but become inadequate to protect against viral challenge. This is known as the "critical period of susceptibility."

8. **c** Peroxides are useful for mechanically cleaning purulent, pocketing wounds but have only mild antiseptic qualities. In addition, when the bubbling ends, so does its action.

9. **d** When used to disinfect instruments, the instruments should first be scrubbed to remove all organic debris and then autoclaved to destroy spores. Quaternary ammonium compounds then help to maintain sterility.

10. **d** Amphoteric compounds, such as alkalinized glutaraldehyde, is known for its activity against spores. Iodophores are not active against spores.

11. **a** The formalin/glutaraldehyde group is more effective against fungi, but amphoteric compounds are more effective against spores.

12. **b** Greyhounds are more sensitive than other breeds to organophosphate insecticides. Cythioate is not approved for use in cats.

13. **e** Transmission of *Toxocara canis* to pups occurs transplacentally and transmammary. In the last trimester of pregnancy, larvae in tissues are reactivated and migrate to the pups *in utero*. The larvae are also shed in the milk.

14. **c** Litterboxes should be cleaned daily. Hookworms of cats (*eg, Ancylostoma braziliense*) are zoonotic and can cause cutaneous larva migrans.

15. **e** Collies may have adverse reactions to ivermectin. Milbemycin oxime also controls hookworms in dogs. Animals should be tested for microfilariae before receiving prophylactic drugs.

16. **a** Intranasal vaccines for feline respiratory viruses have not gained general acceptance by veterinarians in the US.

17. **b** Maternal antibodies provide roughly 1-3 months' protection against the common infectious diseases.

18. **a** Most commercially available vaccines overcome maternal immunity by 12 weeks. Colostrum-deprived pups should be vaccinated beginning at 2-3 weeks of age.

19. **d** The chance of anterior uveitis (blue eye) after adenovirus vaccination is increased if the vaccine is inadvertently given intravenously.

20. **b** Intranasal *Bordetella* and parainfluenza vaccines may confer protection within 3 days of administration. The vaccine may cause mild clinical illness.

21. **e** Bitches should be given a modified-live product at least 2 weeks before breeding. In a pregnant animal with an unknown vaccination history, 2 doses of inactivated vaccine during the last trimester are recommended.

22. **c** Clients should be made aware that intestinally secreted antibodies are short lived and boosters should be considered more often than annually if repeated exposures may occur. Concomitant infections with parvovirus and coronavirus may be more severe than with parvovirus alone. Therefore, vaccination against coronavirus may help prevent serious parvovirus infections.

23. **b** The newer subunit *Leptospira* vaccines being developed may be able to eliminate the carrier state and anaphylaxis problems associated with current products.

24. **b** Boosters should be given annually, regardless of use of modified-live or attenuated products, though modified-live-virus products probably provide longer immunity.

25. **c** Testing for FeLV is encouraged before primary vaccination of all cats whose background or exposure status to FeLV is either at risk or unknown. Kittens from a known FeLV-free or low-risk background may not need to be tested for FeLV before vaccination.

26. **d** Vaccination does not interfere with FeLV diagnostic testing. Vaccines are either inactivated or subunit; hence, vaccine virus does not replicate within the host after vaccination. Diagnostic tests detect viral antigens; immune response to the vaccine is not detected.

27. **e** Splenectomizing of blood donor animals and examining the blood 10 days later for *Hemobartonella* organisms constitute a good screening program.

28. **a** When possible, cats should also be barred from entry into areas where food animals are housed.

29. **d** Borreliosis vaccine has been effective against experimental challenge. Prompt removal of ticks appears to be an effective preventive measure.

30. **d** There are no effective RMSF vaccines available for dogs or people.

31. **b** Cats and dogs may shed organisms from their oral cavity or in feces.

32. **d** Warming devices used should not lead to dehydration. In Europe, immunization with an inactivated product has increased titers but has not provided long-term protection.

33. **a** There is no FIV vaccine currently available. Once clinical signs develop, the long-term prognosis is very poor.

34. **e** Guinea pigs are not involved. Attenuated vaccines can cause reactions as serious as natural infection. The newer subunit vaccines being developed for swine may be of great value for pets in the future.

35. **c** There are no vaccines for salmon disease. Also, metacercariae can remain viable for months in decomposing fish carcasses.

36. **d** Even modified-live products do not entirely prevent colonization of the mucosae and shedding of the organism following exposure.

37. **c** Following oral administration, methenamine is quickly absorbed and excreted in the urine. Antibacterial activity is confined mostly to the urinary bladder.

38. **a** Botulinus toxin is inactivated by heating to 80 degrees C. for 30 minutes or to 100 degrees C. for 10 minutes. Always prevent access to dead carcasses and raw meat.

39. **c** Active immunization with tetanus toxoid is not recommended for dogs and cats.

40. **e** One study reveals that in 69.9% of all households with dermatophyte infected cats, at least one person also became infected.

41. **a** Metronidazole is effective against anaerobes and spirochetes for up to 8 months after administration and may be useful for prevention of periodontal disease and gingivitis. However, side effects may limit its usefulness for this purpose.

42. **b** To help prevent struvite urolithiasis, restrict dietary intake of magnesium and maintain urine pH at 6.0 or less with methionine or ammonium chloride. If infection is present, perform culture and sensitivity tests, and institute appropriate therapy.

43. **d**

44. **c** Initial use of such surgical procedures as abdominal wall muscle flap gastropexy and circumcostal gastropexy may be useful in preventing recurrence.

45. **d** Hairballs are sometimes found secondary to other, more serious ailments. In cats with chronic hairball problems, diagnostics should be performed to rule out primary gastric disease.

46. **e** Fleas are involved in the life cycle of tapeworms. Human dipylidiasis is usually asymptomatic and is seen more commonly in young children.

47. **a** There is no known means of testing cats to see if they are carriers of the cat scratch organism. The ability of a cat to transmit the disease appears to be transient, which makes isolation or euthanasia impractical and unnecessary.

48. **c** Shedding of eggs is sometimes intermittent. Up to 4 negative fecal examinations may be necessary to rule out trichriasis.

49. **c** Cat litter should not be dumped into the environment. Rather, it should be flushed down the toilet, dumped in a septic system,

placed in a landfill or incinerated. Sporulated oocysts may survive in the soil for over 18 months.

50. **e** Coccidial oocysts can survive freezing temperatures. All runs, cages, utensils and other equipment should be disinfected by steam, immersion in boiling water or application of 5% ammonia solutions.

51. **b**

52. **c**

53. **d** The Environmental Protection Agency does not recognize any extra-label use.

54. **a** Euthanize the dog and send the head to the laboratory for rabies testing. Do not wait to confirm the diagnosis.

55. **c**

56. **c**

57. **b**

58. **a**

59. **b**

60. **b**

61. **e** This is adequate time before shipment or entering a boarding facility for a dog or cat.

62. **e** This is the recommendation of the World Health Organization and other governing agencies.

63. **e** It is safest to wait until this age.

64. **b** This is the most common age for initial presentation.

65. **b** This is the most common age for initial presentation.

66. **e** Kittens 6 weeks of age and older can be safely vaccinated.

67. **d** This is the most common site for this mite.

68. **c** The maternal antibodies passed *in utero* can be present in the first 2 weeks of life.

69. **b**

70. **d** The vaccine may contain the wrong strain or type of agent needed for protection of the animal.

71. **a** The other factors listed are more likely to reduce the effectiveness of vaccination.

72. **a** Estrus has no effect on immunization.

73. **c**

74. **b**

75. **b** Check the label of the commercial product.

76. **b**

77. **c** Finding cytoplasmic inclusions confirms chlamydial infection.

78. **b**

79. **e**

80. **d**

81. **c** The white blood cell count is normal in canine coronavirus infection but is decreased in canine parvovirus-2 infection.

82. **d** Check the label of the commercial product.

83. **e** This is the basis of such test kits as Assure, Virachek and Flex II.

84. **d** As soon as puppies begin eating solid food, they can safely begin receiving heartworm preventive.

85. **d** Check the label of the commercial products listed.

86. **e**

87. **b**

Notes

Notes

13

Principles of Surgery

T.P. Colville

Recommended Reading

Knecht CD *et al: Fundamental Techniques in Veterinary Surgery.* 3rd ed. Saunders, Philadelphia, 1987.

Practice answer sheet is on page 355.

Questions

1. Which surgical instrument is primarily used to hold organs and tissues out of the way to facilitate exposure of the operative field?

   a. elevator
   b. forceps
   c. retractor
   d. rongeur
   e. hemostat

2. Which orthopedic instrument has sharp, opposing, cup-shaped jaws used to shape bone by "chewing" out small pieces?

   a. chisel
   b. curette
   c. osteotome
   d. rongeur
   e. trephine

3. Which of the following is the correct surgical term for declawing?

   a. celiotomy
   b. cystotomy
   c. onychectomy
   d. hysterectomy
   e. colpotomy

4. The type of needle most appropriate for suturing internal organs, such as gastrointestinal structures, is the:

   a. blunt
   b. cutting
   c. reverse cutting
   d. tapered
   e. trocar

Correct answers are on pages 251-254.

5. *Which type of needle is most commonly used for suturing in general surgery?*

   a. straight
   b. 3/8 circle
   c. 1/2 circle
   d. 5/8 circle
   e. 1/2 curved

6. *Which of the following surgical procedures is **not** considered an elective procedure?*

   a. correction of a proptosed eye
   b. dew claw removal in a field trial dog
   c. mastectomy to remove a benign tumor
   d. ovariohysterectomy in a healthy 6-month-old cat
   e. tail docking in 3-day-old Boxer puppies

7. *Healing of a properly sutured surgical wound is most appropriately termed:*

   a. first-intention healing
   b. granulation
   c. secondary union
   d. second-intention healing
   e. wound contraction

8. *Which of the following has the **poorest** potential for healing and return to normal function after damage and effective surgical repair?*

   a. bone
   b. intestine
   c. liver
   d. nervous tissue
   e. uterus

9. *Which term describes removal of necrotic tissue from a wound?*

   a. debridement
   b. inspissate
   c. lithotripsy
   d. retraction
   e. ballottement

10. *Which of the following best describes the location of an incision extending from the xiphoid process to the umbilicus of an animal?*

    a. dorsal midline
    b. flank
    c. paracostal
    d. paramedian
    e. ventral midline

For Questions 11 through 13, select the correct answer from the 5 choices below.

    a. autoclave
    b. boiling
    c. dry heat
    d. ethylene oxide gas
    e. liquid chemical disinfectant

11. *Most appropriate for sterilization of an electric drill to be used in an orthopedic surgical procedure.*

12. *Most appropriate for sterilization of a needle holder to be used in a surgical procedure.*

13. *Most appropriate for sterilization of dissecting scissors to be used in a surgical procedure.*

14. *Which of the following describes the minimal exposure time and temperature for autoclaving of a surgical pack?*

    a. 121 C for 15 minutes
    b. 121 F for 15 minutes
    c. 250 F for 5 minutes
    d. 250 C for 20 minutes
    e. 250 F for 20 minutes

15. *Which of the following is the most effective and immediate indicator that the conditions for sterilization have been met in an autoclaved surgery pack?*

    a. appearance of the instruments
    b. autoclave tape

c. chemical indicator

d. culture results

e. melting pellet

16. What is the proper term for entrance of microorganisms to an incision during a surgical procedure?

    a. contamination
    b. debridement
    c. dehiscence
    d. infection
    e. septicemia

17. Which of the following items does **not** have to be sterile during a surgical procedure involving aseptic technique?

    a. drapes
    b. gloves
    c. gown
    d. mask
    e. suture material

18. Which of the following is the agent for sterilization by autoclaving?

    a. chemical disinfectant solution
    b. dry heat
    c. ethylene oxide gas
    d. ionizing radiation
    e. steam

19. Which size of electrical clipper blade is most commonly used for clipping the hair from a surgical site?

    a. #10
    b. #20
    c. #30
    d. #40
    e. #50

20. Which suture size is the **smallest** in diameter?

    a. 0
    b. 0000
    c. 2-0
    d. #2
    e. 3/0

21. Which suture material shows the **least** conduction of fluid by capillary action?

    a. braided cotton
    b. braided polyglycolic acid
    c. braided silk
    d. monofilament nylon
    e. chromic catgut

22. All of the following are nonabsorbable suture materials **except**:

    a. cotton
    b. nylon
    c. silk
    d. stainless-steel wire
    e. chromic catgut

23. Which type of surgical gut is absorbed most rapidly from tissues after surgery?

    a. extra chromic
    b. heavy chromic
    c. medium chromic
    d. mild chromic
    e. plain

24. Which of the following is **not** an effective form of surgical hemostasis?

    a. crushing
    b. curettage
    c. electrocoagulation
    d. ligation
    e. pressure

25. Which of the following is **not** a likely cause of dehiscence of an abdominal incision?

    a. chronic vomiting
    b. excessive physical activity
    c. stormy recovery from anesthesia
    d. surgical wound infection
    e. suture material larger than needed

Correct answers are on pages 251-254.

26. *Concerning aseptic surgical technique, which statement is **least** accurate?*

    a. A sterile item touched by a nonsterile item becomes nonsterile.

    b. If the sterility of an item is in doubt, consider it sterile.

    c. Nonscrubbed personnel can touch only nonsterile items.

    d. Only sterile items can contact exposed patient tissue.

    e. Only sterile items can contact other sterile items.

27. *Which of the following is an everting suture pattern that should only be used to close skin incisions?*

    a. Cushing

    b. Lembert

    c. Parker-Kerr

    d. simple interrupted

    e. vertical mattress

28. *Which of the following is an inverting suture pattern used mainly to suture hollow internal organs?*

    a. horizontal mattress

    b. Lembert

    c. pursestring

    d. simple interrupted or continuous

    e. vertical mattress

29. *Which of the following is most effective in minimizing the scarring from skin sutures and achieving good wound healing?*

    a. leaving sutures permanently in place

    b. removing the sutures 2 days after insertion

    c. removing the sutures 7 days after insertion

    d. using large-diameter suture material

    e. using suture material that produces significant inflammation

30. *Which of the following does **not** enhance healing of an open wound?*

    a. debridement

    b. exuberant granulation tissue

    c. granulation tissue

    d. wound contraction

    e. wound flushing

31. *Which of the following is **not** a characteristic of first-intention wound healing?*

    a. minimal contamination

    b. minimal tissue damage

    c. minimal role of wound contraction

    d. wound edges are not approximated

    e. wound edges are sutured

32. *Which incision is most appropriate for exploratory surgery in a dog's abdomen, in which the precise location of the problem is **not** known?*

    a. dorsal midline

    b. flank

    c. paracostal

    d. paramedian

    e. ventral midline

33. *Which of the following is **not** an early sign of wound dehiscence during the first 24 hours after abdominal surgery?*

    a. body temperature elevation of 1 - 2 F

    b. change in texture of the wound edges

    c. serosanguineous discharge from the incision

    d. swollen incision

    e. very warm incision

34. *The main goal of aseptic surgical technique is to prevent contamination of the:*

    a. operative personnel

    b. sterile fields

    c. sterile zones

    d. surgical instruments

    e. surgical wound

35. *Which factor related to infection of a surgical wound is most significantly affected by aseptic technique?*

a. number of microorganisms entering the wound
b. pathogenicity of microorganisms entering the wound
c. species of microorganisms entering the wound
d. route of exposure to infectious microorganisms
e. susceptibility of the patient

36. The effectiveness of a bactericidal surgical scrub of one's hands and arms depends on the:

a. combination of contact time and scrubbing action
b. length of time the soap is in contact with the skin
c. pH of the skin surface
d. scrubbing action of the brush
e. temperature of the water

37. Which of the following, when used alone as a surgical scrub soap, forms a bacteriostatic film over the skin?

a. chlorhexidine
b. chlorpheniramine
c. hexadimethrine
d. hexachlorophene
e. povidone-iodine

38. Which of the following does **not** normally have to be sterilized as part of good aseptic surgical technique?

a. cap
b. drapes
c. gloves
d. gown
e. scrub brush

39. Liquid chemical sterilization is used primarily for:

a. electrical equipment
b. hemostatic forceps
c. instruments with sharp edges
d. orthopedic equipment
e. surgical drapes

40. The time necessary to achieve disinfection of surgical instruments with liquid chemicals can be shortened by:

a. agitating the solution
b. cooling the solution
c. using a lower concentration than recommended
d. using a higher concentration than recommended
e. warming the solution

41. Which surgical wire size is the **smallest** in diameter?

a. 40 gauge
b. 10 gauge
c. 26 gauge
d. 32 gauge
e. 20 gauge

42. Which surgical drape material prevents passage of bacteria through the drape to the patient's skin by capillary action when the top surface of the drape becomes wet?

a. cloth
b. fenestrated paper
c. muslin
d. paper
e. plastic

43. Which suture size is **smaller** in diameter than 3-0?

a. 2-0
b. #1
c. #3
d. #4
e. 4-0

44. Which suture material is absorbable?

a. cotton
b. nylon
c. polypropylene
d. silk
e. chromic catgut

Correct answers are on pages 251-254.

45. Which surgical instrument should **not** be routinely steam sterilized?

   a. Backhaus towel clamp
   b. Halsted mosquito forceps
   c. Mayo-Hegar needle holder
   d. Metzenbaum scissors
   e. Bard-Parker scalpel handle

46. Castration of a healthy 6-month-old cat is an example of:

   a. cosmetic surgery
   b. elective surgery
   c. emergency surgery
   d. exploratory surgery
   e. first-intention surgery

47. Which solution causes the **least** tissue damage and is most appropriate for wound flushing?

   a. hydrogen peroxide
   b. isotonic saline
   c. povidone-iodine scrub
   d. povidone-iodine solution
   e. tap water

48. Which incision provides the best overall exposure of the abdominal cavity?

   a. dorsal midline
   b. flank
   c. paracostal
   d. paramedian
   e. ventral midline

49. What is the most appropriate suture pattern to close an incision in an animal's stomach?

   a. horizontal mattress
   b. Lembert
   c. pursestring
   d. simple interrupted
   e. vertical mattress

50. Which operating room personnel should try to face away from sterile fields during a surgical procedure?

   a. all personnel
   b. nonscrubbed personnel only
   c. scrubbed personnel only
   d. both nonscrubbed and scrubbed personnel
   e. neither nonscrubbed nor scrubbed personnel

51. What is the significance of dehiscence of the muscle, subcutaneous tissue and skin layers in a ventral midline surgical wound?

   a. acute emergency
   b. cosmetic problem only
   c. minor significance
   d. no significance
   e. serious but not an acute emergency

52. Why is a recent surgical wound usually slightly warmer than the surrounding normal tissues?

   a. contamination
   b. debridement
   c. infection
   d. inflammation
   e. septicemia

53. When does a sutured surgical wound begin to gain significant strength from production of collagen strands, so that the wound edges are beginning to be held together by tissue as well as sutures?

   a. 6-8 hours
   b. 4-6 days
   c. 12-14 days
   d. 24-26 days
   e. 28-30 days

54. Wound contraction is produced by:

   a. movement of only the dermis
   b. movement of only the epidermis
   c. movement of all layers of the skin
   d. reproduction of epidermal cells
   e. reproduction of all skin cells

55. As a part of effective aseptic technique, surgical gowns:

    a. are commonly made of cloth or paper
    b. are put on by touching only the outside
    c. are routinely sterilized by ethylene oxide gas
    d. do not need to be sterile, only clean
    e. protect against contamination from the waist down

56. Which suture size is larger in diameter than size #2?

    a. 0
    b. #1
    c. 2-0
    d. #3
    e. 3-0

57. Which suture material is synthetic?

    a. chromic catgut
    b. cotton
    c. nylon
    d. plain catgut
    e. silk

58. Which of the following is **not** a typical sign of hemorrhagic shock in a postsurgical patient?

    a. deep, slow breathing
    b. pale mucous membranes
    c. slow capillary refill
    d. tachycardia
    e. weakness

59. What is the most appropriate suture pattern to use in closing an incision of the urinary bladder?

    a. Cushing
    b. horizontal mattress
    c. simple continuous
    d. simple interrupted
    e. vertical mattress

60. Suture material used to close a surgical wound represents what kind of irritant to body tissues?

    a. chemical
    b. infectious
    c. photic
    d. physical
    e. thermal

61. What is the usual significance of a small seroma deep to (beneath) the skin suture line after aseptic surgery?

    a. acute emergency
    b. cosmetic problem only
    c. minor significance
    d. no significance
    e. serious but not an acute emergency

62. Which suture pattern is **neither** an inverting **nor** an everting pattern?

    a. Cushing
    b. horizontal mattress
    c. Lembert
    d. simple interrupted or continuous
    e. vertical mattress

63. What is the healing potential of a fractured bone that is properly aligned and kept immobile?

    a. excellent
    b. good
    c. fair
    d. poor
    e. very poor

64. Which of the following indicates the best blood supply to the edges of a wound in unpigmented skin?

    a. black wound edges
    b. bluish-purple wound edges
    c. gray wound edges
    d. pink wound edges
    e. white wound edges

Correct answers are on pages 251-254.

65. What portion of a surgical gown is considered sterile during surgery?

    a. entire outside of the gown
    b. front and sides of the gown, from the neck to the bottom, including the arms
    c. front of the gown, from the neck to the bottom, including the arms
    d. front and sides of the gown, from the neck to the waist
    e. front of the gown, from the waist up, including the arms

66. Which bacterial form is most easily destroyed by common sterilization methods?

    a. spores of aerobes
    b. hyphated form
    c. dormant form
    d. spores of anaerobes
    e. vegetative form

67. The first phase of the wound healing process is the:

    a. epithelial phase
    b. fibroblast phase
    c. inflammatory phase
    d. maturation phase
    e. scarring phase

68. In the first 24 hours of primary union wound healing, most of the resistance to opening of the sutured wound is provided by:

    a. collagen strands
    b. fibrin strands
    c. fibroblasts
    d. granulation tissue
    e. sutures

69. Assuming no complications, how long after surgery should skin sutures generally be removed?

    a. 2-3 days
    b. 4-5 days
    c. 7-10 days
    d. 15-17 days

    e. 18-21 days

70. What is the correct surgical term for incision of the urinary bladder?

    a. cystectomy
    b. cystopexy
    c. cystoscopy
    d. cystostomy
    e. cystotomy

71. What is the correct surgical term for removal of the kidney?

    a. nephrectomy
    b. nephropexy
    c. nephroscopy
    d. nephrostomy
    e. nephrotomy

72. What is the correct surgical term for suturing the stomach to the body wall to fix the stomach in place?

    a. gastrectomy
    b. gastropexy
    c. gastroscopy
    d. gastrostomy
    e. gastrotomy

73. What is the correct surgical term for creation of a permanent artificial opening into the esophagus?

    a. esophagectomy
    b. esophagopexy
    c. esophagoscopy
    d. esophagostomy
    e. esophagotomy

74. With which type of abdominal incision can the abdominal wall be most effectively closed using a single layer of sutures?

    a. high flank
    b. low flank
    c. paracostal
    d. paramedian

e.   ventral midline

75. *Scrubbed surgical personnel become*
     contaminated if they touch:

   a.   objects in sterile fields
   b.   objects outside the sterile zone
   c.   properly sterilized surgical instruments
   d.   sterile objects
   e.   freshly exposed tissues of the patient

76. *Nonscrubbed surgical personnel may properly*
     touch anything that is:

   a.   contaminated
   b.   inside the patient
   c.   inside the sterile zone
   d.   part of a sterile field
   e.   sterile

77. *How should scrubbed personnel pass each*
     other in the operating room?

   a.   any way that is convenient
   b.   back to back
   c.   back to front
   d.   front to back
   e.   front to front

78. *When not otherwise occupied, scrubbed*
     surgical personnel should stand with their:

   a.   arms folded across the chest
   b.   hands held apart and above shoulder level
   c.   hands clapsed between waist and shoulder
        level
   d.   hands held down and to each side
   e.   hands on the surgery table

79. *During surgery, when is it permissible for*
     nonscrubbed surgical personnel to pass
     between scrubbed personnel and the patient?

   a.   at any convenient time
   b.   never
   c.   when opening suture material
   d.   when adjusting the anesthesia machine
   e.   when adjusting the intravenous drip

80. *When aseptically opening a sterile surgical*
     *pack on an instrument stand, it is **not** proper*
     for nonscrubbed surgical personnel to touch
     the:

   a.   autoclave tape
   b.   contents of the pack
   c.   corners of the wrap
   d.   instrument stand
   e.   outside of the wrap

81. *Which characteristic applies to ethylene oxide*
     gas?

   a.   flammable
   b.   exposure is not considered a health hazard
   c.   noncombustible
   d.   nontoxic to tissues
   e.   safe to breathe

82. *Which type of needle is most appropriate for*
     suturing muscle?

   a.   blunt
   b.   cutting
   c.   reverse cutting
   d.   tapered
   e.   trocar

83. *Which type of needle is most appropriate for*
     suturing a ligament?

   a.   blunt
   b.   cutting
   c.   reverse cutting
   d.   tapered
   e.   trocar

84. *Which type of needle is most appropriate for*
     suturing the uterus?

   a.   blunt
   b.   cutting
   c.   reverse cutting
   d.   tapered
   e.   trocar

Correct answers are on pages 251-254.

85. Surgical removal of a ruptured spleen is an example of:

   a. cosmetic surgery
   b. elective surgery
   c. emergency surgery
   d. exploratory surgery
   e. first-intention surgery

86. Removal of a large skin tumor has left a large skin defect to be closed. Which suture pattern is **least** likely to cause skin tearing when large wounds are closed under tension?

   a. Cushing
   b. horizontal mattress
   c. Lembert
   d. pursestring
   e. simple interrupted

87. Which of the following is **not** a likely contributor to dehiscence of an abdominal surgical incision?

   a. chronic vomiting
   b. internal suture ends cut too short
   c. infection
   d. skin sutures left in place too long
   e. suture material of too-small diameter

88. Which type of dressing, when removed, provides the **least** traumatic and **least** irritating means of debriding a wound with extensive tissue damage?

   a. dry gauze
   b. dry nonadhesive pad
   c. gauze dressing with an oily antiseptic
   d. gauze dressing with a water-soluble antiseptic
   e. wet saline dressing

89. Most of the clinical signs seen in animals in shock related to excessive blood loss are attributable to:

   a. acidosis
   b. alkalosis
   c. cell death

   d. redistribution of blood flow
   e. tissue hyperoxia

90. Which of the following is a noncapillary suture material suitable for skin closure?

   a. braided cotton
   b. braided polyglycolic acid
   c. braided silk
   d. monofilament stainless steel
   e. monofilament cotton

91. The main goal of surgery to remove a pus-filled uterus (pyometra) is to:

   a. prevent subsequent pregnancy
   b. alter the behavior of the animal
   c. make a diagnosis
   d. restore the animal to a normal reproductive state
   e. restore health despite loss of normal reproductive function

92. With what kind of knot should sutures be routinely tied?

   a. bowline
   b. granny knot
   c. square knot
   d. slip knot
   e. half hitch

93. Concerning the principles of cryosurgery, which statement is **least** accurate?

   a. Frozen tissues should be thawed slowly.
   b. Little aftercare is required.
   c. Multiple freeze-thaw cycles should be applied.
   d. Tissues should be frozen to -25 C.
   e. Tissues should be frozen rapidly.

94. When does the strength of a sutured surgical skin wound return to its original preoperative strength?

   a. 7-10 days
   b. 21-28 days

c. 60 days

d. 2-3 years

e. never

95. *In second-intention healing, which of the following must be present before wound contraction or epithelial regeneration can occur?*

a. collagen fibers

b. exudative tissue

c. fibrin clot

d. granulation tissue

e. scar tissue

96. *When putting on sterile gloves for aseptic surgery, which of the following is **not** permitted?*

a. touching one gloved thumb with the other gloved thumb

b. touching the outside of the glove with scrubbed fingers

c. touching the outside of the gown cuff with the inside of the glove cuff

d. touching the outside of one glove with the outside of the other glove

e. touching the inside of the glove cuff with scrubbed fingers

97. *How should packs be placed in an autoclave for sterilization?*

a. diagonally

b. horizontally

c. tightly packed

d. unwrapped

e. vertically

98. *The use of extreme cold to destroy unwanted tissue is termed:*

a. cosmetic surgery

b. cryosurgery

c. elective surgery

d. orthopedic surgery

e. prophylactic surgery

Answers

1. **c** The instrument is named for its function of retracting organs and tissues out of the way.

2. **d** None of the other instruments listed has opposing jaws.

3. **c** Declawing involves removal (-ectomy) of the nails or claws (onych-).

4. **d** A tapered-point needle easily passes through soft organs, making a tunnel through which the suture material is drawn.

5. **c** The half-circle needle offers the best compromise of shape, allowing use in both shallow and deep incisions.

6. **a** A proptosed eye must be returned to the eye socket quickly so as to prevent permanent damage to the eye.

7. **a** The basic requirements for healing by first intention are minimal tissue damage and apposition of the edges of the wound, usually with sutures.

8. **d** The basic functional unit of the nervous system, the neuron, is incapable of reproduction, so damage to the nervous system is often repaired by scar tissue. The other organs and tissues listed have excellent healing potential.

9. **a** Debridement of a wound facilitates healing by minimizing the amount of inflammation necessary before filling of the defect can begin.

10. **e** The xiphoid process and umbilicus are both on the animal's ventral midline.

11. **d** An electric drill would be damaged or inadequately sterilized by any of the other methods.

12. **a** Steam sterilization in an autoclave is most commonly used for instruments and equipment not damaged by moisture or heat.

13. **e** The sharp edges of scissors are dulled by steam in an autoclave. Boiling and dry heat are not sufficiently effective. The expense and hazards of ethylene oxide are not warranted.

14. **a** The minimal standard for sterilization of surgical instruments in an autoclave is 121 C (250 F) for at least 15 minutes.

15. **c** Chemical autoclave indicators are the only type listed that can give immediate information on all 3 basic criteria for autoclave sterilization (presence of steam at the proper combination of exposure time and temperature).

16. **a** Microorganisms in a wound during surgery are considered contaminants until, or unless, they multiply and cause damage.

17. **d** A surgical mask does not come in contact with anything sterile during a surgical procedure, so it need only be clean.

18. **e** An autoclave sterilizes by exposing packs to steam under pressure.

19. **d** A #40 clipper blade is a "surgical" blade. It clips the hair off at the skin surface.

20. **b** Numbered suture sizes (*eg*, #2) decrease in size as the number gets smaller, down to size 0. From that point on the sizes get smaller as the number of 0s (or the number in front of the 0) increases.

21. **d** All of the other suture materials listed are either braided or twisted and have the potential for considerable capillary action.

22. **e** Surgical gut is absorbed by the body.

23. **e** Treatment with chromic acid delays absorption of surgical gut by the body.

24. **b** Curettage involves the scraping of a tissue or cavity.

25. **e** Use of overly large suture material would not cause a wound to dehisce. It would actually provide greater holding power than smaller suture material.

26. **b** Contaminated items appear identical to sterile items. If there is any doubt about the sterility of an item, it must be considered contaminated.

27. **e** All of the other patterns are inverting or appositional.

28. **b** The other patterns are inverting (mattress patterns), appositional (simple pattern) or used only to close off an orifice (pursestring).

29. **c** All of the other choices promote increased scarring or early disruption of the wound.

30. **b** Exuberant granulation tissue (proud flesh) acts to block wound healing and epithelial regeneration. The other choices would likely enhance wound healing.

31. **d** One of the most important characteristics of wound healing by first intention is approximation of the wound edges.

32. **e** The ventral midline approach to the abdomen gives the most extensive access to the abdominal cavity.

33. **a** Slight elevation of body temperature for 1-2 days is normal after major surgery. The other choices are all early indicators of wound dehiscence.

34. **e** Prevention of surgical wound contamination is the whole purpose of aseptic technique in the operating room.

35. **a** This is the only choice that can be influenced by aseptic technique. The others are inherent to the patient, the surgical procedure being performed, or the microorganisms in the environment.

36. **a** The antimicrobial effect of a surgical scrub depends on sufficient exposure of the skin to the soap, as well as the scrubbing action that loosens dead skin and debris, and works the soap down into the cracks and crevices of the skin.

37. **d** Hexachlorophene forms a bacteriostatic film on the skin if used exclusively to wash the hands and arms. Other soaps remove the protective film.

38. **a** The surgical cap does not come in contact with tissues of the patient directly or indirectly, so it need only be clean, not sterile.

39. **c** Liquid chemical sterilization does not dull sharp edges.

40. **e** Warming the solution accelerates the chemical reactions necessary to kill microorganisms.

41. **a** The relative size of the wire, as measured by gauge, is inversely proportional to the gauge number. For example, 40-gauge wire is smaller than 32-gauge wire.

42. **e** Cloth and paper drapes are subject to capillary action. Plastic drapes are not.

43. **e** From largest to smallest, these sizes are ranked as follows: #4, #3, #1, 2-0 and 4-0. 3-0 is midway in size between 2-0 and 4-0.

44. **e** All of the other suture materials listed are nonabsorbable.

45. **d** Steam dulls the sharp edges of scissors.

46. **b** Elective surgery is done by choice, so it can be performed when conditions are most appropriate.

47. **b** The other listed solutions are irritating to the tissues or are not isotonic with the patient's tissue fluids.

48. **e** The ventral midline approach provides the most extensive access to the abdominal cavity.

49. **b** Incisions in viscera are best closed with inverting suture patterns. The other listed patterns are everting, appositional or inappropriate for wound closure.

50. **e** All personnel in the operating room should face toward sterile fields so they are aware of their relationship to them.

51. **a** Dehiscence of all layers of the body wall exposes abdominal viscera. Repair must be immediate to prevent serious damage to abdominal structures.

52. **d** Inflammation results from any insult to the body, whether intentional (surgical) or unintentional (traumatic, infectious). Increased blood supply to an inflamed area produces the increased warmth of the area. Good surgical technique minimizes inflammation but does not eliminate it.

53. **b** It takes 4-6 days for production of collagen strands in a wound to reach a significant level. Until that time, the wound is held together by sutures.

54. **c** Wound contraction represents movement of the entire thickness of the skin toward the center of the wound.

55. **a** All of the other choices are incorrect.

56. **d** All of the other choices are smaller.

57. **c** All of the other choices are from natural sources.

58. **a** A patient in shock would show rapid, shallow breathing in an effort to oxygenate the blood as rapidly as possible.

59. **a** The Cushing pattern is the only one listed that is an inverting pattern appropriate for closure of a hollow organ.

60. **d** Suture material acts as a physical irritant until it is absorbed, removed, or encapsulated with scar tissue.

61. **b** Unless very large or ruptured, postoperative seromas are unsightly but of little other importance to the animal's health.

62. **d** The simple pattern is an appositional pattern. It brings the incision edges together without inverting or everting them.

63. **a** Bone has excellent healing capacities, provided the fracture fragments are properly aligned and movement is kept to a minimum.

64. **b** Bluish-purple wound edges indicate that blood vessels in and under the skin are congested with blood.

65. **e** This is the only portion of a surgical gown that is considered sterile during surgery.

66. **e** The vegetative bacterial form is the actively feeding, growing, reproducing form. It is most easily destroyed by common sterilization and disinfection methods.

67. **c** Inflammation is the first step in wound healing. It "cleans up" the damage so the defect can be repaired by the balance of the healing process.

68. **e** Other than sutures, a surgical wound has no appreciable strength until significant numbers of collagen fibers are produced at about 4-6 days.

69. **c** Before 7 days, the wound may not have enough strength to resist separation. After 10 days, inflammatory reaction to the suture material may cause significant scarring.

70. **e** The suffix -otomy means to make an incision into something.

71. **a** The suffix -ectomy means to surgically remove something.

72. **b** The suffix -pexy means to fix something in place.

73. **d** The suffix -ostomy means to create an artificial opening in an organ or tissue.

74. **e** The linea alba, on the ventral midline of the abdominal muscle wall, is the tendinous attachment of the ventral abdominal muscles. One layer of sutures in this area effectively closes the whole thickness of the abdominal wall, after which the skin is closed.

75. **b** Anything outside the sterile zone in an operating room is considered contaminated.

76. **a** Nonscrubbed personnel should only touch things that are not sterile.

77. **b** Passing back to back prevents accidental contamination of the front, sterile portions of their gown.

78. **c** The hands of scrubbed personnel should always be held between waist level and shoulder level to help prevent inadvertent contamination. Clasping the hands, when not otherwise occupied, helps prevent fatigue from compromising the position of the hands and arms.

79. **b** Nonscrubbed personnel should never violate the sterile zone in which scrubbed personnel are working.

80. **b** The sterility of the pack contents would be destroyed if touched by a nonscrubbed person.

81. **a** Ethylene oxide gas is very flammable.

82. **d** A tapered-point needle easily passes through muscle, making a tunnel through which the suture material is drawn.

83. **c** A reverse-cutting needle cuts a tunnel through the tough tissue of a ligament that is less likely to tear through than the tunnel created by a standard (inside-curve) cutting needle. The other needle points would not easily pass through this tough tissue.

84. **d** A tapered-point needle easily passes through muscle, making a tunnel through which the suture material is drawn.

85. **c** Splenic ruture is a potentially life-threatening condition. If surgery is indicated, it must be performed immediately.

86. **b** Mattress suture patterns spread the tension created by each suture over a broad area and are less likely to tear out due to tension on the suture line.

87. **d** Leaving skin sutures in place too long increases scarring but does not directly contribute to breakdown of the surgical wound.

88. **e** Wet saline dressings are useful to help debride wounds with extensive tissue damage. They absorb and remove inflammatory products from the wound.

89. **d** Redistribution of blood flow results in the pale mucous membranes, poor capillary refill and cold extremities seen in shock.

90. **d** The other suture materials listed are braided or twisted and can conduct fluid and microorganisms by capillary action from the surface of the skin to the deeper layers.

91. **e** Removal of the uterus may restore health, but it also precludes future breeding.

92. **c** A square knot is conveniently tied and provides a very secure knot.

93. **b** The principal action of cryosurgery is destruction of unwanted tissue by freezing. This leaves dead tissue that must be liquefied and removed by inflammation. Such areas must be monitored closely and kept clean, and frequently require bandaging.

94. **e** The strength of the scar that results from healing of a surgical skin wound never reaches that of the normal skin around it.

95. **d** After dead and damaged tissue has been removed from a wound by inflammation, a bed of granulation tissue, consisting primarily of collagen fibers and capillaries, must form on the floor of the wound so that the processes that reduce the size of the wound can begin.

96. **b** If the outside of the glove is touched by anything that is not sterile, including freshly scrubbed fingers, it becomes contaminated and must not be used for surgery.

97. **e** Packs placed vertically in the autoclave receive the best circulation of steam around their contents.

98. **b** The prefix cryo- means cold.

Section

14

Surgical Diseases

Recommended Reading

Bojrab MJ: *Current Techniques in Small Animal Surgery.* 3rd ed. Lea & Febiger, Philadelphia, 1990.

Brinker WO *et al: Handbook of Small Animal Orthopedics & Fracture Treatment.* 2nd ed. Saunders, Philadelphia, 1990.

Ettinger SJ: *Textbook of Veterinary Internal Medicine.* 3rd ed. Saunders, Philadelphia, 1989.

Harari J: *Surgical Complications and Wound Healing in the Small Animal Practice.* Saunders, Philadelphia, 1993.

Knecht CD *et al: Fundamental Techniques in Veterinary Surgery.* 3rd ed. Saunders, Philadelphia, 1987.

Piermattei DL and Greeley RG: *An Atlas of Surgical Approaches to the Bones of the Dog and Cat.* 3rd ed. Saunders, Philadelphia, 1992.

Sherding RG: *The Cat: Diseases and Clinical Management.* Churchill-Livingstone, New York, 1989.

Slatter DH: *Textbook of Small Animal Surgery.* Saunders, Philadelphia, 1985.

Swaim SF and Henderson RA: *Small Animal Wound Management.* Lea & Febiger, Philadelphia, 1990.

Practice answer sheets are on page 357-358.

Dogs

J.K. Roush

Questions

1. Which suture pattern provides a continuous inverting closure of hollow organs and does **not** expose suture material to the organ lumen?

   a. Connell
   b. Parker-Kerr
   c. Cushing
   d. vertical mattress
   e. Halsted

For Questions 2 through 6, select the correct answer from the 5 choices below.

   a. povidone-iodine
   b. chlorhexidine gluconate
   c. hexachlorophene
   d. isopropyl alcohol
   e. sodium hypochlorite

Correct answers are on pages 303-314.

Dogs, continued

2. *A biguanide handwash and surgical scrub whose antibacterial action is maintained in the presence of blood.*

3. *Sporicidal as well as bactericidal.*

4. *Kills bacteria by coagulation of proteins.*

5. *Has excellent virucidal action when applied to environmental surfaces, but can dissolve blood clots when applied to wounds.*

6. *Its cumulative antibacterial action is nullified by alcohol.*

Questions 7 through 9

A 6-month-old Rottweiler puppy is presented because of moderate weight-bearing lameness of the left front limb of 2 weeks' duration. There is no history of a traumatic incident. Physical examination findings include pain on flexion of the left elbow joint and effusion in the left elbow joint.

7. *The **least** likely cause of these signs is:*

   a. ununited anconeal process
   b. hypertrophic osteopathy
   c. elbow dysplasia
   d. osteochondrosis of the distal humerus
   e. fragmented medial coronoid process

8. *The diagnostic test most likely to result in definitive diagnosis of the underlying cause of this lameness is:*

   a. thoracic radiography
   b. elbow arthrocentesis
   c. complete blood count and serum chemistry panel
   d. lateral and craniocaudal radiographs of the elbow
   e. bone scintigraphy of the elbow

9. *If the diagnosis is ununited anconeal process, what is the most successful treatment for this disease?*

   a. reattachment of the anconeal process with a bone screw
   b. removal of the anconeal process
   c. cage rest and analgesics for 4 weeks
   d. replacement of the anconeal process with a cortical autograft
   e. reattachment of the anconeal process with cyanoacrylate bone glue

10. *In dogs, osteochondrosis has been reported to affect all of the following **except** the:*

    a. temporomandibular joint
    b. coxofemoral joint
    c. vertebrae (spinous process)
    d. elbow joint
    e. scapulohumeral joint

11. *Where is osteochondrosis most commonly located in the stifle and tarsocrural joints of dogs?*

    a. lateral femoral condyle, medial malleolus of the tibia
    b. medial femoral condyle, medial trochlear ridge of the talus
    c. medial femoral condyle, lateral trochlear ridge of the talus
    d. lateral femoral condyle, lateral trochlear ridge of the talus
    e. lateral femoral condyle, medial trochlear ridge of the talus

12. *In dogs, which of the following is **not** a congenital malformation leading to medial patellar luxation?*

    a. lateral bowing of the femur
    b. medial placement of the tibial crest (tibial deformity)
    c. shallow trochlear groove
    d. coxa valga
    e. increased internal tibial rotation

13. *Persistent patellar luxation that cannot be manually reduced is classified as:*

    a. Grade I
    b. Grade II
    c. Grade III
    d. Grade IV

e. Grade V

14. Which of the following is generally **not** successful in treatment of medial patellar luxation?

    a. lateral retinaculum imbrication
    b. trochlear wedge resection
    c. trocheoplasty
    d. tibial crest transposition
    e. patellectomy

15. Principles of joint arthrodesis include all of the following **except**:

    a. leaving the joint open postoperatively to drain excess joint fluid
    b. autogenous cancellous bone graft
    c. removal of remaining joint cartilage
    d. placement of the joint at a normal anatomic angle for arthrodesis
    e. rigid fixation across the joint

16. Which of the following is **not** a common part of the history of dogs with cranial cruciate ligament rupture?

    a. obese dog
    b. injured while actively playing
    c. 8 months old
    d. overactive dog, always jumping and running
    e. large-breed dog

17. Indications for surgical repair of pelvic fractures include all of the following **except**:

    a. caudal acetabular fracture, with sciatic nerve entrapment
    b. multiple nondisplaced fractures of the pubis
    c. fractured ilium, with a medially displaced caudal fragment
    d. bilateral sacroiliac luxation
    e. acetabular fracture involving the dorsal acetabular rim

For Questions 18 through 22, select the correct answer from the 5 choices below.

    a. asepsis
    b. sterilization
    c. antiseptic
    d. disinfectant
    e. sepsis

18. Absence of pathogenic microbes in living tissue.

19. Chemical agent that kills or inhibits the growth of microorganisms on inanimate objects.

20. Presence of pathogenic microbes or their toxins in living tissue.

21. Process of killing all microorganisms on animate or inanimate materials.

22. Chemical agent that inhibits the growth of microorganisms in living tissue.

23. Which of the following has proven **least** useful in palliative or definitive treatment of hip dysplasia in dogs?

    a. total hip replacement
    b. oral ascorbic acid therapy
    c. intertrochanteric varus osteotomy
    d. triple pelvic osteotomy
    e. oral analgesic therapy

24. A dog with craniodorsal luxation of the right coxofemoral joint may have all the following clinical signs **except**:

    a. right greater trochanter is displaced dorsally as compared with the left
    b. palpable crepitation on manipulation of the right hip joint
    c. left hind limb longer than the right when the hind limbs are fully extended
    d. examiner's thumb pushed out of sciatic notch during external femoral rotation ("thumb test")
    e. lameness of the right hind limb

Correct answers are on pages 303-314.

Dogs, continued

25. *In dogs with avascular necrosis of the femoral head (Legg-Calve-Perthes disease), the history commonly includes all of the following **except**:*

    a. toy or miniature breed
    b. 3-4 years old
    c. no history of trauma
    d. gradual onset with increasing lameness
    e. unilateral or bilateral

26. *In a growing dog, a distal femoral fracture in which the fracture lines runs along the distal physis and exits through the distal metaphysis is classified as:*

    a. Salter I
    b. Salter II
    c. Salter III
    d. Salter IV
    e. Salter V

27. *All of the following describe correct use of twisted cerclage wire in fracture fixation **except**:*

    a. 2 or more full cerclage wires per fracture
    b. wire ends cut off betweeen 2nd and 4th full twist
    c. wire ends bent over
    d. care taken to form symmetric wire twist
    e. ideal fracture configuration is long oblique (obliquity at least 2 times bone diameter)

28. *All of the following are successful treatments for coxofemoral luxation **except**:*

    a. caudal and distal transposition of the greater trochanter
    b. extracapsular suture stabilization
    c. capsulorraphy
    d. transarticular pin fixation
    e. primary suture repair of ligamentum teres

29. *Structures encountered during a medial approach to the midshaft tibia include all of the following **except**:*

    a. long digital extensor muscle
    b. medial saphenous vein
    c. superficial peroneal artery
    d. medial saphenous artery
    e. popliteus muscle

30. *Correct positioning of the hind limb to avoid iatrogenic sciatic nerve injury during retrograde intramedullary pinning of the femur is with the:*

    a. coxofemoral joint extended, hind limb abducted
    b. coxofemoral joint flexed, hind limb abducted
    c. coxofemoral joint flexed, hind limb adducted
    d. coxofemoral joint flexed, hind limb externally rotated
    e. coxofemoral joint extended, hind limb adducted

Questions 31 through 34

A 6-year-old intact male Dachshund is presented 6 hours after acute onset of hind limb paresis. The dog had not been observed during the 2 hours before the onset of clinical signs, and the recent history is unknown. The dog is now quadriplegic. Your neurologic examination shows bilaterally hyperreflexive patellar and withdrawal reflexes, and hyporeflexive biceps and triceps reflexes. Proprioception is absent in all 4 limbs. Deep pain is present in all 4 limbs. Cranial nerve responses are normal.

31. *In what segment of the spinal cord is the lesion most likely located?*

    a. coccygeal (Cy1-10)
    b. lumbosacral (L4-S3)
    c. thoracolumbar (T3-L3)
    d. cervicothoracic (C6-T2)
    e. cervical (C1-C5)

32. *Likely differential diagnoses for this dog's neurologic signs include all of the following **except**:*

    a. intervertebral disk rupture

b.   intradural spinal neoplasm
c.   vertebral body fracture
d.   fibrocartilaginous spinal embolism
e.   traumatic vertebral subluxation/luxation

33. *Diagnostic tests that may aid definitive diagnosis of these conditions include all of the following* **except***:*

a.   survey radiography of the affected area
b.   myelography
c.   magnetic resonance imaging
d.   computed tomography
e.   spinal ultrasonography

34. *If intervertebral disk rupture at C6-7 is diagnosed in this dog, which of the following is an appropriate surgical therapy?*

a.   right hemilaminectomy
b.   left hemilaminectomy
c.   ventral slot decompression
d.   C6-7 stabilization and arthrodesis
e.   cage rest and corticosteroid therapy

35. *In dogs, which intervertebral disk is* **least** *likely to rupture?*

a.   C3-4 (cervical region)
b.   L1-2 (cranial lumbar region)
c.   T12-13 (thoracolumbar region)
d.   T4-5 (thoracic region)
e.   L3-4 (caudal lumbar region)

36. *You are presented with a 10-year-old Labrador Retriever with a noncomminuted, closed, transverse fracture of the midshaft femur. Which fracture fixation method would provide the* **least** *stable fixation?*

a.   single intramedullary pin
b.   Type-I, double-bar external fixator
c.   dynamic compression plate
d.   single intramedullary pin combined with a Type-I, single-bar external fixator
e.   multiple (stacked) intramedullary pins

37. *Which of the following is* **not** *a general goal of modern internal fracture fixation?*

a.   rigid internal fixation
b.   anatomic fracture reduction
c.   early return of limb function
d.   immobilization of the joints proximal and distal to the fractured bone
e.   aseptic/atraumatic surgical technique

For Questions 38 through 42, select the correct answer from the 5 choices below.

a.   polyglycolic acid
b.   polypropylene
c.   stainless steel
d.   nylon
e.   polyglyconate

38. *Nonabsorbable suture material with minimal thrombogenic effects.*

39. *Strongest absorbable suture material at implantation.*

40. *Nonabsorbable suture material with antibacterial degradation products.*

41. *Strongest available suture material.*

42. *Absorbable suture material that should not be exposed to the bladder lumen.*

43. *All of the following are appropriate for treatment of cranial cruciate rupture in a 40-kg Rottweiler* **except***:*

a.   "under and over" fascial strip
b.   "over the top" fascial strip
c.   fibular head transposition
d.   imbrication with extracapsular stainless-steel sutures
e.   6 weeks of cage rest

Correct answers are on pages 303-314.

Dogs, continued

44. *The strongest type of gastropexy used as treatment for gastric dilatation-volvulus in dogs is:*

   a. circumcostal gastropexy
   b. tube gastrostomy
   c. belt-loop gastropexy
   d. gastrocolopexy
   e. gastropexy with scarification of the peritoneum

45. *All of the following are accepted general principles of surgical drain placement **except**:*

   a. aseptic drain placement with drain maintained under sterile bandages
   b. drains should not exit through incision lines
   c. increasing the number of drain lumina decreases wound drainage
   d. fewest drains possible placed through the least number of holes
   e. drains should be removed when drainage becomes negligible

46. *To serve as universal donors, dogs maintained as on-site blood donors should be **negative** for which blood allele?*

   a. DEA 1
   b. DEA 3
   c. DEA 4
   d. DEA 6
   e. DEA 7

47. *All of the following are accepted principles of emergency treatment of an open fracture of the midshaft tibia of 24 hours' duration **except**:*

   a. debride immediately and lavage copiously
   b. culture before and/or after debridement
   c. leave wound open and bandage aseptically
   d. give broad-spectrum antibiotics before culture, then switch to one effective against isolated organisms
   e. apply immediate rigid fixation

48. *The most stable configuration of an external fixation device is:*

   a. Type I, single bar (unilateral)
   b. Type I, double bar (unilateral)
   c. Type II (bilateral, uniplanar)
   d. Type III (bilateral, biplanar)
   e. quadrilateral (unilateral, biplanar)

49. *Which muscle is the only member of the quadriceps group to originate on the ilium?*

   a. semitendinosus
   b. rectus femoris
   c. vastus medialis
   d. vastus intermedius
   e. vastus lateralis

50. *Which of the following approaches to the elbow is appropriate for repair of a comminuted "Y" fracture of the distal humerus in a 6-year-old Cocker Spaniel?*

   a. lateral approach to the lateral humeral epicondyle
   b. olecranon osteotomy (caudal approach to the elbow)
   c. triceps tenotomy (caudal approach to the elbow)
   d. medial approach to the medial humeral epicondyle
   e. caudolateral approach to the elbow joint

51. *You are presented with a 5-year-old Labrador Retriever with acute swelling and joint effusion of the right carpus. Radiographs show minimal degenerative changes of the right carpus and soft tissue swelling surrounding the radiocarpal joint. Arthrocentesis and fluid evaluation of the right carpus show the following results: total cell count 150,000 cells/μl, 90% segmented neutrophils, 10% monocytes, mucin clot friable. What is the most likely cause of these findings?*

   a. traumatic arthritis
   b. degenerative arthritis
   c. septic arthritis

d. systemic lupus erythematosus
e. rheumatoid arthritis

52. *Which developmental bone disease is confirmed by radiographic findings of a radiolucent linear lesion parallel to the physis of affected bones?*

a. panosteitis
b. craniomandibular osteopathy
c. osteochondrosis
d. hypertrophic osteodystrophy
e. retained enchondral bone core

For Questions 53 through 56, select the correct answer from the 4 choices below.

a. autograft
b. allograft
c. isograft
d. xenograft

53. *A graft in which the donor and recipient are individuals of different species.*

54. *A graft in which donor and recipient are genetically unrelated individuals of the same species.*

55. *A graft in which tissue is transferred to a new position on the same individual.*

56. *A graft in which donor and recipient are different individuals but genetically identical.*

57. *Which statement best describes the term "osteoconduction" as it refers to bone grafting?*

a. Living cells within the graft and recipient bed are induced to differentiate and produce bone by a stimulatory factor from the graft.
b. The bone graft acts as a scaffold and is incorporated by creeping substitution.
c. New bone is deposited by viable osteocyte precursors within the graft.
d. The bone graft is revascularized through inosculation (growth of new vessels into former existing vessel lumina).
e. Bone morphogenic protein acts to increase osteoclast resorption and stimulates bone production by osteoblasts.

58. *Concerning limb amputation in dogs, which statement is **least** accurate?*

a. Hind limb amputation is best accomplished by coxofemoral disarticulation for optimal postoperative cosmetic results.
b. Forequarter amputation is the preferred method for front limb amputation.
c. Mid-femoral amputation is adequate for lesions distal to the stifle.
d. Forelimb amputation by scapulohumeral disarticulation results in a less favorable cosmetic appearance due to scapular muscle atrophy.
e. Forelimb amputation by mid-humeral osteotomy produces acceptable results.

Cats

R.M. Bright

59. *Which antimicrobial is most effective for chemoprophylaxis in a cat undergoing colotomy?*

a. trimethoprim-sulfa
b. penicillin
c. tetracycline
d. clindamycin
e. second-generation cephalosporin

Correct answers are on pages 303-314.

Cats, continued

60. *The most common type of dehydration that must be corrected before any surgical procedure is:*

    a. hypotonic dehydration (low serum sodium)
    b. isotonic dehydration (normal serum sodium)
    c. Addison-type dehydration (high potassium, low sodium)
    d. isotonic dehydration with hypokalemia
    e. hypertonic dehydration with hypernatremia

61. *In cats, chronic vomiting associated with pyloric outflow obstruction is likely to cause:*

    a. metabolic alkalosis with hyperkalemia and normochloremia
    b. metabolic alkalosis with hypokalemia and hypochloremia
    c. metabolic acidosis with hyperkalemia and normochloremia
    d. metabolic acidosis with hypokalemia and hypochloremia
    e. respiratory acidosis with compensatory metabolic alkalosis

62. *The fluid of choice for correcting dehydration and metabolic alkalosis before surgical treatment of pyloric stenosis is:*

    a. lactated Ringer's solution
    b. 0.9% saline
    c. hypertonic (7%) saline
    d. 5% dextrose
    e. 10% dextrose

63. *The most common electrolyte disturbance seen in cats after bilateral thyroidectomy is:*

    a. hypokalemia due to aggressive fluid therapy necessary in these cats
    b. hypocalcemia
    c. hypercalcemia
    d. hyperkalemia
    e. hypernatremia

64. *The surgical approach for closure of a patent ductus arteriosus is via:*

    a. the left 4th intercostal space
    b. the left 7th intercostal space
    c. the right 4th intercostal space
    d. median sternotomy
    e. transsternal thoracotomy

65. *Which of the following is **not** an indication for emergency repair of a diaphragmatic hernia (herniorrhaphy)?*

    a. hemopneumothorax
    b. incarcerated intestine within the rent
    c. severe respiratory failure from viscera encroaching on the lungs
    d. stomach entrapment within the thorax, with enlarging gas accumulation
    e. persistent cyanosis despite oxygen and fluid therapy

66. *In treatment of chronic frontal sinusitis in cats, the frontal sinuses can be obliterated using:*

    a. a cancellous bone graft
    b. a fat graft implant
    c. a musculocutaneous graft
    d. temporalis muscle (free graft)
    e. synthetic mesh (polypropylene)

67. *What is the most likely source of intrathoracic hemorrhage following median sternotomy?*

    a. the internal thoracic artery
    b. the bronchoesophageal artery
    c. the intercostal arteries
    d. the marrow of split sternebrae
    e. the subclavian artery

68. *To facilitate removal of the left caudal lung lobe, which structure attaching the lung lobe to the mediastinal pleura should be severed?*

    a. hilar-mediastinal band
    b. diaphragmatic tendon
    c. pulmonary ligament
    d. sternopericardial ligament
    e. pneumopericardial ligament

69. *Lymphangiography to diagnose chylothorax is best performed by placing a catheter in a mesenteric lymphatic via:*

    a. the right 9th intercostal space
    b. the left 9th intercostal space
    c. a midline ventral abdominal incision
    d. a right paracostal incision
    e. a left paracostal incision

70. *Thoracic duct leakage of chyle into the pleural cavity is thought to be most often related to:*

    a. thymoma
    b. lung lobe torsion
    c. cardiomyopathy
    d. thoracic duct obstruction/lymphangiectasia
    e. thoracic duct tear secondary to trauma

71. *In cats, one of the most severe postoperative complications associated with repair of a chronic diaphragmatic hernia is:*

    a. liver failure
    b. renal infarcts
    c. artrial fibrillation
    d. pulmonary edema
    e. hemorrhage from the diaphragmatic wound

72. *The structure that can be used in lieu of a synthetic mesh implant to repair caudal thoracic wall defects following* en-bloc *resection of tumors is:*

    a. the pericardium made into an advancement flap
    b. the diaphragm used as an advancement flap
    c. an intercostal muscle flap
    d. a bone allograft
    e. the rhomboideus muscle belly

73. *The agent of choice for anesthetic induction and maintenance of cats undergoing surgery for correction of a portosystemic shunt is:*

    a. methoxyflurane
    b. halothane
    c. ether

    d. thiamylal sodium
    e. isoflurane

74. *What muscle is associated with laryngeal paralysis secondary to trauma of the recurrent laryngeal nerve during thyroidectomy?*

    a. thyropharyngeal
    b. cricothyroideus dorsalis
    c. arytenoideus ventralis
    d. cricoarytenoideus dorsalis
    e. intrinsic adductor muscles of the larynx

75. *The most medially located muscle that is separated bluntly on ventral approach to the trachea is the:*

    a. sternothyroideus
    b. sternohyoideus
    c. sternocephalicus
    d. cleidomastoideus
    e. thyrohyoideus

76. *Which of the following is most likely to contribute to postoperative aspiration pneumonia in a cat subjected to surgery for correction of severe pyloric outflow disease caused by a benign or neoplastic tumor?*

    a. concurrent megaesophagus due to vagal nerve involvement by the tumor
    b. gastric retention of fluids
    c. dysphagia
    d. impingement on the diaphragm by the distended stomach
    e. postoperative use of a vagolytic agent

77. *In cats, megacolon is most commonly associated with:*

    a. an extraluminal mass, such as adenocarcinoma
    b. an intraluminal mass, such as a foreign body
    c. unknown factors
    d. lumbosacral trauma
    e. pelvic fractures

Correct answers are on pages 303-314.

Cats, continued

78. In cats, oral surgery is done primarily to treat which type of tumor?

  a. fibrosarcoma
  b. osteosarcoma
  c. lymphosarcoma
  d. squamous-cell carcinoma
  e. malignant melanoma

79. A foreign body lodged in the thoracic esophagus between intercostal spaces 2 and 3 is best approached via:

  a. the right sixth intercostal space
  b. the left fourth intercostal space
  c. the right second or third intercostal space
  d. the left second or third intercostal space
  e. median sternotomy

80. An oronasal defect created by partial maxillectomy is most often repaired/closed with a:

  a. lingual-facial rotating flap
  b. buccal flap
  c. hard palate rotating flap
  d. free graft with microvascular technique
  e. bilateral hard palate mucosal overlay

81. In hemimandibulectomy for treatment of oral neoplasia, where is the mandibular artery encountered and ligated?

  a. lateral aspect of the temporomandibular joint
  b. on the buccal mucosa just caudal to the third premolar
  c. between the mylohyoid and geniohyoid muscles
  d. as it enters the medial aspect of the caudal end of the mandible
  e. on the lateral aspect of the digastricus muscle, running parallel with the mandible

82. If a squamous-cell carcinoma involves the middle segment of the mandible but has not metastasized to the lungs or lymph nodes, what is the most appropriate surgical procedure to decrease the chances of tumor recurrence?

  a. bilateral rostral mandibulectomy
  b. hemimandibulectomy
  c. segmental mandibulectomy with a cortical bone graft
  d. complete mandibulectomy
  e. excision of the mass, limited to soft tissue structures overlying the hemimandible

83. In a cat with suspected esophageal foreign body, a contrast esophagogram also reveals contrast material in the trachea. Preoperative planning for treatment of this cat should consider the possibility of encountering:

  a. an esophagotracheal fistula
  b. pneumomediastinum
  c. mediastinitis
  d. an oronasal fistula
  e. stricture of the esophagus

84. What is the most likely cause of regurgitation in a cat 4-8 weeks after ovariohysterectomy?

  a. megaesophagus due to the residual effects of preanesthetic drugs
  b. megaesophagus due to transient generalized esophageal hypomotility
  c. esophageal stricture secondary to reflux esophagitis
  d. dysautonomia due to a vagal nerve disorder
  e. hypersensitivity to the food given at home because it is different than that given in the hospital

85. The layer of the esophagus that is the most likely to retain sutures is the:

  a. surrounding adventitia
  b. mucosa
  c. submucosa
  d. smooth muscle layer
  e. skeletal muscle

86. As seen through the right third intercostal space at thoracotomy, the large blood-filled structure running transversely over the esophagus is the:

   a. confluence of the external and internal jugular veins
   b. major deep thoracic artery branching from the bronchoesophageal artery
   c. azygos vein
   d. left subclavian vein
   e. thymus vein, seen only in cats under 1 year of age

87. A surgical technique designed to correct spraying or inappropriate urination in cats is:

   a. perineal urethrostomy
   b. scrotal urethrostomy
   c. transection of the ischiourethralis musculature
   d. ischiocavernosus myectomy
   e. muscle sling technique to reposition the course of the penile urethra

88. During laparotomy in an icteric cat from Florida, you find extensive scar tissue around the bile ducts. The most likely cause of this scar tissue is:

   a. toxoplasmosis
   b. liver fluke (Platynosomum)
   c. hepatic amyloidosis
   d. hepatic lipidosis
   e. portosystemic shunt with secondary biliary lithiasis

89. In cats, granulomatous masses found during surgical exploration of the nasal cavity are most likely associated with:

   a. histoplasmosis
   b. cryptococcosis
   c. blastomycosis
   d. coccidioidomycosis
   e. aspergillosis

90. A unilateral chain mastectomy includes removal of which lymph node lying dorsal to the fifth mammary gland?

   a. pudendal
   b. superficial perineal
   c. inguinal
   d. pudendo-epigastric
   e. popliteal

91. The paired artery and vein that must be located, isolated, ligated and transected during removal of the fifth mammary gland in cats is the:

   a. caudal superficial epigastric
   b. pudendo-epigastric
   c. caudal deep epigastric
   d. inguinal
   e. external pudendal

92. A surgical incision into the respiratory tract is classified as:

   a. clean
   b. clean-contaminated
   c. contaminated
   d. dirty
   e. purulent

93. During exploration of the nasal cavity, the turbinate structures located most caudal and contiguous with the cribriform plate are the:

   a. maxilloturbinates
   b. ethmoturbinates
   c. cribroturbinates
   d. septoturbinates
   e. sinonasal turbinates

94. A common postoperative complication of rhinotomy in cats is:

   a. weakness of the rear quarters
   b. pyothorax
   c. subcutaneous emphysema
   d. pneumothorax
   e. Horner's syndrome

Correct answers are on pages 303-314.

Cats, continued

95. *Though rare, which pleural-related problem may be associated with rhinotomy in cats?*

    a. hydrothorax
    b. pneumothorax
    c. chylothorax
    d. pyothorax
    e. pleuritis

96. *If nasopharyngeal polyps involve the osseous bullae, which surgical treatment is recommended?*

    a. soft palate splitting and traction on the pharyngeal component
    b. bulla osteotomy via a lateral approach
    c. bulla osteotomy following total ear ablation
    d. ventral bulla osteotomy
    e. intraoral approach to each bulla

97. *Surgical management of laryngeal paralysis in cats includes:*

    a. ventriculocordectomy and arytenoidopexy via a ventral approach
    b. bilateral arytenoidopexy
    c. partial laryngectomy and vocal fold removal
    d. bilateral "tie-back" procedure
    e. vocal cord removal and partial amputation of the epiglottis

98. *A traumatic tear of the cranial portion of the thoracic trachea is approached surgically via:*

    a. a ventral midline caudal cervical approach, with cranial traction on the trachea
    b. thoracotomy through the left third intercostal space
    c. thoracotomy through the right third intercostal space
    d. a transsternal approach between the third and fourth sternebrae
    e. median sternotomy

99. *The most important complication related to use of tracheostomy tubes in cats is:*

    a. subcutaneous emphysema
    b. pneumomediastinum
    c. laryngeal paralysis due to recurrent laryngeal nerve entrapment
    d. obstruction of the tube with mucus
    e. serous drainage from the skin wound

100. *Tracheal stenosis secondary to anastomosis of 2 tracheal segments is most often due to:*

    a. poor perfusion of the tracheal segments
    b. tension across the suture line
    c. use of nonabsorbable sutures
    d. bacteria in the lumen of the trachea
    e. sutures placed too far apart

101. *The tracheostomy incision **least** likely to result in tracheal stricture is a:*

    a. longitudinal paramedian incision involving 6 tracheal rings
    b. longitudinal midline incision involving 6 tracheal rings
    c. transverse incision between tracheal rings 4 and 5
    d. longitudinal paramedian incision involving tracheal rings 3 through 6
    e. midline incision creating a triangular opening

102. *A thoracic wall chondrosarcoma is best treated surgically by:*

    a. "fillet" excision of the mass to the level of the rib cage
    b. resection of the mass and associated rib
    c. *en-bloc* excision involving one rib cranial and one rib caudal to the extent of the mass
    d. wide *en-bloc* excision involving a minimum of 4 ribs
    e. electrosurgical resection, followed by cryosurgery

103. *Thoracic wall defects repaired with a mesh implant sometimes do not have enough muscle to overlay the mesh and fill the defect. Which technique can be used to fill the remaining defect?*

a. diaphragmatic advancement flap
b. omental pedicle flap
c. rib rotation
d. ox fascia implant
e. rotational muscle flap using iliopsoas muscle

104. *When using synthetic mesh to repair a thoracic wall defect, it is best to place it:*

a. as an extrapleural single-layer onlay implant
b. as a double-layer onlay implant
c. intrapleurally, with the edges doubled over
d. between the layers of muscle adjacent to the defect
e. overlying the muscle and subcutaneous tissue initially used to close the defect

105. *Correction of a salivary mucocele manifested as a cervical swelling requires removal of the:*

a. parotid gland
b. lacrimal and parotid glands
c. monostomatic and polystomatic portions of the mandibular salivary gland
d. mandibular and parotid glands
e. sublingual and mandibular glands

106. *Which salivary gland is most often associated with a salivary mucocele?*

a. mandibular
b. sublingual
c. parotid
d. acromial
e. zygomatic

107. *Which vessels serve as important landmarks for the skin incision used in the lateral approach to salivary-gland resection?*

a. sublingual and submandibular arteries
b. parotid and maxillary veins
c. submaxillary and facial veins
d. maxillary and linguofacial veins
e. deep mandibular and superficial lacrimal veins

108. *In what areas is a salivary mucocele likely to be manifested?*

a. sublingual (ranula), pharyngeal and cervical
b. cervical, subauricular and intermandibular
c. retrobulbar, pharyngeal and cervical
d. sublingual (ranula), cervical and sublaryngeal
e. retrolaryngeal, retropharyngeal and sublingual

109. *A term used to describe a salivary mucocele located ventral to the tongue is:*

a. linguoma
b. frenulocele
c. ranula
d. myoglossal cyst
e. thyroglossal duct cyst

110. *Omental patching techniques used to reinforce primary suture lines have been described for use primarily in:*

a. adrenalectomy
b. partial splenectomy
c. partial hepatectomy
d. enterotomy and end-to-end anastomosis
e. choleenterostomy

111. *The portion of the gastrointestinal tract that is used as a serosal patch to reinforce primary closure of the bowel is the:*

a. ileum
b. cecum
c. greater curvature of the stomach
d. jejunum
e. ascending colon

112. *Intestinal malabsorption with diarrhea and malnutrition that may follow resection of a large portion of the small intestine is called the:*

a. Zollinger-Ellison syndrome
b. Branham reflex
c. steatorrhea complex
d. short-bowel syndrome
e. lymphangiectasia

Correct answers are on pages 303-314.

Cats, continued

113. *Removal of the ileocolic valve may result in malabsorption and diarrhea. This is most likely related to:*

    a. bacterial overgrowth
    b. disruption of lymphatic drainage
    c. increased possibility of eosinophilic enteritis
    d. decreased transit time of ingesta coursing through the small and large bowel
    e. increased intestinal motility

114. *Two segments of esophagus can be anastomosed with a horizontal mattress suture pattern, which is:*

    a. an everting suture pattern
    b. an inverting suture pattern
    c. an approximating suture pattern
    d. a simple appositional suture pattern
    e. a "crushing" suture pattern

115. *Cushing or Lembert sutures used to close a gastrotomy incision are an example of:*

    a. an inverting suture pattern
    b. an everting suture pattern
    c. a simple-continuous suture pattern
    d. an approximating suture pattern
    e. a "crushing" suture pattern

116. *A pancreatic mass and an ulcer involving the duodenum are most likely associated with:*

    a. an insulinoma
    b. the Zollinger-Ellision syndrome (gastrinoma)
    c. an islet-cell tumor of the pancreas
    d. a hepatoma
    e. exocrine pancreatic insufficiency

117. *When doing some routine blood tests in a cat before surgery for resection of an intestinal mass in cats, you detect hypercalcemia. This finding is most likely related to:*

    a. adenocarcinoma
    b. leiomyosarcoma

    c. lymphosarcoma
    d. plasmacytoma
    e. leiomyoma

118. *After resection of an intestinal adenocarcinoma, the average survival time is approximately:*

    a. 4-6 months
    b. 4-6 weeks
    c. 1 year
    d. 2-3 years
    e. 1 week

119. *At exploratory laparotomy on a cat, you find an intestinal lesion that is both nodular and diffuse. This lesion is most likely:*

    a. a leiomyosarcoma
    b. an adenocarcinoma
    c. a carcinoid
    d. lymphosarcoma
    e. an adenomatous polyp

120. *A cat with a complete mid-duodenal obstruction has frequent episodes of profuse vomiting. Before surgery to remove the obstruction, the cat should be treated to correct:*

    a. respiratory acidosis with compensatory metabolic alkalemia
    b. metabolic acidosis
    c. metabolic alkalosis
    d. respiratory alkalosis with compensatory metabolic acidemia
    e. metabolic alkalosis with compensatory respiratory acidemia

121. *The muscle in the cervical region that is most often used to reinforce esophageal suture lines is the:*

    a. sternobrachialis
    b. sternocephalicus
    c. cleidomastoideus
    d. sternothyroideus
    e. sternohyoideus

122. *Esophageal strictures due to reflux esophagitis following surgery or general anesthesia usually are located:*

a. in the mid-cervical region
b. in the mid-thoracic region
c. just cranial to the diaphragm
d. just caudal to the cricopharyngeal muscle (upper esophageal sphincter)
e. at the thoracic inlet

123. *The most common vascular ring anomaly causing regurgitation in cats is:*

a. aberrant left subclavian artery
b. right subclavian artery originating from the aorta
c. double aorta
d. persistent right aortic arch
e. right caudal vena cava

124. *Most hiatal hernias are:*

a. axial-type sliding hernias
b. related to gastroesophageal intussusceptions
c. related to type-II esophageal hypoplasia
d. strangulating hernias
e. paraesophageal hernias

125. *Sometimes a fundoplication procedure is necessary to prevent gastroesophageal reflux associated with hiatal hernia. The fundoplication procedure recommended for use in cats is the:*

a. Ellison 270-degree fundoplication
b. Markhaun 180-degree fundoplication
c. Leonardi fundoplication
d. Nissen 360-degree fundoplication
e. Boerma fundoplication

126. *The most common indication for gastrotomy in cats is:*

a. gastric parasitism (*Physaloptera*)
b. neoplasia
c. gastric ulcers
d. chronic hypertrophic pyloric gastropathy
e. foreign bodies

127. *The most common sign related to pyloric stenosis in cats is:*

a. ptyalism
b. anorexia
c. emesis
d. abdominal pain
e. hematemesis

128. *The surgical procedure that uses an antral flap to increase the diameter of the pyloric outflow tract is the:*

a. Heineke-Mikuliciz pyloroplasty
b. Y-U pyloroplasty
c. Fredet-Ramstedt pyloroplasty
d. Finney pyloroplasty
e. MacPherson submucosal resection/sliding flap technique

129. *The Gambee suture pattern used in intestinal surgery is:*

a. everting
b. continuous
c. approximating
d. inverting
e. crushing

130. *Which set of criteria is used to assess the viability of small intestine involved in intussusception?*

a. serosal texture, venous congestion, color
b. color, arterial pulsations, venous congestion
c. peristalsis, arterial pulsations, venous congestion
d. decreased bowel contractility when occluding the portal vein (Bella-Wein reflex), serosal texture, venous congestion
e. color, peristalsis, arterial pulsations

131. *The invaginated portion of the bowel in an intussusception is called the:*

a. intussusceptum
b. intussuscipiens
c. inverted segment
d. invaginatiens
e. inaperistalicum

Correct answers are on pages 303-314.

Cats, continued

132. The portion of the bowel most commonly involved in intussusception is the:

a. duodenocolic segment
b. distal jejunum
c. transverse/proximal colon
d. ileocolic valve area
e. duodenojejunal junction

133. In cats, adenocarcinomas most often involve which portion of the gastrointestinal tract?

a. duodenum
b. ileum
c. jejunum
d. stomach
e. distal colon

134. The surgical procedure of choice for relieving chronic constipation associated with idiopathic megacolon is:

a. segmental colectomy
b. removal of a longitudinal strip of colon to decrease lumen diameter
c. multiple colotomy incisions
d. colopexy
e. subtotal colectomy

135. The microbes of most concern in colorectal surgery are:

a. Gram-positive aerobes
b. Gram-negative enterics
c. anaerobes and Gram-positive aerobes
d. Gram-negative enterics and anaerobes
e. anaerobes only

136. The antimicrobial of choice for perioperative use in colotomy is:

a. metronidazole
b. erythromycin
c. neomycin
d. second-generation cephalosporin
e. ampicillin

137. The most important postoperative complication related to liver biopsy or lobectomy is:

a. liver abscess
b. bile leakage peritonitis
c. vomiting
d. hemorrhage
e. arteriovenous fistula

138. In animals with a portosystemic shunt, the sign seen far more frequently in affected cats than in affected dogs is:

a. emesis
b. ascites
c. ptyalism
d. headpressing
e. diarrhea

139. Ascites during the early postoperative period following occlusion of a portosystemic shunt suggests:

a. right-sided heart failure
b. endotoxemia
c. peritonitis
d. hypoglobinemia
e. portal hypertension

140. When evaluating the portal vein for anomalous shunts to the systemic circulation, the surgeon should know the vein normally contributing the most blood to portal flow is the:

a. caudal mesenteric vein
b. cranial mesenteric vein
c. gastric vein
d. splenic vein
e. pancreaticoduodenal vein

141. In normal cats, intraoperative portal vein pressure is approximately:

a. 8-10 cm H_2O
b. 20-40 cm H_2O
c. 8-10 mm Hg
d. 1-2 mm Hg

e. 3-5 mm Hg

142. As a preoperative measure, the blood ammonia level in cats with a portosystemic shunt is best reduced by:

a. periodic phlebotomy
b. administration of ammonium chloride
c. administration of sodium bicarbonate and lactulose
d. administration of penicillin G and feeding a low-protein diet
e. administration of lactulose and neomycin, and feeding a low-protein diet

143. Which drug should be avoided preoperatively in a cat with ascites and encephalopathy associated with a portosystemic shunt?

a. injectable penicillin G
b. prednisolone
c. furosemide
d. lactulose
e. neomycin

144. The most important anatomic feature to be considered during partial or complete pancreatectomy is the:

a. major papilla
b. minor papilla
c. common bile duct
d. common blood supply with the duodenum
e. splenic vein draining the left lobe

145. A day after exploratory laparotomy, a cat develops acute abdominal pain localized to the cranial right quadrant of the abdominal cavity and vomiting. These signs are most likely related to:

a. pyelonephritis
b. hepatic hematoma
c. pancreatitis
d. intestinal volvulus
e. ileus

146. The cranial thyroid artery is the primary blood supply to each lobe of the thyroid gland. From which artery does this vessel arise on the left side?

a. internal carotid artery
b. common carotid artery
c. sternohyoideus artery
d. supracervical artery
e. ventral psoas artery

147. In cats, the most serious complication following bilateral thyroidectomy is:

a. hypocalcemia
b. hyperkalemia
c. hemorrhage from the major arterial supply
d. hypercalcemia
e. laryngeala paralysis secondary to recurrent laryngeal nerve trauma

148. In cats, the most important disadvantage related to the intracapsular technique of thyroidectomy is:

a. hypoparathyroidism and hypocalcemia
b. hemorrhage
c. recurrence of hyperthyroidism
d. recurrent laryngeal nerve damage
e. thrombosis of the cranial thyroid artery

149. Clinical signs of hypocalcemia that may develop following bilateral thyroidectomy usually occur within:

a. 30 minutes
b. 1-3 hours
c. 7-10 days
d. 24-72 hours
e. 3 weeks

150. Careless application of a tourniquet to the limb during onychectomy may result in:

a. ulnar neuropraxis
b. temporary radial nerve paralysis
c. permanent brachial nerve damage
d. permanent median nerve paralysis
e. severance of the ulnar nerve

Correct answers are on pages 303-314.

Cats, continued

151. *Which nerve is most likely to become entrapped during surgery to repair a proximal femoral fracture or pelvic fracture?*

    a. obturator nerve
    b. perineal nerve
    c. internal pudendal nerve
    d. external pudendal nerve
    e. ischiatic nerve

152. *Fibrosarcoma involving the scapula is best treated with:*

    a. limb-sparing techniques, including resection of the tumor mass followed by cisplatin therapy
    b. cisplatin injections into the major artery leading to the scapula
    c. amputation of the limb
    d. wide *en-bloc* excision with 3-cm margins
    e. *en-bloc* excision and hyperthermia

153. *A cat develops ureteral obstruction after erroneous ureteral ligature during ovariohysterectomy. This cat is likely to lose 80% of the ipsilateral kidney's function within:*

    a. 48 hours
    b. 4-6 hours
    c. 30-35 days
    d. 1 week
    e. 2 weeks

154. *How long (total time) can the renal artery be occluded during nephrolithotomy without damage to the kidney?*

    a. 3-5 minutes
    b. 20-25 minutes
    c. 2 hours
    d. 1 hour
    e. 5 hours

155. *If the paired fan-shaped muscle covering the crus of the penis is not excised during perineal urethrostomy, urethral obstruction may recur. This muscle is the:*

    a. retractor penis
    b. rectococcygeus
    c. sacrotuberous
    d. bulbocavernosus
    e. ischiocavernosus

156. *In male cats with complete urethral obstruction, the most common metabolic derangements that must be corrected before urethrostomy are:*

    a. metabolic alkalosis, hyperkalemia and azotemia
    b. metabolic acidosis, hypokalemia and azotemia
    c. metabolic acidosis, hyperkalemia and azotemia
    d. respiratory alkalosis, hypokalemia and hypernatremia
    e. hypernatremia, metabolic acidosis and hyperchloremia

157. *An inverting suture pattern suitable for closure of a cystotomy incision is the:*

    a. Gambee
    b. simple continuous
    c. continuous mattress
    d. Lembert
    e. simple-interrupted crushing

158. *During perineal urethrostomy, the most caudal extent of the pelvic urethra is located by finding the:*

    a. corpus cavernosus muscle
    b. prostate gland
    c. ischiourethralis muscle
    d. bulbourethral glands
    e. bulbocavernosus muscle

159. *The most common and serious complication following perineal urethrostomy is:*

    a. urethral stricture
    b. urinary incontinence
    c. fecal incontinence

d. rectal prolapse

e. urine scalding

160. *Extensive damage or stricture to the urethra is best treated definitively with:*

a. tube cystostomy

b. urine diversion via a Stamey prepubic catheter

c. urethral metal prosthesis

d. marsupialization of the bladder

e. antepubic urethrostomy

161. *Vulvar bleeding persisting after 3 weeks postpartum is most likely associated with:*

a. excessive use of oxytocin

b. endometritis

c. hyperestrogenism

d. subinvolution of placental sites

e. postpartum hypocalcemia

162. *In cats, empiric antimicrobial therapy following ovariohysterectomy for pyometra should be directed against which commonly isolated organism?*

a. *Staphylococcus aureus*

b. *Staphylococcus epidermidis*

c. *Streptococcus pyogenes*

d. *Escherichia coli*

e. *Pseudomonas aeruginosa*

163. *Of the following antibacterials, which is the best choice for perioperative use in a cat with pyometra?*

a. erythromycin

b. metronidazole

c. tetracycline

d. cefoxitin

e. clindamycin

164. *Unilateral ablation of the ear canal is most often performed in treatment of:*

a. end-stage otitis externa

b. middle-ear infection

c. neoplasia

d. chronic yeast infection

e. traumatic avulsion of the base of the ear

165. *When incised, which tunic differentiates a "closed" castration from an "open" castration?*

a. visceral vaginal tunic

b. double vaginal tunic

c. spermatic tunic

d. parietal vaginal tunic

e. parietal testicular tunic

166. *Which of the following is most helpful in determining if a male cat is bilaterally cryptorchid and still producing androgenic hormones?*

a. urine spraying behavior

b. territorial behavior

c. presence of fully developed spines on the penis

d. no history of urethral obstruction

e. prominent retractor penis muscle on palpation

167. *Following vasectomy, a tomcat may have viable sperm in its ejaculate for up to:*

a. 50 days

b. 15 days

c. 3 days

d. 6 months

e. 1 year

168. *Which ligament of the female reproductive tract courses caudally along the free edge of the mesometrium and through the inguinal canal, and, when broken down, allows better exteriorization of the uterine body during ovariohysterectomy?*

a. suspensory ligament

b. proper ligament

c. uteroovarian ligament

d. round ligament

e. broad ligament

Correct answers are on pages 303-314.

Cats, continued

169. *If a prolapsed uterus is corrected via laparotomy and the owner wishes the cat to remain intact for breeding purposes, the most appropriate couse of action is to:*

    a. perform a unilateral hysterectomy to decrease uterine volume so prolapse is less likely to recur
    b. perform a unilateral ovariohysterectomy
    c. perform a hysterocolopexy
    d. suture the uterine body or each uterine horn to the lateral body wall
    e. place pursestring sutures (nonabsorbable) in the vaginal vault via episiotomy

170. *Which surgical procedure is designed to enlarge the vulvar opening?*

    a. hysterotomy
    b. vaginotomy
    c. episiotomy
    d. celiotomy
    e. stomostomy

171. *The surgical procedure of choice for treatment of a mammary tumor present in one gland is:*

    a. simple mastectomy, with removal of lymph nodes nearest the affected gland
    b. resection of the tumor mass only ("lumpectomy")
    c. regional mastectomy
    d. ovariohysterectomy
    e. ipsilateral chain mastectomy, with regional lymph node removal

172. *The 4 components forming the "module of wound repair" are the:*

    a. tissue macrophage, lymphocyte, monocyte and granulocyte
    b. tissue macrophage, fibroblast, granulocyte and capillary bud
    c. capillary bud, tissue macrophage, plasmacyte and granulocyte
    d. tissue macrophage, capillary bud, prostaglandins and granulocyte
    e. leukotrienes, prostaglandins, serotonin and histamine

173. *The cell that directs events in early wound repair, such as fibroplasia and angiogenesis, is the:*

    a. small lymphocyte
    b. granulocyte
    c. macrophage
    d. plasma cell
    e. fibroblast

174. *The specialized cells responsible for wound contraction are the:*

    a. fibrilloblasts
    b. macrophages
    c. myofibroblasts
    d. monofibroblasts
    e. chondrofibroblasts

175. *Stretching and thinning of the skin surrounding a contracted wound is called:*

    a. bolstered growth
    b. epithelial migration
    c. intussusceptive growth
    d. collagenolysis
    e. epidermolytic migration

176. *The mineral sometimes given to help mobilize vitamin A from the liver in an effort to stimulate wound epithelialization following corticosteroid therapy is:*

    a. magnesium
    b. copper
    c. zinc
    d. calcium
    e. manganese

177. *A pedicle graft that incorporates a direct cutaneous artery and vein is the:*

a. circular flap graft
b. random pedicle flap
c. direct cutaneous flap
d. rotating flap
e. axial-pattern flap

178. *An example of a compound or composite flap for reconstructive surgery is the:*

a. axial pattern flap
b. myocutaneous flap
c. sliding H-pattern flap
d. random-pattern flap
e. thoracic pouch flap

179. *An axial-pattern flap that can be used to close a skin defect on the medial aspect of the thigh is the:*

a. thoracodorsal flap
b. caudal superficial epigastric flap
c. omocervical flap
d. craniala tibialis flap
e. caudal deep epigastric flap

180. *Surgery in the neck region of cats may result in Horner's syndrome, which is associated with trauma to the:*

a. recurrent laryngeal nerve
b. cranial laryngeal nerve
c. auriculopalpebral nerve
d. sympathetic chain

e. vagus nerve

181. *When performing a disarticulating amputation of a pelvic limb for treatment of osteosarcoma of the proximal femur, which muscle group is left intact to provide some coverage of the coxofemoral joint and hemipelvis?*

a. rotator muscle group
b. semimembranosus, semitendinosus
c. sartorius (cranial and caudal bellies)
d. gluteal
e. quadriceps

182. *With complete avulsion of the scapula, the scapula can be reattached to which muscle?*

a. latissimus dorsi
b. rhomboideus
c. external abdominal oblique
d. serratus ventralis
e. intercostal

183. *Osteomyelitis following fracture repair is most commonly due to infection with:*

a. *E coli*
b. *Staphylococcus*
c. *Streptococcus*
d. *Pasteurella*
e. *Klebsiella*

Dogs and Cats

P.A. Bushby, J. Harari

184. *The most common cause of degenerative osteoarthritis of the canine stifle joint is:*

a. medial patellar luxation
b. lateral patellar luxation

c. rupture of the cranial cruciate ligament
d. rupture of the caudal cruciate ligament
e. lateral meniscal tear

Correct answers are on pages 303-314.

Dogs and Cats, continued

185. *Which Putnam classification of medial patellar luxation is characterized by femoral and tibial bone deformations, persistent lameness and inability to manually reduce the luxation?*

   a. Grade I
   b. Grade II
   c. Grade III
   d. Grade IV
   e. Grade V

186. *In repairing patellar luxations, what is the name of the technique in which the trochlear groove is deepened and covered by a triangular osteochondral fragment?*

   a. lateral imbrication
   b. retinacular plication
   c. derotation suture
   d. tibial tuberosity transplantation
   e. wedge recession

187. *The stifle joint is classified as a:*

   a. condylar joint
   b. ball-and-socket joint
   c. ellipsoid joint
   d. hinge joint
   e. plane joint

188. *What is the most common concurrent injury in dogs with cranial cruciate ligament rupture?*

   a. medial patellar luxation
   b. medial meniscal tear
   c. lateral meniscal tear
   d. gastrocnemius tendon avulsion
   e. long digital extensor tendon avulsion

189. *Rupture of the cranial cruciate ligament is characterized clinically by:*

   a. external tibial rotation
   b. cranial drawer motion of the tibia
   c. caudal drawer motion of the tibia
   d. valgus deviation of the stifle joint
   e. varus deviation of the stifle joint

190. *Medial luxation of the patella in dogs is most appropriately treated with:*

   a. a partial medial meniscectomy
   b. a medial relief incision and lateral tightening procedures
   c. a lateral relief incision and medial tightening procedures
   d. a partial patellectomy
   e. intraarticular corticosteroid injections

191. *Which of the following is an extracapsular repair for rupture of the cranial cruciate ligament?*

   a. fabella to tibial tuberosity derotation suture
   b. fascia lata autograft
   c. medial one-third of the patellar tendon autograft
   d. middle one-third of the patellar tendon autograft
   e. lateral one-third of the patellar tendon autograft

192. *In general, surgical treatments for repair of cranial cruciate ligament injury are classified as:*

   a. extracapsular and intracapsular procedures
   b. arthrodesis or amputation procedures
   c. corrective osteotomy procedures
   d. limb-lengthening procedures
   e. limb-shortening procedures

193. *Lateral luxation of the patella in large dogs is often associated with:*

   a. lateral meniscal tear
   b. lateral collateral ligament injury
   c. avulsion of the tibial tuberosity
   d. medial meniscal tear
   e. hip dysplasia

194. *The surgical approach that provides the greatest exposure to organs in the thoracic cavity is via:*

a. lateral intercostal thoracotomy
b. rib resection
c. rib pivot
d. median sternotomy
e. ventral celiotomy and incision through the diaphragm

195. *The most common surgical approach for treatment of a patent ductus arteriosus or persistent right aortic arch is:*

a. left 4th intercostal thoracotomy
b. right 4th intercostal thoracotomy
c. median sternotomy
d. left 10th rib resection
e. right 10th rib pivot

196. *A pathognomonic sign of a persistent right aortic arch is:*

a. fever
b. machinery murmur
c. postprandial regurgitation at weaning
d. caudal paresis
e. thoracic pain

197. *The most common congenital cardiac anomaly in dogs is:*

a. persistent right aortic arch
b. ventricular septal defect
c. tetralogy of Fallot
d. patent ductus arteriosus
e. aortic stenosis

198. *The most common congenital cardiac defect in cats is:*

a. ventricular septal defect
b. cardiomyopathy
c. patent ductus arteriosus
d. persistent right aortic arch
e. pulmonic stenosis

199. *The most common congenital cardiac anomaly in dogs that produces cyanosis is:*

a. cardiomyopathy
b. tetralogy of Fallot
c. pulmonic stenosis
d. pulmonic insufficiency
e. aortic stenosis

200. *Treatment for patent ductus arteriosus requires:*

a. ligation of the ductus
b. beta-adrenergic blockers
c. a low-protein diet
d. arterial embolectomy
e. cardiac patch grafting

201. *Which of the following is **not** an appropriate treatment for chylothorax?*

a. thoracostomy tube drainage
b. pleuroperitoneal shunting
c. pleurodesis
d. short- and medium-chain fatty acid dietary supplementation
e. long-chain fatty acid dietary supplementation

202. *Instability of a thoracic chest wall segment, associated with trauma, that causes paradoxic chest motions is called:*

a. flail chest
b. hemothorax
c. pneumothorax
d. peritoneopericardial hernia
e. chylothorax

203. *An abnormal patent communication between an artery and vein is termed:*

a. hemangioma
b. hemangiosarcoma
c. arteriovenous fistula
d. Eck's fistula
e. arterioma

Correct answers are on pages 303-314.

Dogs and Cats, continued

204. *Neoplasia of the spleen is best treated by:*

a. irradiation
b. chemotherapy
c. arterial bypass procedures
d. splenectomy
e. debulking procedures

205. *A large dog with sudden, gaseous abdominal distention associated with exercise after eating most likely has:*

a. rectal prolapse
b. infectious hepatitis
c. splenic rupture
d. esophageal neoplasia
e. gastric dilatation-volvulus

206. *The most common neurologic disorder in small animals is:*

a. cervical vertebral instability
b. spinal cord neoplasia
c. intervertebral disk disease
d. diskospondylitis
e. atlantoaxial subluxation

207. *Which of the following is **not** an appropriate treatment for lumbosacral stenosis in dogs?*

a. analgesics
b. vitamin E/selenium injections
c. antiinflammatories
d. dorsal laminectomy
e. foraminotomy

208. *A thoracolumbar spinal cord lesion associated with disk herniation produces:*

a. upper motor neuron lesions of the hind limbs
b. lower motor neuron lesions of the hind limbs
c. cervical pain
d. upper motor neuron lesions of the front limbs
e. lower motor neuron lesions of the front limbs

209. *Progressive cervical vertebral instability in Doberman Pinschers requires:*

a. cervical disk fenestration
b. cervical decompression and stabilization
c. cervical facetectomy
d. chemonucleolysis of the cervical disks
e. vitamin E/selenium and dimethyl sulfoxide injections

210. *A progressive, nonpainful condition that causes hind limb paresis in German Shepherds is:*

a. lumbosacral stenosis
b. lumbosacral instability
c. thoracolumbar disk herniation
d. degenerative myelopathy
e. cervical vertebral instability

211. *In Dachshunds, the most common site of intervertebral disk disease is:*

a. C1-C2
b. T1-T2
c. T12-13
d. L1-L2
e. L7-S1

212. *Which of the following lesions is **not** involved in the "brachycephalic airway syndrome"?*

a. eustachian tube dilatation
b. stenotic nares
c. elongated soft palate
d. everted laryngeal saccules
e. hypoplastic trachea

213. *Which of the following is **not** a likely complication of laryngeal surgery?*

a. scar formation
b. inhalation pneumonia
c. laryngeal edema
d. cervical ventroflexion
e. dyspnea

214. *The most common surgical approach for debulking of the nasal cavity is termed:*

a. dorsal craniotomy
b. dorsal rhinotomy
c. ventral rhinotomy

d. ventral sinotomy

e. ventral laryngotomy

d. medial meniscal tear

e. epiphysitis

215. *Which surgical procedure can provide immediate relief of upper airway obstruction?*

a. ventriculocordectomy

b. arytenoidectomy

c. tracheostomy

d. thoracostomy

e. pneumonectomy

216. *An abnormal communication between the mouth and nasal sinuses is termed:*

a. arteriovenous shunt

b. oronasal fistula

c. odontoplastic diverticulum

d. sinopharyngeal tube

e. brachygnathism

217. *Osteochondritis dissecans is **not** usually associated with which joint?*

a. shoulder

b. elbow

c. carpus

d. stifle

e. hock

218. *Surgical treatment for osteochondritis dissecans involves:*

a. cancellous bone autografts

b. arthrodesis of the affected joint

c. cartilage flap removal and curettage of subchondral bone

d. joint stabilization with an external fixator

e. synovectomy

219. *A young, rapidly growing, large dog is being fed a high-energy diet and has forelimb lameness associated with the elbow joint. Which lesion is likely to require surgical intervention in this dog?*

a. panosteitis

b. retained cartilagenous cores

c. fragmented medial coronoid process

220. *Traumatic hip luxation occurs most commonly in which direction?*

a. craniodorsal

b. caudoventral

c. caudodorsal

d. lateral

e. cranioventral

221. *Which of the following is a surgical treatment for traumatic hip luxation?*

a. intramedullary pinning

b. tension-band wiring

c. cerclage wiring

d. bone plating

e. De Vita pinning

222. *Which physeal injury (based on the Salter-Harris classification) has the **poorest** prognosis for recovery?*

a. Type I

b. Type II

c. Type III

d. Type IV

e. Type V

223. *In repair of epiphyseal fractures, what is the primary aim of surgical intervention?*

a. bone alignment

b. articular cartilage congruency

c. periosteal stripping

d. physeal compression

e. physeal distraction

224. *An intramedullary pin used for repair of a long bone fracture provides:*

a. interfragmentary compression

b. rotational stability

c. metaphyseal compression

d. tension-band stabilization

e. axial alignment

Correct answers are on pages 303-314.

Dogs and Cats, continued

225. Which orthopedic device provides the greatest degree of compression across a fracture line?

   a. dynamic compression plate
   b. Kirschner wires
   c. intramedullary pins
   d. cerclage wire
   e. external skeletal fixation

226. Primary bone union is most likely to occur in a fracture being treated with:

   a. bone plate and screws
   b. hemicerclage and full cerclage wires
   c. multiple intramedullary pins
   d. external fixator
   e. plaster cast

227. Which condition should be treated before orthopedic surgery in a trauma patient?

   a. fractured phalanges
   b. fractured, nondisplaced ribs
   c. muscle bruising
   d. ruptured urinary bladder
   e. epistaxis

228. Which lesion could cause depression, poor growth and central nervous system disorders in a young dog being fed a high-protein diet?

   a. patent ductus arteriosus
   b. persistent right aortic arch
   c. portosystemic shunt
   d. persistent urachus
   e. congenital megaesophagus

229. Surgical treatment for unilateral ectopic ureter consists of:

   a. urinary diversion using a segment of ileum
   b. perineal urethrostomy
   c. prepubic urethrostomy
   d. cystopexy
   e. ureteral reimplantation

230. In obese female dogs, chronic perivulvar dermatitis associated with redundant tissue can be treated with:

   a. episiotomy
   b. episioplasty
   c. ovariohysterectomy
   d. vaginotomy
   e. typhlectomy

231. Which of the following is most appropriate for treatment of a transverse midshaft radial fracture in a large dog?

   a. intramedullary pinning
   b. cerclage wires
   c. external skeletal fixator
   d. Kirschner pins
   e. Robert Jones bandage

232. At what time should prophylactic antibiotics be given to prevent surgical wound infections?

   a. 1-2 days before surgery
   b. 1 week before surgery
   c. 12 hours after surgery is terminated
   d. 1-2 hours after surgery is terminated
   e. immediately before surgery

233. The highest concentrations of antibiotics in serum, plasma and tissues are achieved when prophylactic antibiotics are given:

   a. orally
   b. intravenously
   c. intramuscularly
   d. subcutaneously
   e. topically in lavage fluid

234. In a dog with hypoglycemia, you identify a solitary pancreatic tumor during laparotomy. The most likely cause of this dog's hypoglycemia is:

   a. diabetes insipidus
   b. hemangioma
   c. acute hemorrhagic pancreatitis
   d. chronic fibrosing pancreatitis
   e. insulinoma

235. *To reduce swelling and provide temporary fracture stability, which device should be applied to a tibial fracture in a dog?*

 a. external fixator
 b. Schroeder-Thomas splint
 c. Robert Jones bandage
 d. Mason meta splint
 e. padded limb bandage

236. *Which drug is useful for treatment of spinal cord swelling due to trauma of disk herniation?*

 a. aspirin
 b. phenylbutazone
 c. acetaminophen
 d. dexamethasone
 e. acepromazine

237. *Chronic obstipation associated with megacolon in cats is effectively treated by:*

 a. staphylectomy
 b. colopexy
 c. colectomy
 d. cystotomy
 e. gastropexy

238. *Chronic multifocal abscessation around the anus and base of the tail in German Shepherds is termed:*

 a. perianal fistulae
 b. perineal hernia
 c. stud tail
 d. circumanal metaplasia
 e. pilonidal cysts

239. *A 6-month-old female Irish Setter is presented to your clinic with a 3-day history of vomiting. Following physical examination, laboratory workup and abdominal radiographs, you confirm a diagnosis of intestinal obstruction due to a radiopaque foreign body. For surgical exploration and correction of this problem, what is the most appropriate incisional approach?*

 a. ventral abdominal midline, xyphoid to umbilicus
 b. ventral abdominal midline, umbilicus to pubis
 c. ventral abdominal midline, xyphoid to pubis
 d. right paramedian, xyphoid to pubis
 e. right paramedian, umbilicus to pubis

240. *You are performing surgery to remove an intestinal foreign body from a 6-month-old female Irish Setter. You find the foreign body in the distal jejunum. Visual inspection reveals that the intestine proximal (cranial) to the foreign body is distended. Palpation suggests that the intestinal contents are fluid and gas. The foreign body is rough and irregular. The intestines at the site of the foreign body are intact but discolored. Upon digital manipulation, the serosa at the site of the lesion begins to tear, but does not bleed. The most appropriate course of action is to:*

 a. digitally manipulate the foreign body proximally, then perform an enterotomy
 b. digitally manipulate the foreign body distally, then perform an enterotomy
 c. perform an enterotomy at the site of the foreign body
 d. perform an intestinal resection and anastomosis of devitalized intestine, including removal of the foreign body
 e. flush the lumen of the distal intestine with sterile saline to move the foreign body proximally, then perform an enterotomy

241. *In performing an intestinal resection and anastomosis, you remember that the blood supply to the remaining intestine is critical. To ensure adequate blood supply to the remaining intestine, you must make your intestinal incisions at an angle. Which of the following is most likely to maintain an adequate blood supply to remaining intestine?*

 a. leave the mesenteric surface longer than the antimesenteric
 b. leave the antimesenteric surface longer than the mesenteric
 c. leave the mesenteric and antimesenteric surfaces the same length
 d. leave the medial surface longer than the lateral surface
 e. leave the proximal surface longer than the distal surface

Correct answers are on pages 303-314.

Dogs and Cats, continued

242. *Which suture pattern is most appropriate for closure of the small intestine in a dog after intestinal resection?*

    a. Cushing
    b. Bunnell
    c. Parker-Kerr
    d. simple interrupted
    e. vertical mattress

Question 243

You are presented with a 6-year-old male Poodle with acute onset of caudal paresis. Physical examination reveals abnormalities only in the nervous system. Neurologic examination reveals the following:

Mental Status: alert, with no abnormalities noted
Cranial Nerves: no abnormalities noted
Posture and Gait: paraplegia
Postural Reactions:

	Left Front	Left Rear	Right Front	Right Front
Wheelbarrowing	2	0	0	2
Ext Post Thrust	2	0	0	2
Hemiwalk	2	0	0	2
Consc Proprio	2	0	0	2
Hopping	2	0	0	2

Spinal Reflexes:

	Left Front	Left Rear	Right Front	Right Rear
Biceps	2	–	–	2
Triceps	2	–	–	2
Patellar	–	3	3	–
Cranial Tibial	–	3	3	–
Gastrocnemius	–	3	3	–
Flexor	2	2	2	2
Anal Sphincter	–	2	2	–
Panniculus	absent caudal to thoracolumbar area			

Sensation: hyperesthesia over thoracolumbar area, superficial pain absent caudal to thoracolumbar area, deep pain present in all 4 limbs

243. *Which neurologic pathway is most likely affected?*

    a. upper motor neuron to the front limbs
    b. upper motor neuron to the rear limbs
    c. lower motor neuron to the front limbs
    d. lower motor neuron to the rear limbs
    e. upper motor neuron to all 4 limbs

244. *A 6-year-old male Poodle is presented to your clinic with acute onset of caudal paresis.*

Radiographs confirm intervertebral disk protrusion at L1-2. You plan to perform a decompressive hemilaminectomy combined with intervertebral disk fenestration. After making the incision in the skin, subcutaneous tissue and thoracolumbar fascia, you must elevate the epaxial muscles off one side of the vertebra. Starting dorsally, you perform subperiosteal elevation of these muscles. You must continue this dissection until you find what landmark?

    a. dorsal spinous processes
    b. articular processes
    c. transverse spinous processes
    d. ventral spinous processes
    e. accessory process

245. *You wish to perform spinal decompression in a 6-year-old male Poodle with spinal cord compression associated with intervertebral disk disease. Radiographs confirm an intervertebral disk rupture at L1-2. Assuming normal anatomy, what is the most appropriate landmark to use during surgery to identify the first lumbar vertebra (L1)?*

    a. the last rib
    b. dorsal spinous process of L1
    c. L1 is the anticlinal vertebra
    d. T10 and count backward to L1
    e. L1 has a large ventral process off the transverse spinous process

246. *You are performing a hemilaminectomy on a 6-year-old male Poodle with an intervertebral disk rupture that is causing spinal compression at L1-2. You begin your decompression at the L2-3 articular processes and proceed cranially. You find intervertebral disk material under the spinal cord at L1-2 and carefully remove the material. You must determine the most cranial and caudal extent for your decompression. Which of the following is most helpful in making that decision?*

    a. condition of the dura mater
    b. absence of cord swelling
    c. presence of epidural hematoma
    d. absence of intervertebral disk material
    e. presence of epidural fat

247. *Surgical castration of cats requires:*

   a. 1 incision in the prescrotal skin
   b. 2 incisions in the scrotum
   c. 2 incisions in the prescrotal skin
   d. 1 incision in the scrotum
   e. scrotal ablation

248. *Surgical castration of dogs requires:*

   a. 1 incision in the prescrotal skin
   b. 2 incisions in the scrotum
   c. 2 incisions in the prescrotal skin
   d. 1 incision in the scrotum
   e. scrotal ablation

249. *For ovariohysterectomy in a cat, the skin incision is made:*

   a. caudally from the umbilicus
   b. from the umbilicus to the pubis
   c. cranially from the umbilicus
   d. midway between the umbilicus and pubis
   e. midway between the xyphoid and umbilicus

250. *For ovariohysterectomy in a dog, the skin incision is made:*

   a. caudally from the umbilicus
   b. from the umbilicus to the pubis
   c. cranially from the umbilicus
   d. midway between the umbilicus and pubis
   e. midway between the xyphoid and umbilicus

251. *You are performing a perineal urethrostomy in a 7-year-old castrated cat to correct recurrent urinary obstruction. You remember that the bulbourethral glands are a critical landmark for determining the site of the new urethral orifice. What is the anatomic basis for slitting the dorsal wall of the urethra to the location of the bulbourethral glands?*

   a. it is located at the junction of the vascular and avascular urethra
   b. it represents the site of least hemorrhage
   c. it represents the site of control of urinary continence

   d. proximal to this point, the urethra is narrowed
   e. it is located at the junction of the pelvic and penile urethra

252. *In transplantation of the ureter into the urinary bladder, what is the purpose of tunneling through the bladder wall so the ureter passes obliquely through the bladder wall?*

   a. increases surface area for healing of ureter to bladder
   b. minimizes stricture by increasing ureteral lumen diameter
   c. minimizes back flow of urine by acting as a 1-way valve
   d. prevents hydronephrosis by facilitating urine flow
   e. encourages emptying of the ureter due to muscular action of the bladder

253. *Concerning the relationship between skin incisions and skin tension lines in dogs, which statement is most accurate?*

   a. Incisions parallel to tension lines decrease healing time.
   b. Incisions perpendicular to tension lines decrease healing time.
   c. Incisions perpendicular to tension lines decrease the chance of dehiscence.
   d. Incisions parallel to tension lines decrease the chance of dehiscence.
   e. Skin tension lines have no relationship to wound healing or closure.

254. *In closure of the urinary bladder following cystotomy, sutures must **not** penetrate the lumen of the bladder. Why is this so?*

   a. Sutures in the bladder lumen increase the chance of ascending urinary tract infection.
   b. Sutures in the bladder lumen increase the chance of urine leakage into the abdomen.
   c. Sutures in the bladder lumen increase the chance of cystic calculi formation.
   d. Sutures in the bladder lumen impede healing.
   e. Sutures in the bladder lumen increase the chance of bladder dehiscence.

Correct answers are on pages 303-314.

Dogs and Cats, continued

255. *You are presented with a 3-year-old, 30-kg dog with a large (12-cm-long) laceration of the skin on the right side in the midthoracic region. The dog had been missing for 3 days and the owners are not sure what happened. On physical examination you detect a significant amount of debris in the wound. You judge the laceration to be at least 2 days old (if not older). Your goal is to minimize infection, scarring and healing time. Which plan of management would best accomplish your goals?*

a. clean and debride the wound, implant a drain and suture the wound

b. clean, debride and suture the wound

c. leave the wound open to heal by granulation

d. clean and debride the wound and leave open to heal by granulation

e. give oral broad-spectrum antibiotics, and clean, debride and suture the wound

256. *Your associate performed an ovariohysterectomy on a 6-month-old Irish Setter last week. He is out of the office today and the owners are now returning the dog for suture removal. On examination you note serosanguineous drainage from the suture line. On closer inspection you palpate an obvious defect in the abdominal wall, with what you believe is small intestine palpable under the skin. What is the most appropriate course of action?*

a. as long as the skin incision is healed, remove the sutures and send the dog home; this situation should pose no problem

b. leave the skin sutures intact, manipulate the abdominal contents back into the abdominal cavity, place a belly band around the animal, and reexamine the dog in a week

c. leave the skin sutures intact, manipulate the abdominal contents back into the abdominal cavity, place a belly band around the animal, hospitalize the dog for a week of cage rest, and recheck after that time

d. hospitalize the animal for surgery to repair the defect in the abdominal wall

e. leave the sutures in place, send the dog home and recheck in 1 week

257. *In an adult dog, the amount of callus formed in healing of a fractured long bone is:*

a. inversely proportional to the degree of stability of the fracture site

b. directly porportional to the amount of hemorrhage at the time of fracture

c. dependent upon the age of the animal

d. inversely proportional to the amount of soft tissue injury associated with the fracture

e. directly proportional to the amount of soft tissue injury associated with the fracture

258. *Concerning bone healing and callus formation in a fracture repaired with an intramedullary pin versus with a plate and screws, which statement is most accurate?*

a. Callus formation with either stabilization technique is essentially the same.

b. With an intramedullary pin, healing occurs primarily by periosteal bridging callus, while with the plate and screws, healing occurs primarily by medullary bridging callus.

c. With an intramedullary pin, healing occurs by periosteal, intercortical and medullary bridging callus, while with the plate and screws, healing occurs primarily by medullary bridging callus.

d. With an intramedullary pin, healing occurs by periosteal, intercortical and medullary bridging callus, while with the plate and screws, healing occurs primarily by intercortical bridging callus.

e. With an intramedullary pin, healing occurs by intercortical bridging callus, while with the plate and screws, healing occurs primarily by medullary bridging callus.

259. *You are repairing a closed comminuted femoral fracture in a 2-year-old, 20-kg male mongrel. A butterfly fragment, 2 cm long and entirely devoid of blood supply, is present at the midshaft of the femur. What is the most appropriate course of action?*

a. the fragment should be discarded; with no blood supply, the risk of bone sequestration far outweighs the value of including the fragment in the repair

b. the fragment should be discarded; the best approach to management of a comminuted fracture is removal of small fragments and stabilization of the proximal and distal fragments of the femoral shaft

c. the fragment should be placed loosely in the defect during the repair; it will revascularize and contribute to callus formation

d. the fragment should be incorporated into the repair and secured in place; it will function as a cancellous bone graft during healing

e. the fragment should be incorporated into the repair and secured in place; it will function as an autogenous bone graft during healing

260. *In the surgical approach to the left hemithorax for repair of a patent ductus arteriosus, which muscle is **not** encountered?*

a. cutaneous trunci
b. latissimus dorsi
c. serratus dorsalis
d. serratus ventralis
e. scalenus

261. *You are performing resection and anastomosis of a section of cervical esophagus. The preferred method of closure is a:*

a. 2-layer closure, with 1 layer in the mucosa/submucosa and the second layer in the muscularis/adventitia

b. 2-layer closure, with 1 layer in the musosa and the second layer in the submucosa

c. single-layer crushing suture passing full-thickness through the wall of the esophagus

d. single-layer closure, with sutures not entering the esophageal lumen

e. 3-layer closure, with 1 layer in the mucosa, the second in the submucosa, and the third in the muscularis

262. *Surgical correction and prevention of recurrence of salivary mucoceles generally involve excision of the:*

a. cyst and mandibular salivary gland
b. cyst and sublingual salivary gland
c. parotid and mandibular salivary glands
d. mandibular and sublingual salivary glands

e. parotid and sublingual salivary glands

263. *Cushing and Connell suture patterns are used primarily for closure of hollow organs. Which of the following best differentiates between Cushing and Connell sutures?*

a. Cushing sutures are everting, while Connell sutures are inverting

b. Connell sutures enter the lumen, while Cushing sutures do not enter the lumen

c. Cushing sutures are absorbable, while Connell sutures are nonabsorbable

d. Connell sutures are interrupted, while Cushing sutures are continuous

e. Cushing sutures parallel the incision line, while Connell sutures are perpendicular to the incision line

264. *Alteration of the lumen diameter of the pylorus is advocated for surgical correction of pyloric stenosis in dogs. Which technique is **not** appropriate for surgical management of pyloric stenosis?*

a. Heller's myotomy
b. Fredet-Ramstedt myotomy
c. Heineke-Mikulicz procedure
d. Finney procedure
e. Y-V pyloroplasty

265. *You have performed an enterotomy through a longitudinal incision in the jejunum of an 8-kg dog. As you begin to close the enterotomy, you suspect that there may be a significant reduction in lumen diameter. What is the most appropriate course of action?*

a. perform a resection and anastomosis at the site of the enterotomy

b. suture the longitudinal enterotomy transversely

c. suture the enterotomy longitudinally using an everting suture pattern

d. do not worry about the reduction in diameter; the intestine will expand to normal diameter during healing

e. make sure that the enterotomy incision is at a 60-degree angle to the longitudinal axis of the intestine

Correct answers are on pages 303-314.

Dogs and Cats, continued

266. *To minimize the risk of leakage of intestinal contents into the abdomen after single-layer closure of an enterotomy of the small intestine in a dog, you should:*

  a. wrap the involved intestine in omentum
  b. wrap the involved intestine in mesentery
  c. oversew the enterotomy with a second layer of sutures
  d. place a Penrose drain in the abdomen at the site of the enterotomy
  e. oversew the enterotomy with a second layer of sutures and wrap the involved intestine in omentum

267. *Brachycephalic dogs may develop upper airway obstruction due to one or more anatomic abnormalities. Which abnormality **cannot** be corrected surgically?*

  a. elongated soft palate
  b. laryngeal collapse
  c. tracheal hypoplasia
  d. stenotic nares
  e. everting laryngeal saccules

268. *A 9-month-old Golden Retriever has been lame on its right forelimb for approximately 3 weeks. The dog is bearing weight only partially on the right forelimb and shows pain on extension of the right shoulder. What is the most likely cause of this dog's lameness?*

  a. panosteitis
  b. osteochondritis dissecans
  c. ununited anconeal process
  d. fragmented coronoid process
  e. scapulohumoral luxation

269. *Accidental wounds can be classified as open or closed. Which of the following is considered a closed wound?*

  a. contusion
  b. abrasion
  c. laceration
  d. incision
  e. puncture

270. *Assuming identical environmental conditions and identical risks of contamination, which wound is most likely to result in infection?*

  a. contusion
  b. abrasion
  c. laceration
  d. incision
  e. puncture

271. *A 6-year-old, 32-kg male mongrel is presented to your office 6 days after being involved in a fight with another dog. The dog has a 3-cornered laceration on the left lateral thoracic wall with a 4-cm horizontal tear and a 6-cm vertical tear in the skin. You find the skin flap to be necrotic and discover purulent discharge from the wound. Your goal is to manage the infection and minimize scarring. Which of the following would best meet these goals?*

  a. clean and debride the wound, implant a drain, and suture the wound
  b. clean, debride and suture the wound
  c. leave the wound open to heal by granulation
  d. clean and debride the wound, and leave it open to heal by granulation
  e. clean and debride the wound, leave it open until healthy granulation appears, and then suture the wound

272. *Which of the following accurately describes an allograft?*

  a. the recipient and donor sites are on the same animal
  b. the recipient and donor sites are on genetically different animals of the same species
  c. the recipient and donor sites are on animals of different species
  d. the recipient and donor are identical twins
  e. the recipient and donor are F1 hybrids produced by crossing inbred strains

273. In declawing a cat (oncychectomy), the surgeon must be careful to prevent regrowth of the claw. This is done by removing the:

a. entire third phalanx
b. germinal cells in the ungual process
c. germinal cells in the ungual crest
d. digital pad
e. bilateral dorsal ligaments

274. You are planning for correction of patent ductus arteriosus in a 6-month-old mongrel. The most appropriate site for the thoracotomy is the:

a. right 4th intercostal space
b. left 4th intercostal space
c. right 6th intercostal space
d. left 6th intercostal space
e. ventral midline sternum

275. You are planning for correction of a persistent right aortic arch in a 6-month-old mongrel. The most appropriate site for the thoracotomy is the:

a. right 4th intercostal space
b. left 4th intercostal space
c. right 6th intercostal space
d. left 6th intercostal space
e. ventral midline sternum

276. What is the primary objective in surgical management of persistent right aortic arch?

a. establish normal patency of the thoracic esophagus
b. prevent shunting of blood from pulmonary vessels to the aorta
c. prevent shunting of blood from the aorta to pulmonary vessels
d. establish normal patency of the aorta
e. prevent eventual congestive heart failure

277. Sialoliths are relatively rare in dogs. They are usually found in the ducts of the parotid salivary glands. Which of the following most accurately represents appropriate surgical management of unilateral parotid sialolithiasis?

a. excise the involved parotid salivary gland and leave the stone in the duct
b. incise the duct through a ventral cervical incision, remove the stone, and leave the wound open to drain
c. incise the duct through a lateral cervical incision, remove the stone and leave the wound open to drain
d. incise the duct through a lateral cervical incision, remove the stone, and suture the wound
e. incise the duct through an oral incision, remove the stone and leave the wound open to drain

278. A 4-year-old female Irish Setter with a history of regurgitation for 3 days has an irregularly shaped radiopaque foreign body in the caudal thoracic esophagus. You elect to perform a thoracic esophagotomy for removal of the foreign body. The most appropriate location for the thoracic approach is the:

a. right 4th intercostal space
b. right 8th intercostal space
c. left 4th intercostal space
d. left 8th intercostal space
e. ventral midline sternum

279. A 6-year-old male Bassett Hound is presented to your clinic with acute onset of restlessness, salivation, retching without vomition, and abdominal distention. You confirm gastric dilatation/torsion. In management of this patient, which of the following is **least** appropriate?

a. treatment for shock
b. correction of acid-base and electrolyte imbalances
c. gastropexy
d. pyloroplasty
e. gastrotomy

Correct answers are on pages 303-314.

Dogs and Cats, continued

280. *The preferred approach for percutaneous hepatic biopsy is:*

   a. transthoracic, with needle entry at the right 7th intercostal space
   b. transthoracic, with needle entry at the left 7th intercostal space
   c. transabdominal, with needle entry at the left caudal costochrondral junction
   d. transabdominal, with needle entry at the right caudal costochondral junction
   e. transthoracic, with needle entry at the right 12th intercostal space

281. *The appropriate site of trocar insertion for bone marrow aspiration in a 20-kg mongrel is the:*

   a. tuber ischii
   b. tibial crest
   c. sternum
   d. iliac crest
   e. greater tubercle of the humerus

282. *Which of the following is an indication for partial splenectomy, as opposed to total splenectomy?*

   a. splenic tumor confined to one end of the spleen
   b. splenic rupture confined to one end of the spleen
   c. splenic torsion
   d. gastric torsion
   e. generalized splenic trauma

283. *Concerning classification of intervertebral disk disease, which statement is most accurate?*

   a. Chondroid metaplasia occurs in young chondrodystrophoid dogs and may result in extensive mechanical rupture of one or more disks.
   b. Chondroid metaplasia occurs primarily in old chondrodystrophoid dogs and may result in extensive mechanical rupture of one or more disks.

   c. Chondroid metaplasia occurs in nonchondrodystrophoid dogs and results in partial rupture of the annular band.
   d. Massive ruptures of the disk are generally associated with fibroid metaplasia in chondrodystrophoid dogs.
   e. Massive ruptures of the disk are generally associated with fibroid metaplasia in nonchondrodystrophoid dogs.

284. *The surgeon confronted with a patient with cervical intervertebral disk disease must choose between medical management, surgical fenestration, surgical decompression or a combination of these techniques. Which of the following is the most appropriate candidate for fenestration only?*

   a. a 2-year-old chondrodystrophoid dog with radiographic evidence of nuclear mineralization and no clinical signs
   b. a 1-year-old chondrodystrophoid dog with radiographic evidence of nuclear mineralization and protrusion, with intermittent hyperesthesia
   c. a 2-year-old nonchondrodystrophoid dog with radiographic evidence of mineralized disk material in the spinal canal, and hyperesthesia with motor deficits
   d. a 6-year-old nonchondrodystrophoid dog with radiographic evidence of mineralized disk material in the spinal canal, and motor and sensory deficits
   e. a 10-year-old chondrodystrophoid dog with radiographic evidence of mineralized disk material in the spinal canal, and hyperesthesia with motor deficits

285. *A 12-year-old Cocker Spaniel is presented to your clinic with a history of vomiting and anorexia. You confirm bilateral renal calculi with significant impairment of renal function and elect to remove the calculi by nephrotomy. This procedure involves:*

   a. incision of the renal pelvis to expose the calculi in the pelvis
   b. removal of one pole of the kidney to expose the calculi in the pelvis

c. longitudinal incision through the renal parenchyma to expose the calculi in the pelvis

d. surgical removal of the kidney

e. transverse incision through the renal parenchyma to expose the calculi in the pelvis

286. *An 8-year-old male Beagle with stranguria and hematuria has radiopaque calculi in the urinary bladder and in the urethra just caudal to the os penis. What is the most appropriate management of this dog?*

a. urethrotomy to remove urethral calculi, and dietary management to dissolve the cystic calculi

b. urethrostomy at the site of urethral calculi, and cystotomy

c. urethrostomy at the site of the urethral calculi, and dietary management to dissolve the cystic calculi

d. dietary management to dissolve all of the calculi

e. backflush of the urethral calculi into the bladder for removal of all calculi by cystotomy

287. *Forces acting upon a fractured long bone have been classified as rotational, bending, shearing or appositional. Which fixation technique is most likely to neutralize all of these forces?*

a. compression plate

b. single intramedullary pin

c. multiple intramedullary pins

d. lag screw fixation

e. cerclage wire

288. *Forces acting upon a fractured long bone have been classified as rotational, bending, shearing or appositional. Which fixation technique is **least** likely to overcome rotational forces?*

a. compression plate

b. single intramedullary pin

c. multiple intramedullary pins

d. lag screw fixation

e. hemi-cerclage wire

289. *A 1-year-old mongrel is brought to your clinic immediately after being hit by a car. Radiographs confirm a diaphragmatic hernia on the left side, with abdominal contents in the thoracic cavity. The most common surgical approach for repair of this type of hernia is:*

a. thoracotomy through the left 4th intercostal space

b. thoracotomy through the left 8th intercostal space

c. left paracostal approach

d. left paramedian approach

e. ventral abdominal midline approach

290. *Five days previously, you spayed a 6-month-old mongrel through a ventral abdominal midline approach. Today the dog is presented to your clinic with a breakdown of the abdominal closure. The skin suture line is intact, but you palpate an incisional hernia in the abdominal wall. Which statement describes appropriate surgical correction of this incisional hernia?*

a. A skin incision should be made lateral to the original incision, and the edges of the linea alba should be debrided before closure.

b. An elliptic skin incision should be made excising the tissue bordering the original incision line, and the edges of the linea alba should be debrided before closure.

c. The original incision should be opened, and the linea alba stripped of any adhesions but not debrided before closure.

d. The original incision should be opened, the linea alba stripped of any adhesions, and the edges of the skin incision should be debrided before closure.

e. An elliptic incision should be made in the skin encompassing the original skin incision, and a second elliptic incision should be made in the linea alba encompassing the original linea incision before closure.

Correct answers are on pages 303-314.

Dogs and Cats, continued

291. Surgical repair of a perineal hernia may incorporate all of the following structures *except* the:

    a. rectococcygeus muscle
    b. coccygeus muscle
    c. levator ani muscle
    d. external anal sphincter
    e. internal obturator muscle

292. Perineal hernia is most likely to occur in:

    a. an 8-month-old male Boston Terrier
    b. a 2-year-old female Poodle
    c. a 4-year-old male mongrel
    d. a 6-year-old female Cocker Spaniel
    e. a 12-year-old male Collie

293. In surgical correction of patent ductus arteriosus with a left-to-right shunt, the surgeon must be extremely cautious during the dissection necessary to pass ligatures around the ductus. What is the reason for this caution?

    a. The ductus arteriosus is generally dilated, weakened and at risk of tear or rupture.
    b. The aorta is generally dilated, weakened and at risk of tear or rupture.
    c. The pulmonary artery is generally dilated, weakened and at risk of tear or rupture.
    d. The subclavian artery is generally dilated, weakened and at risk of tear or rupture.
    e. The vagus nerve passes deep to the ductus arteriosus and must be avoided.

294. Which of the following most accurately describes the proper technique for retrograde placement of an intramedullary pin for stabilization of an irregular oblique midshaft femoral fracture?

    a. The pin is inserted at the trochanteric fossa and directed distally, crosses the fracture site and is secured in the distal cancellous bone.

    b. The pin is inserted at the site of the fracture and directed distally to protrude from the femur at the stifle. The chuck is reversed and the pin driven proximally, crossing the fracture site and lodging in the proximal cancellous bone.
    c. The leg is held in a normal weight-bearing position and slightly abducted. The pin is inserted at the fracture site and directed proximally to protrude from the femur at the trochanteric fossa. The chuck is reversed and the pin is driven distally, crossing the fracture site to lodge in the distal cancellous bone.
    d. The leg is held in a normal weight-bearing position and slightly adducted. The pin is inserted at the fracture site and directed proximally to protrude from the femur at the trochanteric fossa. The chuck is reversed and the pin is driven distally, crossing the fracture site to lodge in the distal cancellous bone.
    e. The hip is extended maximally and the leg slightly adducted. The pin is inserted at the fracture site and directed proximally to protrude from the femur at the trochanteric fossa. The chuck is reversed and the pin is driven distally, crossing the fracture site to lodge in the distal cancellous bone.

295. Screws should be placed through the center of bone fragments to ensure maximal compression. What is the effect if a screw is placed eccentrically rather than centrally in bone fragments?

    a. fragments are distracted rather than compressed
    b. shearing forces impair fracture reduction
    c. rotational forces impair fracture reduction
    d. bending forces deform the bone
    e. there is no adverse effect

296. A plate used to bridge a diaphyseal defect is referred to as a:

    a. tension-band plate
    b. neutralization plate
    c. double-hooked plate

d. dynamic compression plate

e. buttress plate

297. *A plate that converts distractional forces into compressive forces is considered a:*

a. tension-band plate

b. neutralization plate

c. double-hooked plate

d. dynamic compression plate

e. buttress plate

298. *A 6-year-old mongrel is presented with a nonunion fracture of the midshaft right femur. The original transverse fracture had been treated with a single intramedullary pin 4 months previously. The pin was removed after 10 weeks and the animal has been very lame since then. Radiographs reveal callus formation and a persistent fracture gap. There is no evidence of infection. What is the most appropriate treatment protocol?*

a. compression plating, with or without cancellous bone grafting

b. compression plating, with cortical bone grafting

c. debridement of the ends of the nonunion with rongeurs, cancellous bone grafting and compression plating

d. tension-band plating, with or without cancellous bone grafting

e. intramedullary pin fixation, with cancellous bone grafting

299. *Concerning management of animals with osteomyelitis and nonhealing of a fracture treated with an orthopedic implant, which statement is most accurate?*

a. All orthopedic implants should be removed from the site until the infection is eliminated; at that time the fracture should be rigidly stabilized.

b. If the orthopedic implants are providing rigid stability to the fracture, they should be left intact.

c. Bone plates should be removed, but intramedullary pins should remain in place.

d. Intramedullary pins should be removed, but bone plates should remain in place.

e. All internal fixation devices should be removed and replaced with external fixation devices.

300. *Physeal fractures have been classified by Salter and Harris. A transverse fracture through the region of cartilage hypertrophy is considered a:*

a. Salter-I fracture

b. Salter-II fracture

c. Salter-III fracture

d. Salter-IV fracture

e. Salter-V fracture

301. *A transverse fracture through the region of cartilage hypertrophy and extending into the metaphysis is considered a:*

a. Salter-I fracture

b. Salter-II fracture

c. Salter-III fracture

d. Salter-IV fracture

e. Salter-V fracture

302. *A fracture that crushes the chondroblastic cell layer is considered a:*

a. Salter-I fracture

b. Salter-II fracture

c. Salter-III fracture

d. Salter-IV fracture

e. Salter-V fracture

303. *A 5-month-old German Shepherd sustains a Salter-V fracture of the distal ulnar epiphysis. What is the most likely complication?*

a. nonunion due to limited blood supply to the distal radius

b. nonunion due to rotational forces

c. radius curvis due to premature closure of the ulnar physis

d. radius curvis due to premature closure of the radial physis

e. osteomyelitis due to sequestration

Correct answers are on pages 303-314.

Dogs and Cats, continued

304. After a 5-year-old mongrel is hit by a car, you confirm a fracture of the left humeral diaphysis at the junction of the middle and distal thirds. Which nerve is most likely to be injured when the fracture occurs or during surgical repair?

    a. humeral nerve
    b. lateral cutaneous brachial nerve
    c. musculocutaneous nerve
    d. radial nerve
    e. ulnar nerve

305. A 6-month-old Sheltie is presented to your clinic with a fracture of the lateral condyle of the right humerus. The fracture line extends from the articular surface, through the epiphysis and into the metaphysis. Which treatment offers the greatest chance for return of full function?

    a. closed reduction and a coaptation splint
    b. open reduction and a single intramedullary pin
    c. open reduction and a bone plate
    d. open reduction and cancellous bone screws
    e. open reduction and full-pin splintage

306. A 4-year-old Pointer is presented to your clinic with a comminuted fracture of the left acetabulum. Which approach provides the best exposure for repair of this fracture by plating?

    a. trochanteric osteotomy
    b. gluteal "roll-up" procedure
    c. separation of the vastus lateralis and rectus femoris muscles
    d. ventral approach to the hip
    e. dorsal intergluteal incision

307. The most definitive indication of cranial cruciate ligament rupture in a dog is:

    a. the Ortoloni sign
    b. the cranial drawer sign
    c. the caudal drawer sign
    d. nonweight-bearing lameness
    e. the Balani sign

308. What type of meniscal damage is most likely to occur in conjunction with rupture of the cranial cruciate ligament?

    a. tear of the caudal body of the medial meniscus
    b. tear of the cranial body of the medial meniscus
    c. tear of the caudal body of the lateral meniscus
    d. tear of the cranial body of the lateral meniscus
    e. tear of the intermeniscal ligament

309. A noninflammatory, nonneoplastic, proliferative bone disease with a predilection for endochondral bone is:

    a. hypertrophic osteodystrophy
    b. osteochondritis dissecans
    c. panosteitis
    d. hypertrophic osteoarthropathy
    e. craniomandibular osteopathy

310. A young growing dog is presented to you with a history of shifting-leg lameness of 3 weeks' duration. Physical examination reveals pain on compression of the long bones. The most likely cause of these signs is:

    a. hypertrophic osteodystrophy
    b. osteochondritis dissecans
    c. panosteitis
    d. hypertrophic osteoarthropathy
    e. craniomandibular osteopathy

311. A dog with a fragmented coronoid process is best treated by:

    a. external immobilization with a cast, and cage rest
    b. removal of the process via medial arthrotomy
    c. stabilization with a bone screw
    d. removal of the process via lateral arthrotomy
    e. dietary supplementation with calcium, and limited exercise

312. You review a radiograph of a dog's fractured femur. Multiple fracture lines converge on one point. This fracture is appropriately classified as:

a. oblique
b. spiral
c. segmental
d. comminuted
e. bicondylar

313. *You review the radiograph of a dog's fractured tibia. The cortex on one side of the bone is broken and the other is bent. This fracture is appropriately classified as a:*

a. fissure fracture
b. greenstick fracture
c. physeal fracture
d. comminuted fracture
e. impacted fracture

314. *Which fracture is best treated with a tension-band wire?*

a. avulsion fracture of the olecranon
b. compression fracture of the distal femoral physis
c. spiral fracture of the humeral diaphysis
d. segmental fracture of the femoral diaphysis
e. greenstick fracture of the distal ulnar metaphysis

315. *Concerning the difference between osteochondrosis and osteochondritis dissecans, which statement is most accurate?*

a. Osteochondrosis is an abnormality of endochondral ossification, with asymmetric maturation into bone. Osteochondritis dissecans is a sequel to osteochondrosis in which a cartilaginous flap pulls loose from underlying bone.
b. Osteochondrosis is an abnormality of nutrition to the articular cartilage. Osteochondritis dissecans occurs when the articular cartilage becomes inflamed and separates from the underlying bone.
c. Osteochondrosis is a developmental defect of bone. Osteochondritis dissecans refers specifically to osteochondrosis of the humeral head.
d. Osteochondrosis does not result in a cleft that separates cartilage from bone, while osteochondritis dissecans does.

e. Osteochondrosis must be treated surgically, while osteochondritis dissecans can be treated with antiinflammatories and cage rest.

316. *Most coxofemoral luxations in dogs are the result of vehicular trauma. Which type of coxofemoral luxation is most common in dogs?*

a. lateral
b. caudoventral
c. craniodorsal
d. caudodorsal
e. ventral

317. *While performing small intestinal resection and anastomosis in a cat, you discover that the proximal segment of bowel has a diameter of approximately 20% greater than that of the distal segment of bowel. The easiest way to solve this problem is to:*

a. perform an end-to-side anastomosis
b. perform a side-to-side anastomosis
c. cut the distal segment of the intestine at an oblique angle
d. cut the proximal segment of the intestine at an oblique angle
e. perform a Bilroth-2 anastomosis

318. *An 8-month-old St. Bernard puppy is rushed to your clinic as an emergency at 11 PM. The owners saw the dog swallow a marble 1.5 cm in diameter. What is the most appropriate course of action?*

a. make radiographs to confirm the presence of the foreign body, then administer general anesthesia and remove the foreign body with a gastroscope
b. make radiographs to confirm the presence of the foreign body, then administer general anesthesia and remove the foreign body by gastrotomy or enterotomy
c. administer apomorphine to induce vomiting
d. hospitalize the dog for observation
e. send the dog home and instruct the owners to watch for vomiting or lack of appetite

Correct answers are on pages 303-314.

Dogs and Cats, continued

319. *During intestinal resection, the mucosa frequently everts from the cut surfaces of the intestinal wall. What is the most appropriate way to manage such mucosal eversion in a small-breed dog?*

a. suture the intestine with an inverting pattern
b. trim the everted mucosa with a scissors before suturing
c. suture the mucosal layer first, then oversew the serosal layer
d. repeat the resection to remove bowel segment with the everted mucosa
e. suture the intestine with a modified Bunnell-Meyer pattern

Question 320

A 4-year-old mongrel develops acute onset of neurologic signs. Physical examination reveals abnormalities only in the nervous system. Neurologic examination reveals the following:

Mental Status: alert, with no abnormalities noted
Cranial Nerves: no abnormalities noted
Posture and Gait: paraplegia
Postural Reactions:

	Left Front	Left Rear	Right Front	Right Front
Wheelbarrowing	0	0	0	0
Ext Post Thrust	0	0	0	0
Hemiwalk	0	0	0	0
Consc Proprio	0	0	0	0
Hopping	0	0	0	0

Spinal Reflexes:

	Left Front	Left Rear	Right Front	Right Rear
Biceps	1	–	–	1
Triceps	1	–	–	1
Patellar	–	1	1	–
Cranial Tibial	–	1	1	–
Gastrocnemius	–	1	1	–
Flexor	1	1	1	1
Anal Sphincter	–	1	1	–
Panniculus	absent caudal to thoracolumbar area			

Sensation: superficial pain absent in all 4 limbs, deep pain present in all 4 limbs

320. *Which neurologic pathway is most likely affected?*

a. upper motor neuron to all 4 limbs
b. upper motor neuron to the rear limbs, lower motor neuron to the front limbs

c. lower motor neuron to all 4 limbs
d. lower motor neuron to the rear limbs, upper motor neuron to the front limbs
e. upper motor neuron to the front limbs

Questions 321 and 322

A 2-year-old female Poodle suddenly refuses to stand or walk. Physical examination reveals abnormalities only in the nervous system. Neurologic examination reveals the following:

Mental Status: alert, with no abnormalities noted
Cranial Nerves: no abnormalities noted
Posture and Gait: paraplegia
Postural Reactions:

	Left Front	Left Rear	Right Front	Right Front
Wheelbarrowing	0	0	0	0
Ext Post Thrust	0	0	0	0
Hemiwalk	0	0	0	0
Consc Proprio	0	0	0	0
Hopping	0	0	0	0

Spinal Reflexes:

	Left Front	Left Rear	Right Front	Right Rear
Biceps	3	–	–	3
Triceps	3	–	–	3
Patellar	–	3	3	–
Cranial Tibial	–	3	3	–
Gastrocnemius	–	3	3	–
Flexor	3	3	3	3
Anal Sphincter	–	3	3	–
Panniculus	absent caudal to thoracolumbar area			

Sensation: hyperesthesia over thoracolumbar area, superficial pain absent caudal to thoracolumbar area, deep pain present in all 4 limbs

321. *Which neurologic pathway is most likely affected?*

a. upper motor neuron to all 4 limbs
b. upper motor neuron to the rear limbs, lower motor neuron to the front limbs
c. lower motor neuron to all 4 limbs
d. lower motor neuron to the rear limbs, upper motor neuron to the front limbs
e. lower motor neuron to the front limbs

322. *What is the most likely location of the lesion causing neurologic signs in this dog?*

a. brainstem
b. C1-C4 segment of the spinal cord

c. C5-T2 segment of the spinal cord

d. T2-L3 segment of the spinal cord

e. L3-S2 segment of the spinal cord

323. *Which anatomic landmarks best help determine vertebral location during ventral decompressive surgery in a Dachshund with a ruptured intervertebral disk at the C3-4 spinal cord segment?*

a. wings of the atlas and ventral tubercle

b. wings of the atlas and ventral protuberance of the transverse spinous process of C7

c. wings of the atlas and ventral protuberance of the transverse spinous process of C6

d. ventral tubercle of C6 and wings of C1

e. intervertebral disk space of C1-C2 and ventral protuberance of the transverse spinous process of C7

324. *Which of the following is **not** appropriate for hemostasis in castration of a cat?*

a. tying the vas deferens to the venous plexus on each side

b. tying the venous plexus on itself

c. ligating the venous plexus with absorbable suture

d. pulling the vas deferens and venous plexus until they stretch and break

e. applying hemostatic clips to the venous plexus

325. *Concerning ovariohysterectomy in dogs, which statement is most accurate?*

a. The left ovary is located farther cranially in the abdominal cavity than the right ovary, increasing the difficulty in exteriorizing the left ovary.

b. The right ovary is located farther cranially in the abdominal cavity than the left ovary, increasing the difficulty in exteriorizing the right ovary.

c. The ovaries are freely movable, but the cervix is difficult to exteriorize.

d. The ovarian arteries are small and rarely require ligation.

e. The uterine arteries are small and rarely require ligation.

326. *To maximize the chances of future fertility in an adult dog, the incision for cesarean section should be made:*

a. in the dorsal wall of the uterine body

b. in the ventral wall of the uterine body

c. in the ventral wall of the uterine horn containing more pups

d. in the dorsal wall of the uterine horn containing more pups

e. transversely in the ventral wall of the uterine body, extending from one horn to the other

327. *Concerning perineal urethrostomy, which statement is most accurate?*

a. A stent should be placed in the new urethral orifice to minimize the risk of stricture formation.

b. A stent is generally contraindicated because of the increased risk of ascending infection and interference with healing.

c. An indwelling urethral catheter is indicated until primary healing occurs.

d. The urethra should be flushed daily for the first 3 days to prevent clot formation that could cause urinary obstruction.

e. Topical corticosteroids should be applied to the suture line to minimize the risk of stricture.

328. *While performing an ovariohysterectomy, your associate releases the stump of the right ovarian pedicle before it is ligated. He reaches into the abdomen with a hemostat and is about to clamp all the tissue in the vicinity of the bleeder. You stop him from doing this because of the risk of damage to the:*

a. right ureter

b. caudal pole of the right kidney

c. caudal vena cava

d. pancreas

e. right ovary

Correct answers are on pages 303-314.

Dogs and Cats, continued

329. *You have previously diagnosed a left-sided perineal hernia in an 11-year-old mongrel. For financial reasons, the owners have delayed surgical repair. The dog is now presented to your clinic with a 24-hour history of anuria and distention in the left perineal area. You suspect that the urinary bladder has herniated into the perineal defect. Which technique will allow you to manually return the bladder to its normal anatomic position while preparing the animal for primary correction of the hernia?*

  a. urethral catheterization to remove urine
  b. administration of a diuretic to facilitate urine production
  c. perineal incision over the bladder
  d. caudoventral compression of the abdomen
  e. cystocentesis to remove urine

330. *Which of the following is **not** an appropriate site for urethrostomy in dogs?*

  a. preputial
  b. prescrotal
  c. scrotal
  d. perineal
  e. prepubic

331. *Dogs with portal vascular anomalies have a high incidence of which type of cystic calculi?*

  a. cystine
  b. struvite
  c. ammonium urate
  d. calcium oxalate
  e. silica

332. *The Zepp procedure and modifications of the Zepp procedure have been used in management of chronic otitis externa refractory to medical therapy. Which of the following best describes the Zepp procedure?*

  a. resection of the pinna to improve ventilation
  b. resection of the lateral cartilaginous wall of the vertical ear canal, with formation of a ventral cartilaginous flap

  c. ablation of the external ear canal
  d. resection of the ventral cartilaginous wall of the horizontal ear canal
  e. resection of the cartilaginous wall of the vertical and horizontal ear canals, with formation of cartilaginous flaps

333. *Drainage of the middle ear in animals with chronic or recurrent middle ear infections is best achieved via:*

  a. myringotomy
  b. pharyngeal bulla osteotomy
  c. penetration of the tympanic membrane and ventral floor of the bulla with a Steinmann pin
  d. Zepp procedure
  e. ventral bulla osteotomy

334. *Surgical correction of a patent ductus arteriosus requires:*

  a. resection of the ductus arteriosus
  b. ligation of the ductus arteriosus
  c. transection of the ductus arteriosus
  d. anastomosis of the ductus arteriosus
  e. transposition of the ductus arteriosus

335. *Surgical correction of a persistent right aortic arch requires:*

  a. resection of the ligamentum arteriosus
  b. ligation of the ligamentum arteriosus
  c. transection of the ligamentum arteriosus
  d. anastomosis of the ligamentum arteriosus
  e. transposition of the ligamentum arteriosus

336. *Concerning traumatic diaphragmatic hernias in dogs, which statement is most accurate?*

  a. The muscular portion of the diaphragm is more frequently torn than the central tendon.
  b. The prevalence of left-sided hernias is significantly greater than the prevalence of right-sided hernias.

c. The spleen is the abdominal organ that most commonly herniates into the thorax.

d. Traumatic diaphragmatic hernias represent an emergency situation requiring immediate surgical correction.

e. Surgical correction of traumatic diaphragmatic hernias is not indicated unless signs of respiratory distress are evident.

337. *In routine ovariohysterectomy of dogs, exteriorizing the ovaries is facilitated by:*

a. transection of the ovarian pedicle

b. stretching or breaking the suspensory ligament

c. extending the skin incision caudally

d. incision of the broad ligament

e. retraction of the colon on the left side and the duodenum on the right side

338. *A perineal hernia is most likely to occur in a:*

a. 4-year-old intact female Beagle

b. 10-year-old spayed Collie

c. 12-year-old intact male Boxer

d. 4-year-old castrated Sheltie

e. 16-year-old intact female Boston Terrier

339. *What type of suture material is polydioxanone?*

a. synthetic nonabsorbable

b. synthetic absorbable

c. natural nonabsorbable

d. natural absorbable

e. monofilament nonabsorbable

340. *What type of suture material is polypropylene?*

a. synthetic nonabsorbable

b. synthetic absorbable

c. natural nonabsorbable

d. natural absorbable

e. monofilament absorbable

341. *What type of suture material is chromic catgut?*

a. synthetic nonabsorbable

b. synthetic absorbable

c. natural nonabsorbable

d. natural absorbable

e. monofilament nonabsorbable

342. *Which suture material produces the **least** tissue reaction?*

a. chromic catgut

b. plain catgut

c. polyglycolic acid

d. polyester fiber

e. stainless steel

343. *Which suture material produces the most tissue reaction?*

a. chromic catgut

b. plain catgut

c. polyglycolic acid

d. polyester fiber

e. stainless steel

344. *Which suture pattern is considered everting?*

a. Cushing

b. simple continuous

c. vertical mattress

c. cross mattress

e. Ford interlocking

345. *Which suture pattern is considered inverting?*

a. Cushing

b. simple continuous

c. vertical mattress

d. cross mattress

e. Ford interlocking

Correct answers are on pages 303-314.

Dogs and Cats, continued

346. In a 1-year-old, 12-kg mongrel, which condition is most appropriately treated with a Schroeder-Thomas splint?

a. irregular oblique midshaft fracture of the humerus
b. fracture of the distal femoral epiphysis
c. craniodorsal coxofemoral luxation
d. comminuted mid-diaphyseal tibial fracture
e. avulsion fracture of the olecranon

347. A 3-year old female Golden Retriever is brought to your clinic with a severely comminuted, highly unstable fracture of the left radius. Which of the following would provide the best temporary immobilization while you prepare for surgical repair?

a. Schroeder-Thomas splint
b. fiberglass cast
c. Valpeau bandage
d. Ehmer sling
e. Robert Jones bandage

348. The Heineke-Mikulicz procedure has been recommended for surgical management of pyloric stenosis. Which of the following best describes this procedure?

a. longitudinal incision through all layers of the pylorus, except the mucosa
b. longitudinal incision through all layers of the pylorus, sutured transversely
c. Y-shaped incision in the pylorus, sutured as a V
d. gastroduodenostomy
e. longitudinal incision through all layers of the pylorus, with the mucosa sutured longitudinally

349. The goal of surgical correction of an elongated soft palate is to have the caudal border of the soft palate located:

a. 1 cm caudal to the tip of the epiglottis
b. at the tip of the epiglottis
c. 1 cm rostral to the tip of the epiglottis
d. at the level of the lateral saccules

e. at the level of the fourth upper premolar

350. A 12-month-old German Short-Haired Pointer is presented to your clinic with left forelimb lameness of 6 months' duration. You suspect osteochondritis dissecans, and radiographs reveal a defect in the caudal aspect of the left humeral head. What is the most appropriate treatment for this dog?

a. cage rest for 2 months
b. administration of corticosteroids as needed
c. surgical exploration of the joint and curettage of the lesion, with removal of any joint mice
d. surgical exploration of the joint, with removal of any joint mice
e. intraarticular injection of corticosteroids, combined with cage rest

351. In a 10-month-old German Shepherd with acute onset of right forelimb lameness, radiographs reveal panosteitis. What is the most appropriate treatment for this dog?

a. daily administration of antiinflammatory dosages of corticosteroids for 2 months
b. excision of the anconeal process
c. culture of bone marrow aspirates, with administration of appropriate antibiotics
d. reevaluation after 2 months of cage rest
e. administration of aspirin as needed

352. In routine elective surgery of small animals, which of the following does **not** increase the likelihood of wound infection?

a. prolonged operative time
b. administration of corticosteroids
c. crushing muscle tissue with hemostats
d. rough handling of tissues
e. good hemostasis

Questions 353 and 354

A dog sustained a laceration of the right metatarsal area 15 minutes previously. The owner presents the dog and has the leg wrapped in a tee shirt that is now soaked with blood. On removing the shirt, you find bright *red blood spurting from the wound under pressure.*

353. *In regard to source and time of occurrence, how is this dog's hemorrhage classified?*

   a. arterial, primary
   b. venous, primary
   c. capillary, primary
   d. arterial, intermediate
   e. venous, intermediate

354. *You plan to repair the laceration. Before closing the wound, you must stop the hemorrhage. What is the most appropriate way to stop the hemorrhage from this wound, without likelihood of recurrence?*

   a. crushing the vessels with hemostats
   b. ligating any bleeders
   c. applying a tourniquet
   d. applying astringents
   e. applying gentle manual or digital pressure

Questions 355 and 356

A cat is admitted for elective surgery. After making the skin incision, you note that blood oozes from the subcutaneous tissue under very low pressure.

355. *In regard to source and time of occurrence, how is this cat's hemorrhage classified?*

   a. arterial, primary
   b. venous, primary
   c. capillary, primary
   d. venous, intermediate
   e. capillary, intermediate

356. *Before proceeding with the surgery, you decide to stop the bleeding. What is the most appropriate way to stop the hemorrhage at the surgical site, without likelihood of recurrence?*

   a. crushing the vessels with hemostats
   b. ligating any bleeders
   c. applying an ice pack

   d. applying astringents
   e. applying gentle manual or digital pressure

357. *Placing subcutaneous sutures during closure of a routine skin incision is most likely to:*

   a. improve hemostasis
   b. decrease skin apposition
   c. decrease dead space
   d. improve strength of the healed wound
   e. decrease contamination of the wound

358. *A dog sustains a skin laceration but is not presented for treatment until 24 hours later. The 4-inch wound exposes subcutaneous tissue only. How is this wound classified?*

   a. clean
   b. clean-contaminated
   c. contaminated
   d. dirty
   e. necrotic

359. *Concerning function of electrosurgical units, which statement is most accurate?*

   a. No current passes through the patient's body.
   b. Current is concentrated at the active electrode.
   c. Current is concentrated at the passive electrode.
   d. Heat is produced in the transformer.
   e. Heat is concentrated at the passive electrode.

360. *Why is a surgical drape considered contaminated if it becomes wet during a surgical procedure?*

   a. fluid diminishes the antibacterial action of the drape
   b. the fluid may contain disinfectants
   c. fluid on the skin rinses away the disinfectant solutions
   d. capillary action can draw bacteria through the material of the drape
   e. the space between threads of the drape increases with wetting

---

Correct answers are on pages 303-314.

Dogs and Cats, continued

361. During a routine celiotomy, you discover a fatty structure adhered to the peritoneal surface of the linea alba, just cranial to the umbilicus. What is this structure?

   a. ligamentum arteriosus
   b. falciform ligament
   c. greater omentum
   d. lesser omentum
   e. gastrohepatic ligament

362. In nephrectomy, the ipsilateral ureter should be ligated and transected:

   a. as close to the bladder as possible
   b. as close to the renal pelvis as possible
   c. at the midpoint of the ureter
   d. 4 cm distal to the renal pelvis
   e. 4 cm proximal to the ureterovesicular junction

363. Cryosurgery has been advocated as treatment for perianal fistulas, superficial tumors and other lesions in small animals. The most common cryogenic agent used in veterinary medicine is:

   a. nitrous oxide
   b. freon
   c. liquid nitrogen
   d. liquid helium
   e. carbon dioxide

364. During cryosurgery, the frozen tissue is termed an "ice ball." Not all tissue within the ice ball dies. Which tissue in the ice ball becomes necrotic after cryosurgery?

   a. the most superficial two-thirds of the tissue
   b. tissue that reaches -20 C or colder
   c. tissue in direct contact with the cryogen
   d. the most poorly perfused tissue
   e. the inner one-third of the ice ball

365. Laser surgery has predictable effects on soft tissue. In relation to the tip of the laser instrument, which area of tissue shows reversible changes?

   a. zone of vaporization
   b. zone of carbonization
   c. zone of coagulation
   d. zone of edema
   e. zone of necrosis

366. When using laser surgical instruments, the surgeon must carefully avoid "collateral" thermal injury. Collateral thermal injury is best avoided by:

   a. using a carbon dioxide laser
   b. setting the laser at "high" power (60-100 watts)
   c. holding the instrument perpendicular to the tissue
   d. setting the laser at "low" power (20-40 watts)
   e. quickly making the incision

367. In the surgical approach to the **right** kidney, what structure can be used to help retract the abdominal contents and facilitate visualization of the kidney?

   a. spleen
   b. omentum
   c. descending colon
   d. descending duodenum
   e. broad ligament

368. In the surgical approach to the **left** kidney, what structure can be used to help retract the abdominal contents and facilitate visualization of the kidney?

   a. spleen
   b. omentum
   c. descending colon
   d. descending duodenum
   e. broad ligament

369. Different tissues have differing reactions to cryosurgery. The factor that most influences a tissue's reaction to application of cold is:

a. proximity to major blood vessels
b. amount of intracellular and extracellular water
c. metabolic rate
d. degree of perfusion
e. surface area subjected to application of cold

370. Which procedure is most effective in management of a descemetocele?

a. conjunctival flap
b. third eyelid flap
c. superficial keratectomy
d. transposition of the parotid duct
e. corneal eburnation

371. An untreated skin wound heals by a process of granulation, contraction and reepithelialization. This type of healing is best termed:

a. first-intention healing
b. second-intention healing
c. third-intention healing
d. fourth-intention healing
e. delayed primary closure

372. In treatment of keratoconjunctivitis sicca, which surgical technique maintains corneal hydration?

a. transplantation of the mandibular duct
b. transplantation of the zygomatic duct
c. transplantation of the parotid duct
d. conjunctival flap
e. superficial keratectomy

373. In routine application of a bone plate for fixation of a long-bone fracture, how many screws should anchor the plate proximal and distal to the fracture line?

a. at least 1 screw proximally and 2 distally
b. at least 2 screws proximally and 1 distally
c. at least 3 screws proximally and 3 distally
d. at least 4 screws proximally and 2 distally
e. at least 5 screws proximally and 5 distally

374. A cat is presented to you with a laceration several days old. You elect to debride the wound, let it granulate for several days and only suture the wound closed when all evidence of infection is gone. This type of wound healing is referred to as:

a. first-intention healing
b. second-intention healing
c. third-intention healing
d. fourth-intention healing
e. primary closure

375. In performing a paramedian abdominal approach in a dog, you enter the abdomen through an incision 1 cm to the right of the linea alba. In this approach, the fibers of what muscle must be separated?

a. external abdominal oblique
b. internal abdominal oblique
c. scalenus
d. rectus intermedius
e. rectus abdominis

376. A cat is presented to your clinic with upper motor neuron signs to the rear limbs and lower motor neuron signs to the front limbs. What do these signs indicate?

a. generalized neurologic disease
b. a lesion at C5-T2
c. a lesion at T2-L3
d. lesions at C1-5 and L4-S3
e. lesions at C5-T2 and L4-S3

377. A dog is presented to your clinic with lower motor neuron signs to the rear limbs and upper motor neuron signs to the front limbs. What do these signs indicate?

a. generalized neurologic disease
b. a lesion at C5-T2
c. a lesion at T2-L3
d. lesions at C1-5 and L4-S3
e. lesions at C5-T2 and L4-S3

Correct answers are on pages 303-314.

Dogs and Cats, continued

378. *Which suture pattern is **not** considered appositional?*

   a. simple interrupted
   b. cross mattress
   c. Ford interlocking
   d. simple continuous
   e. Connell

379. *A 5-year-old Pointer is brought to your clinic with a craniodorsal luxation of the left coxofemoral joint. You attempt closed reduction. Which of the following should be applied after closed reduction of a coxofemoral luxation?*

   a. Schroeder-Thomas splint
   b. fiberglass cast
   c. Valpeau bandage
   d. Ehmer sling
   e. Robert Jones bandage

380. *A 7-year-old mongrel is brought to your clinic with a fracture of the left scapula. The fracture parallels the spine of the scapula. Which of the following should be applied in **initial** management of this fracture?*

   a. Schroeder-Thomas splint
   b. fiberglass cast
   c. Valpeau bandage
   d. Ehmer sling
   e. Robert Jones bandage

381. *Which suture pattern is most appropriate for closure of the uterine stump after ovariohysterectomy for pyometra?*

   a. Cushing
   b. Bunnell
   c. Parker-Kerr
   d. simple interrupted
   e. vertical mattress

382. *Which technique does **not** help stabilize the stifle joint after rupture of the cranial cruciate ligament?*

   a. Paatsama technique
   b. over-the-top technique
   c. cranial transposition of the fibular head
   d. tibial crest transplantation
   e. imbrication of the lateral joint capsule

383. *Cushing and Lembert suture patterns are used primarily for closure of hollow organs. Which of the following most accurately describes the difference between Cushing and Lembert sutures?*

   a. Cushing sutures are everting, while Lembert sutures are inverting.
   b. Cushing sutures enter the lumen, while Lembert sutures do not enter the lumen.
   c. Cushing sutures are absorbable, while Lembert sutures are nonabsorbable.
   d. Lembert sutures are interrupted, while Cushing sutures are continuous.
   e. Cushing sutures parallel the incision line, while Lembert sutures are perpendicular to the incision line.

384. *Neurologic signs associated with rupture of intervertebral disks between T2 and T10 are very rare in dogs. Why is this so?*

   a. the dorsal longitudinal ligament prevents dorsal rupture
   b. the disks from segment T2 to T10 do not degenerate
   c. the intercapital ligaments prevent dorsal rupture
   d. there are no disks from segment T2 to T10
   e. the ventral longitudinal ligament prevents dorsal rupture

385. *A 2-year-old mongrel is presented to your clinic with a luxation between the 3rd sacral vertebra and 1st coccygeal vertebra. The dog has no voluntary motion of the tail and no deep pain sensation in the tail, but exhibits extreme pain on manual elevation of the tail. Urinary and bowel function remains normal. What is the most appropriate treatment for this animal?*

   a. amputation of the tail at the site of the luxation

b. amputation of the tail at the junction of the 3rd and 4th coccygeal vertebrae

c. open reduction of the luxation and stabilization with a plate

d. open reduction of the luxation and stabilization with pins and wires

e. conservative therapy consisting of corticosteroids and cage rest

386. *For repair of a mid-diaphyseal femoral fracture, the fascia lata is incised and the femur is exposed by retraction of the:*

a. rectus femoris and biceps femoris

b. vastus lateralis and biceps femoris

c. rectus femoris and vastus lateralis

d. vastus intermedius and rectus femoris

e. vastus intermedius and biceps femoris

387. *For removal of a gastric foreign body, the stomach should be incised in an avascular area:*

a. midway between the greater and lesser curvatures of the stomach

b. of the lesser curvature of the stomach

c. of the greater curvature of the stomach

d. of the pylorus

e. of the cardia

388. *In routine surgery of the urinary bladder and stomach, use of "stay" or retention sutures is recommended. Which of the following most accurately describes a "stay" suture?*

a. suture placed to prevent other sutures from slipping

b. suture placed to allow atraumatic manipulation of tissue

c. nonabsorbable suture that is not removed from the tissue

d. suture that is not removed from the tissue, but that is eventually absorbed

e. suture placed to oversew the primary suture line

Answers

1. **c** The Cushing pattern is continuous and inverting, and does not expose suture material to the lumen. The Connell pattern exposes suture material to the lumen. The Halsted pattern is not a continuous pattern.

2. **b** Chlorhexidine's activity is maintained in the presence of blood.

3. **a** Povidone-iodine has sporicidal action in addition to its Gram-positive and Gram-negative antibacterial activity.

4. **d** Isopropyl alcohol kills bacteria by coagulation of proteins.

5. **e** Sodium hypochlorite (Clorox) is more commonly used to disinfect environmental surfaces.

6. **c** Alcohol eliminates the cumulative antibacterial action of hexachlorophene.

7. **b** Hypertrophic osteopathy is characterized by multiple-limb lameness and pain on palpation of distal limbs. It usually occurs in older animals secondary to a space-occupying mass in the thoracic or abdominal cavity.

8. **d** Radiographs of the elbow would be sufficient to display the likely lesions. Resolution of bone scintigraphy is not sufficient to differentiate these diseases. Fluid from elbow arthrocentesis might be normal or indicate only mild degenerative change.

9. **b** Removal of the anconeal process through a lateral arthrotomy results in quick resolution of clinical signs.

10. **a** Osteochondrosis has not been reported in the temporomandibular joint of dogs.

11. **e** Osteochondrosis is most commonly found on the medial aspect of the lateral condyle of the femur and on the medial trochlear ridge of the talus.

12. **d** Coxa valga leads to lateral patellar luxation, while coxa vara predisposes to medial patellar luxation.

13. **d** Grade-IV patellar luxation is characterized by a patella that remains luxated and cannot be manually reduced.

14. **e** Patellectomy generally results in severe stifle degenerative changes and should only be used for severe patellar fractures that cannot be repaired.

15. **a** Sound principles of joint arthrodesis include primary closure of the joint to maintain aseptic conditions postoperatively.

16. **c** Cranial cruciate ligament ruptures are rare in dogs less than 1 year of age. Ligaments are generally stronger than the bone in young dogs, so injuries in young dogs are more commonly physeal fractures.

17. **b** Fractures of the pubis are not commonly repaired in dogs unless they result in a caudal abdominal hernia.

18. **a**

19. **d**

20. **e**

21. **b**

22. **c**

23. **b** Vitamin C is not useful for treatment of hip dysplasia, either in growing or adult animals.

24. **d** The thumb is not displaced when the hip is luxated craniodorsally and the limb is externally rotated.

25. **b** Avascular necrosis commonly occurs in young (8-12 months old) toy-breed dogs.

26. **b** A Salter-II physeal fracture is one in which the distal fragment includes all of the epiphysis and a portion of the metaphysis.

27. **c** Bending over the twist results in loss of tension in the wire (loosens the wire).

28. **e** The remnants of the ligamentum teres are generally inadequate to hold sutures or provide support.

29. **a** The long digital extensor muscle traverses the lateral aspect of the tibia.

30. **e**

31. **d** This dog shows lower motor neuron front limb signs and upper motor neuron rear limb signs.

32. **b** An intradural spinal neoplasm would be an unlikely cause for these signs due to the acute onset noted.

33. **e** Ultrasonography cannot be used to adequately evaluate spinal structures due to the bony structures surrounding them.

34. **c** Ventral slot decompression would allow removal of disk material from the spinal canal at C6-7.

35. **d** The intervertebral disk at T4-5 is unlikely to rupture because of the added stability provided by the intercapital ligaments in that region.

36. **a** A single intramedullary pin would not provide any rotational stability in a midshaft transverse fracture.

37. **d** Joint immobilization leads to joint contracture, muscle atrophy, and other aspects of "fracture disease."

38. **b** Polypropylene is a nonabsorbable, very inert suture material.

39. **e** Polyglyconate is the strongest absorbable material at implantation but degrades faster than polydiaxanone.

40. **d** Nylon is considered nonabsorbable but does slowly degrade, releasing antibacterial degradation products.

41. **c** Stainless steel is the strongest available suture material.

42. **a** Degeneration of polyglycolic acid is accelerated on exposure to urine.

43. **e** Nonsurgical treatment of cranial cruciate ruptures in large dogs generally results in severe, progressive degenerative joint disease.

44. **a** Circumcostal gastropexy provides the strongest adhesion of stomach to body wall and decreases recurrence.

45. **c** Increasing the number of drain lumina (*eg*, from single-lumen tube drains to triple-lumen sump drain for example) increases the drainage of fluid.

46. **a** Dogs that are DEA 1 negative (40% of the population) can serve as universal donors.

47. **e** Immediate rigid fixation is not necessary for proper treatment of open fractures. If the wound is adequately cleaned, debrided, lavaged and bandaged, definitive fracture repair may be postponed.

48. **d** The Type-III configuration of external fixation devices provides rigid stability for most applications.

49. **b** The rectus femoris originates on the ilium just cranial to the acetabulum. The semitindinosus is not a member of the quadriceps group. The 3 vastus muscles originate on the proximal femur.

50. **b** Olecranon osteotomy provides excellent visualization of the distal articular surface of the humerus, and allows for more secure fixation in a mature dog than triceps tenotomy.

51. **c** The cell count, differential count and mucin clot strongly implicate septic arthritis as a cause.

52. **d** Hypertrophic osteodystrophy is characterized by hot, swollen metaphyses, multiple-limb lameness, and a "double physeal line" on radiographs.

53. **d**

54. **b**

55. **a**

56. **c** Isografts are grafts between identical twins or cloned individuals.

57. **b** Osteoconduction is the process by which the former bone graft acts as a scaffold for the construction of new bone.

58. **a** Hind limb amputation by coxofemoral disarticulation is cosmetically undesirable, as it leaves little muscle coverage for pelvic prominences after muscle atrophy, and results in exposure of the genitals in male dogs.

59. **e** Examples include cefmetazole and cefoxitin.

60. **e**

61. **b**

62. **b**

63. **b**

64. **a**

65. **a** Diaphragmatic hernia rarely needs to be surgically corrected on an emergency basis. Initial treatment of these patients should include fluid and electrolyte support and supplemental oxygen as needed. Many affected cats have underlying lung lesions, such as hemothorax or pulmonary contusions. Fluids should be infused very cautiously to these patients, as they are predisposed to pulmonary edema. It is ideal to wait at least 49-72 hours before performing surgery. Occasionally, life-threatening situations, such as those posed by strangulated bowel, encroachment of the lungs by abdominal viscera, stomach dilatation, or failure of the cat to respond to initial therapy, dictate the need for earlier surgical intervention (herniorrhaphy). The prognosis in these cases is generally worse.

66. **b**

67. **a**

68. **c**

69. **e**

70. **d**

71. **d**

72. **b**

73. **e** Ultrashort-acting barbiturates, such as thiamylal sodium, require biotransformation by the liver for elimination. Methoxyflurane, halothane and ether require a greater amount of hepatic biotransformation than isoflurane and, therefore, are not as ideal for use in a patient with liver disease.

74. **d**

75. **b**

76. **b**

77. **c**

78. **d**

79. **c**

80. **b**

81. **d**

82. **b**

83. **a**

84. **c** When an animal spontaneously begins to regurgitate, an acquired esophageal disorder should be suspected. If the animal has no history of regurgitation before an anesthetic or surgical episode but shows these signs after such an experience, reflux esophagitis must be a primary differential diagnosis. Reflux of gastric contents into the esophagus during anesthesia can result in prolonged contact of gastric contents (acid, bile, pancreatic juices) with the esophageal mucosa. This can cause extensive mucosal damage and, if severe enough, could result in a stricture once healing is complete. Contrast esophagography and endoscopy will confirm the diagnosis of stricture.

85. **b**

86. **c**

Correct answers are on pages

87. **d**

88. **b**

89. **b**

90. **c**

91. **e**

92. **b**

93. **b**

94. **c**

95. **b** Lack of an air-tight seal following rhinotomy may allow air to escape into the subcutaneous tissues around the head and neck. This subcutaneous emphysema may extend through the thoracic inlet and collect within the mediastinal space. If air continues to accumulate, the mediastinal barrier will be lost and air will escape into the pleural space, resulting in pneumothorax.

96. **d**

97. **c**

98. **b**

99. **d**

100. **b**

101. **c**

102. **c**

103. **b**

104. **c**

105. **e**

106. **b**

107. **d**

108. **a**

109. **c**

110. **d**

111. **d**

112. **d**

113. **d**

114. **a**

115. **a**

116. **b**

117. **c**

118. **a**

119. **d**

120. **b** A mid-duodenal obstruction results in a tremendous loss of the bicarbonate present in pancreatic juices and bile. This also decreases the amount of bicarbonate ion available for absorption from the intestinal tract. This loss of bicarbonate ion may result in metabolic acidosis if vomiting is severe.

121. **e**

122. **e**

123. **d**

124. **a**

125. **d**

126. **e**

127. **c**

128. **b**

129. **c**

130. **e**

131. **a**

132. **d**

133. **b**

134. **e**

135. **d**

136. **d** The microbes targeted in the colon are Gram-negative enterics and anaerobes. Of the drugs listed, the one that will cover the spectrum of activity needed is a second-generation cephalosporin, such as cefoxitin or cefmetazole.

137. **d**

138. **c**

139. **e**

140. **b**

141. **a**

142. **e** Lactulose, neomycin and a low-protein diet are all contributory to decreasing the hyperammonemia present in affected animals. Lactulose changes the pH to a more acidic environment, preventing conversion of ammonium ions to ammonia, which is freely diffusable across the enteric mucosa. Neomycin kills colonic urease-producing bacteria that are responsible for converting intraluminal urea to ammonia. A low-protein diet makes fewer amino acids available, which act as a substrate for production of ammonia and other nitrogenous toxins.

143. **c** Furosemide use may result in hypokalemia and alkalosis. Excessive loss of potassium increases renal output of ammonia. Alkalosis enhances transfer of ammonia into the central nervous system, which may worsen hepatoencephalopathy.

144. **d** When isolating the pancreas for removal, the blood supply common to both the duodenum and the pancreas is the pancreaticoduodenal artery and vein. Disruption of these vessels during pancreatotomy may result in loss of viability of the adjacent duodenum.

145. **c** Pancreatic trauma may result from rough handling of the pancreas by the surgeon. A potential sequela is pancreatitis.

146. **b**

147. **a** If an extracapsular technique of bilateral thyroidectomy is used, parathyroid tissue may be removed as well. Loss of the parathyroid glands can result in hypoparathyroidism and decreased serum calcium levels.

148. **c** The intracapsular technique for thyroidectomy is used so as to preserve parathyroid tissue and prevent hypocalcemia. While this more conservative approach may preserve parathyroid function, it may result in incomplete removal of thyroid tissue, which could lead to recurrence of signs related to hyperthyroidism.

149. **d**

150. **b**

151. **e**

152. **c**

153. **c**

154. **b**

155. **e**

156. **c**

157. **d**

158. **d**

159. **a**

160. **e**

161. **d**

162. **d**

163. **d** *E coli* is most likely to be involved with pyometra. The drug with the most efficacy against this microbe should be chosen. Of the choices available, a second-generation cephalosporin would be most effective.

164. **c**

165. **d**

166. **c** Urine spraying behavior and territoriality are inconsistent and may be present even in castrated cats. Castration has no effect on the prevalence of urethral obstruction. Similarly, the retractor penis muscle is not affected by the absence or presence of male hormones. Therefore, the only consistently predictable sign of retained testicles is the spines on the penis.

167. **a**

168. **d**

169. **d** Removing a portion of the genital tract is not likely to correct a uterine prolapse. Suturing the uterus to the colon is not likely to help because the colon is moveable. The technical difficulty of placing a pursestring suture in the vaginal vault, combined with the unpredictable results, makes this a poor choice of therapy for this condition. Hysteropexy gives good results and is relatively simple to perform.

170. **c**

171. **e** Mammary tumors in cats are usually highly malignant. For this reason, increased disease-free intervals and longevity are best served by an aggressive surgical approach. This involves a complete chain mastectomy with regional lymph node removal, followed by removal of the opposite chain 3-4 weeks later.

172. **b**

173. **c**

174. **c**

175. **c**

176. **c** Zinc methionine can be given orally at 15 mg/10 kg of body weight.

177. **e**

178. **b**

179. **b**

180. **d**

181. **d**

182. **d**

183. **b**

Correct answers are on pages

184. **c** Traumatic rupture of the cranial cruciate ligament is the most common cause of degenerative osteoarthritis of the canine stifle joint.

185. **d** Grade-IV medial patellar luxation is the classification characterized by the most severe bone lesions and clinical signs.

186. **e** Wedge resection of the trochlear groove deepens the femoral sulcus and maintains articular cartilage contact between the patella and femur.

187. **a** The stifle joint is a complex, condylar, synovial joint.

188. **b** A medial meniscal tear occurs in 40-60% of the cases involving rupture of the cranial cruciate ligament.

189. **b** Rupture of the cranial cruciate ligament causes cranial drawer motion of the tibia relative to the femur.

190. **b** Treatment for medial luxation of the patella requires a medial relief incision and lateral tightening procedures.

191. **a** A derotation, nonabsorbable suture between the lateral fabella and tibial tuberosity is classified as an extracapsular repair.

192. **a** Surgical treatments for cranial cruciate ligament injury include extracapsular or intracapsular repairs.

193. **e** Lateral patellar luxation in large dogs can be associated with ipsilateral hip dysplasia.

194. **d** A median sternotomy provides the greatest exposure for organs in the thoracic cavity.

195. **a** A left 4th intercostal thoracotomy is used most frequently for repair of a patent ductus arteriosus or patent ductus venosus.

196. **c** A persistent right aortic arch produces postprandial regurgitation at weaning.

197. **d** The most common congenital cardiac anomaly in dogs is patent ductus arteriosus.

198. **a** The most common congenital cardiac anomaly in cats is ventricular septal defect.

199. **b** Tetralogy of Fallot is the most common congenital cardiac disease causing cyanosis in dogs.

200. **a** Treatment for patent ductus arteriosus includes ligation of the shunt.

201. **e** Treatment for chylothorax includes avoidance of long-chain fatty acids in the diet.

202. **a** Flail chest is an unstable thoracic wall segment associated with paradoxic chest motions.

203. **a** An arteriovenous fistula or shunt is an abnormal communication between an artery and vein.

204. **d** Splenic neoplasia is most often and most easily treated by splenectomy.

205. **e** Gastric dilatation-volvulus occurs most frequently in large dogs that have exercised after eating.

206. **c** Intervertebral disk degeneration (disease) commonly produces signs of neurologic dysfunction, including pain, paresis and paralysis.

207. **b** The signs of lumbosacral stenosis, including caudal pain and paresis, are not affected by vitamin E or selenium injections.

208. **a** Thoracolumbar disk herniation causes upper motor neuron signs (hyperreflexia and spasticity) in the hind limbs.

209. **b** Progressive cervical vertebral instability requires spinal cord decompression and vertebral stabilization.

210. **d** Degenerative myelopathy of German Shepherds is a progressive, nonpainful condition characterized by hind limb paresis.

211. **c** The caudal thoracic intervertebral disks are frequently associated with degeneration and disease in chondrodystrophic dogs.

212. **a** Eustachian tube dilatation is not associated with the brachycephalic syndrome.

213. **d** Ventral flexion of the neck is not associated with laryngeal surgery.

214. **b** Dorsal rhinotomy is the most common surgical procedure of the nasal cavity.

215. **c** Tracheostomy provides a passage for movement of air into the trachea and lungs, circumventing an upper air obstruction.

216. **b** An oronasal fistula associated with severe periodontal disease most frequently produces a communication between the oral and nasal cavities.

217. **c** Osteochondritis dissecans has not been reported in the carpal joints.

218. **c** Treatment for osteochondritis dissecans includes cartilage flap removal and subchondral bone curettage to stimulate fibrocartilage formation.

219. **c** A fragmented medial coronoid process associated with lameness in a rapidly growing dog should be excised.

220. **a** Traumatic hip luxations usually occur in a craniodorsal direction due to the pull of the gluteal muscles.

221. **e** A De Vita pin can be used to stabilize a traumatic hip luxation.

222. **e** A Type-V Salter-Harris physeal injury associated with crushing of germinal cells warrants the poorest prognosis.

223. **b** In repair of epiphyseal fractures, the primary goal is articular cartilage congruency producing joint stability.

224. **e** An intramedullary pin can only provide axial alignment and resistance to bending forces.

225. **a** A dynamic compression plate secured by screws provides the greatest degree of compression across a fracture line.

226. **a** Primary bone union most frequently occurs when a fracture is stabilized with a bone plate and screws.

227. **d** A ruptured urinary bladder produces metabolic acidosis, hyperkalemia and azotemia, and should be repaired before definitive orthopedic surgery.

228. **c** A portosystemic shunt produces central nervous system derangements due to excessive accumulation of toxic metabolites normally handled by a liver perfused by the portal vein and its tributaries.

229. **e** Ectopic ureters are treated by ligation and reimplantation into the urinary bladder.

230. **b** Episioplasty refers to excision of redundant skin around the vulva that has caused a perivulvar dermatitis, especially in overweight dogs.

231. **c** Of the choices listed, only an external fixator can provide axial alignment, rotational stability and interfragmentary compression.

232. **e** Prophylactic antibiotics should be administered intravenously immediately before surgery, after induction of general anesthesia.

233. **b** Of the choices listed, intravenous antibiotics provide the highest drug concentration in serum, plasma and tissues.

234. **e** An insulinoma is a solitary tumor of the pancreas that causes profound hypoglycemia.

235. **c** A Robert Jones bandage can reduce soft tissue swelling and provide temporary stability for a fractured tibia.

236. **d** Corticosteroids, such as dexamethasone, can effectively reduce inflammation and spinal cord swelling in traumatic or disk-associated injuries.

237. **c** Chronic obstipation and megacolon in cats can be effectively treated by removal of the affected segment of colon.

238. **a** Perianal fistulae are abscesses around the anus and tail base in German Shepherds. They require surgical treatment.

239. **c** This approach provides the greatest possible exposure to explore the abdominal contents.

240. **d** If the viability of small intestines is in question, resection and anastomosis are the preferred surgical approach. Attempting to move an irregularly shaped foreign body within devitalized intestine risks significant intestinal damage.

241. **a** The antimesenteric surface should be shorter than the mesenteric surface. This maximizes the blood supply to the antimesenteric surface.

242. **d** The simple-interrupted pattern placed in a crushing manner is simple and effective. The suture locks on the submucosa, which is the layer with the greatest holding strength.

243. **b** Upper motor neuron lesions cause loss of inhibitory function. Reflexes are exaggerated while postural reactions are depressed to the rear limbs.

244. **c** Exposure to the level of the transverse spinous processes allows fenestration.

245. **a** The last rib originates at the 13th thoracic vertebra and is directed caudally. The transverse spinous process of the 1st lumbar vertebra is directed cranially. It is easy to palpate and visualize these structures.

246. **e** Fat disappears from the epidural space at sites of spinal cord compression. Decompression should proceed both cranially and caudally until epidural fat is observed.

Correct answers are on pages

247. **b** In cats, castration is performed through 2 scrotal incisions, one directly over each testicle.

248. **a** In dogs, castration is performed through 1 prescrotal incision. The testicles are pushed cranially into the prescrotal subcutaneous tissue and the incision is made in the midline just cranial to the scrotum.

249. **d** The skin incision for ovariohysterectomy in cats is made midway between the umbilicus and pubis. The anatomic structure that is most difficult to exteriorize is the uterine body; therefore, the incision must be made more caudally (as compared with the incision for ovariohysterectomy in dogs) to allow exposure of the uterus.

250. **a** The skin incision for ovariohysterectomy in dogs is started at the umbilicus and continued caudally. The anatomic structure that is most difficult to exteriorize is the right ovary; therefore, the incision must be made more cranially (as compared with the incision for ovariohysterectomy in cats) to allow exposure of the ovaries.

251. **e** The bulbourethral glands represent the junction of the dilated pelvic urethra and the constricted penile urethra. The new urethral orifice must be constructed using dilated pelvic urethral tissue.

252. **c** The ureter, passing obliquely through the bladder wall, is compressed as the bladder fills with urine. This reduces back flow of urine into the ureter and renal pelvis with increasing bladder pressure.

253. **d** When incisions parallel skin tension lines, only a minimal gap is created because of less tension pulling the wound apart. This reduces the likelihood of dehiscence.

254. **c** Suture material in the bladder lumen can serve as a nidus for formation of cystic calculi.

255. **a** A drain minimizes the chances of infection and scarring.

256. **d** This represents a dehiscence of the abdominal wall and requires repair. It will not heal without treatment.

257. **a** The degree of callus formation is inversely related to the stability of a fracture.

258. **d** Callus formation in bone healing is classified on the basis of location. Callus can be periosteal, intercortical or medullary. With intramedullary pin stabilization, all 3 types of callus may form. With plate and screw fixation, the primary callus formed is intercortical. There may be some medullary callus formed with plate/screw fixation.

259. **e** Bone fragments should be incorporated into the repair. They should only be discarded if the wound is contaminated and the risk of infection is great. Fragments of cortical bone, even devoid of blood supply, function as autogenous bone grafts.

260. **c** The serratus dorsalis would not be in the surgical field in this procedure. It is located dorsal to the surgical field.

261. **a** The preferred closure of the esophagus is 2 layers. The first layer captures the mucosa and submucosa. The second layer closes the muscularis and adventitia.

262. **d** Correcting and preventing recurrence of salivary mucocele generally do not involve excision of the cyst itself. The responsible salivary glands (mandibular and sublingual) are excised and the cyst is drained.

263. **b** Connell sutures penetrate all layers and enter the lumen. Cushing sutures do not enter the lumen.

264. **a** Heller's myotomy is used to expand the esophageal-gastric junction. The other 4 procedures may be used to expand the lumen of the pyloric-intestinal junction.

265. **b** Suturing a longitudinal incision transversely expands the diameter of the intestine at that site and reduces the risk of intestinal obstruction.

266. **a** Omentum adheres to the intestinal incision rapidly, creating a fluid-tight seal.

267. **c** Elongated soft palate, laryngeal collapse, stenotic nares, and everting laryngeal saccules can all be managed surgically. There is no effective surgical management for tracheal hypoplasia.

268. **b** Osteochondritis dissecans of the right humeral head is the most likely cause, considering pain on extension of the shoulder and partial weight bearing.

269. **a** Contusions are classified as closed wounds.

270. **e** Puncture wounds are most likely to result in infection due to impeded egress of foreign material or exudates from the wound.

271. **e** Delayed closure of this wound would minimize scarring. Debridement and leaving the wound open until a healthy bed of granulation tissue develops would minimize infection.

272. **b** Allografts (also called homografts) are grafts between different animals of the same species.

273. **c** The stratum basale of the ungual crest contains germinal cells that give rise to the claw. These cells must be removed to prevent regrowth of the claw.

274. **b** A patent ductus arteriosus is best approached through the left 4th intercostal space.

275. **b** The thoracotomy approach for PRAA is the same as for PDA (left 4th).

276. **a** The problem associated with PRAA is that the ligamentum arteriosus creates a constriction of the thoracic esophagus. Your objective is to remove that constriction.

277. **e** Sialoliths are removed through an oral incision. The incisions are left open to drain saliva into the mouth.

278. **b** The caudal thoracic esophagus is best approached through a right 8th intercostal thoracotomy.

279. **d** Recent studies have failed to confirm the value of pyloroplasty in preventing recurrence of gastric dilatation torsion.

280. **a** The transthoracic approach is generally preferred and is performed at the right 7th intercostal space. The transabdominal approach involves needle entry on the left between the xyphoid and the coastal arch.

281. **d** The most common sites for bone marrow aspiration are the iliac crest and the proximal femur.

282. **b** Partial splenic rupture is an indication for partial splenectomy. Partial splenectomy is contraindicated in splenic neoplasia, regardless of the location of the tumor.

283. **a** Hansen's type-I classification is chondroid metaplasia. It occurs in young chondrodystrophoid dogs and results in massive rupture.

284. **b** Many factors influence selection of the appropriate techniques for management of cervical intervertebral disk disease. Absence of clinical signs generally precludes surgical management, while the presence of motor or sensory deficits indicates the need for decompression.

285. **c** The calculi are exposed by longitudinal incision through the renal parenchyma.

286. **e** Cystotomy, combined with urethral backflushing, allows use of only one surgical procedure. The backflushing may be unsuccessful, at which point urethrotomy or urethrostomy may be indicated.

287. **a** Bone plates are most likely to neutralize all forces acting upon a fracture.

288. **b** A single intramedullary pin by itself will not neutralize rotational forces.

289. **e** Diaphragmatic hernias, especially acute hernias with little chance of adhesion formation, are repaired through a ventral abdominal midline approach.

290. **c** The approach to incisional hernias should take advantage of the tissue already actively involved in the healing process. Debridement or excision of the existing wounds removes this advantage.

291. **a** The coccygeus, levator ani, external anal sphincter and internal obturator muscle may all be used in repair of a perineal hernia. Of the muscles mentioned, only the rectococcygeus would not be involved.

292. **e** Perineal hernias occur most commonly in older male dogs. Several breeds, including Collies and Boston Terriers, are overrepresented.

293. **c** A left-to-right shunt causes dilation of the pulmonary artery, predisposing it to tearing or rupturing.

294. **d** Retrograde pinning implies that the pin is initially inserted at the fracture site, driven out the proximal end of the femur and redirected distally. Positioning the limb in a normal weight-bearing position with slight adduction is necessary to minimize soft tissue injury and prevent impingement on the sciatic nerve.

295. **b** Eccentrically placed screws result in shear and loss of reduction.

296. **e** Buttress plates bridge defects in diaphyseal bone.

297. **a** Tension-band plates convert tensile forces into compressive forces.

Correct answers are on pages

298. **a** Compression plating to establish rigid fixation is the most appropriate choice. Debridement is not necessary as long as the bone ends are viable.

299. **b** In cases of nonhealing fractures complicated by osteomyelitis, implants providing rigid stability should not be removed unless they are keeping a sequestrum in place.

300. **a** Salter-I fractures are transverse fractures through the region of cartilage hypertrophy.

301. **b** Salter-II fractures are transverse fractures through the region of cartilage hypertrophy that extend into the metaphysis.

302. **e** Salter-V fractures are compression fractures of the epiphysis.

303. **c** Compression fractures of the ulnar epiphysis most likely result in radius curvis due to premature closure of the ulnar physis.

304. **d** The radial nerve crosses the humerus at the site of the fracture and must be reflected during surgical repair.

305. **d** The joint should be opened to visualize the reduction. The fracture should be stabilized with cancellous bone screws.

306. **a** Trochanteric osteotomy allows elevation of the gluteals and complete exposure of the dorsal aspect of the acetabulum.

307. **b** The cranial drawer sign is observed with cranial cruciate ligament damage.

308. **a** Tearing of the caudal body of the medial meniscus is the most common injury and the most difficult to detect on exploration of the stifle.

309. **e** Craniomandibular osteopathy is a noninflammatory, nonneoplastic proliferative bone disease occurring in young animals. It has a predilection for endochondral bone.

310. **c** Panosteitis causes shifting-leg lameness and long-bone pain in young growing dogs.

311. **b** The coronoid process is removed through a medial approach to the elbow joint.

312. **d** A comminuted fracture involves splintering or fragmentation, with multiple fracture lines converging on one point.

313. **b** Fractures on one side of the bone, with bending of the opposite side, are called greenstick fractures. They occur primarily in young growing dogs.

314. **a** Tension-band wires are applied in situations in which the bone fragments are distracted due to the pull of tendinous insertions of muscles.

315. **a** Osteochondrosis refers to an abnormality of endochondral ossification, with asymmetric maturation to bone. It may result in a horizontal cleft separating the articular cartilage from bone. Osteochondritis dissecans is a sequel to osteochondrosis, in which a vertical cleft arises and a cartilaginous flap pulls loose from underlying bone.

316. **c** Craniodorsal luxation is most common, with reports of 75% or greater incidence.

317. **c** The lumen diameter of the distal segment can be increased by cutting it at a more oblique angle.

318. **e** This foreign body should pass through the alimentary system of a large-breed dog with no problem. Good client education is important.

319. **b** Trimming the excess mucosa facilitates tissue apposition during the anastomosis.

320. **c** All 4 limbs show decreased proprioception and decreased reflexes.

321. **a** All 4 limbs show decreased proprioception and increased reflexes. The lesion is in the upper motor neuron to all 4 limbs.

322. **b** Upper motor neuron signs for all 4 limbs indicate a high cervical lesion.

323. **c** The wings of the atlas and the large ventral protuberance of the sixth cervical vertebra allow you to determine location. These landmarks can then be used to count cranially and caudally.

324. **d** While some veterinarians use this technique, it is the most prone to complications.

325. **b** The right ovary is located more cranially than the left. Some surgeons prefer a right paramedian approach in canine ovariohysterectomy to reduce the difficulty in exteriorizing the right ovary.

326. **a** A dorsal incision in the uterine body is recommended. Incisions in the uterine horn may result in enough scarring to reduce future fertility.

327. **b** Stents can interfere with primary healing and increase the risk of ascending infection.

328. **a** It is important to isolate and specifically clamp and ligate the bleeding vessel. The ureter is located in this area and gross ligation could occlude the ureter.

329. **e** Cystocentesis reduces the size of the bladder and allows repositioning of the bladder back into a normal anatomic position.

330. **a** There is no technique described for preputial urethrostomy in dogs.

331. **c** Ammonium urate uroliths are associated with portal vascular anomalies.

332. **b** The Zepp procedure involves resection of the lateral cartilaginous wall of the vertical ear canal and formation of a ventral cartilaginous flap.

333. **e** Ventral bulla osteotomy provides the best means for drainage of the middle ear.

334. **b** The purpose of surgical management of PDA is to stop the left-to-right flow of blood. This is accomplished by ligation of the ductus.

335. **c** The purpose of surgical management of PRAA is transection of the ligamentum arteriosus, which forms a restrictive band of tissue occluding the esophagus.

336. **a** The central tendon of the diaphragm is stronger than the muscular portion and, therefore, tears less frequently.

337. **b** Stretching or breaking of the suspensory ligament is usually necessary for delivery of the ovaries into the surgical field.

338. **c** The incidence of perineal hernias is highest in older intact male dogs. Several breeds appear predisposed, including Boxers.

339. **b** Polydioxanone is a monofilament synthetic absorbable suture material.

340. **a** Polypropylene is a monofilament synthetic nonabsorbable suture material.

341. **d** Surgical catgut is a natural absorbable suture material.

342. **e** Stainless steel is inert in tissue.

343. **b** Plain catgut incites the most tissue reacion. Chromic catgut causes much less tissue reaction.

344. **c** The vertical mattress suture is everting.

345. **a** The Cushing pattern is an inverting pattern used on hollow organs.

346. **d** One of the basic principles of external fixation of fractures is immobilization of the joints proximal and distal to the fracture. Of the fractures listed, only the mid-diaphyseal fracture of the tibia could be treated with a Schroeder-Thomas splint.

347. **e** The Robert Jones bandage is the best technique to minimize soft tissue damage and provide temporary stability to a fracture distal to the stifle or elbow.

348. **b** The lumen diameter of the pylorus is increased by suturing a longitudinal incision transversely.

349. **b** The caudal border of the soft palate should be at the tip of the epiglottis.

350. **c** If a radiographically visible defect is present, surgical management is indicated. Curettage of the lesion is believed to stimulate filling of the defect.

351. **e** Panosteitis is a self-limiting disease of undetermined etiology. Analgesics are given as needed.

352. **e** The length of the surgical procedure, amount of tissue damage, amount of hemorrhage, and immunocompetence of the animal all influence the incidence of wound infection.

353. **a** A lacerated artery spurts blood under pressure.

354. **b** Arterial bleeders should be ligated.

355. **c** Bleeding in which blood oozes under low pressure at the time of incision is considered capillary/primary hemorrhage.

356. **e** Capillary bleeding can generally be stopped by applying light pressure with gauze sponges.

357. **c** Careful placement of subcutaneous sutures decreases dead space and can improve tissue apposition.

358. **d** An accidental wound, created in a nonsterile environment and of this duration, should be considered dirty.

359. **b** Current is concentrated at the active electrode and either cuts or coagulates tissue.

360. **d** Capillary action may draw bacteria from the underlying environment through the drapes.

361. **b** The falciform ligament is a fatty structure adherent to the linea alba just cranial to the umbilicus. Many surgeons recommend removal of this structure upon closure of the abdominal wall.

362. **a** The ureter should be left with little or no blind stump. Ligation and transection should be done as close to the bladder as possible.

363. **c** Liquid nitrogen is the most commonly used cryogen in veterinary medicine because of its temperature, availability and cost.

364. **b** Tissue that reaches -20 C or colder is most likely to undergo necrosis.

365. **d** The zone of edema is farthest from the tip of the laser instrument and eventually recovers.

366. **c** Holding the instrument perpendicular to the tissue prevents thermal injury in collateral tissues.

367. **d** The descending duodenum can be gently elevated and retracted to the left, providing improved exposure of the right kidney.

368. **c** The descending colon can be gently elevated and retracted to the right, providing improved exposure of the left kidney.

369. **b** Cellular death occurs by intracellular and extracellular formation of ice. Water content, therefore, is the factor that influences a tissue's reaction to cryosurgery.

370. **a** A conjunctival flap protects the inner layer of the cornea and provides a blood supply for more rapid healing.

371. **b** Second-intention healing is the process whereby the wound heals by granulation, contraction and reepithelialization, without human intervention.

372. **c** Transplantation of the parotid duct is frequently effective in management of keratoconjunctivitis sicca.

373. **c** Current recommendations are for placement of 3 screws proximal and 3 distal to the fracture line.

374. **c** Third-intention healing involves delayed primary closure.

375. **e** The fibers of the rectus abdominis muscle parallel the linea alba and must be separated.

376. **b** A single lesion at C5-T2 would account for both sets of neurologic signs.

377. **d** A lesion at C1-5 would cause upper motor neuron signs to the front limbs. A lesion at L4-S3 would cause lower motor neuron signs to the rear limbs.

378. **e** The Connell suture pattern is inverting.

379. **d** The Ehmer sling prevents weight bearing and produces medial rotation of the femoral head into the acetabulum.

380. **c** The Valpeau bandage prevents weight bearing and holds the scapula firmly against the body wall.

381. **c** The Parker-Kerr pattern is an inverting continuous suture pattern used for closing transected tubular structures.

382. **d** Transplantation of the tibial crest may be indicated in patellar luxations, but not in rupture of the cranial cruciate ligament.

383. **e** The Cushing suture pattern is placed parallel to the incision line. In the Lembert pattern, the bites in the tissue are perpendicular to the incision line.

384. **c** The intercapital ligaments extend from the head of one rib to the head of the contralateral rib, passing ventral to the spinal cord and dorsal to the intervertebral disk. These ligaments prevent dorsal rupture of disk material.

385. **b** Amputation of the tail at Cy3-4 prevents fecal and urine soiling of the tail, minimizes the possibility of pain associated with motion of the tail, and preserves the origin of the muscles of the pelvic diaphragm.

386. **b** The femur is approached between the vastus lateralis and the biceps femoris.

387. **a** The incision should be made in an avascular area midway between the greater and lesser curvatures of the stomach and paralleling the long axis of the stomach.

388. **b** Stay sutures allow relatively atraumatic manipulation of tissue.

15

Theriogenology

S.D. Van Camp, C.B. Waters

Recommended Reading

Feldman EC and Nelson RW: *Canine and Feline Endocrinology and Reproduction*. Saunders, Philadelphia, 1987.

Frandson RD and Spurgeon TL: *Anatomy and Physiology of Domestic Animals*. 5th ed. Lea & Febiger, Philadelphia, 1992.

McDonald LE: *Veterinary Endocrinology and Reproduction*. 4th ed. Lea & Febiger, Philadelphia, 1989.

Morrow DA: *Current Therapy in Theriogenology 2*. Saunders, Philadelphia, 1986.

Roberts SJ: *Veterinary Obstetrics and Genital Diseases*. 3rd ed. David & Charles, North Pomfret, VT, 1986.

Practice answer sheet is on page 361.

Questions

1. *The ejaculate of male dogs consists of 3 fractions. Concerning the fractions of canine ejaculates, which statement is **least** accurate?*

   a. The second fraction is the sperm-rich fraction.

   b. A pause often occurs between the semen fractions being collected.

   c. The most voluminous fraction is the third fraction.

   d. The third fraction consists mainly of prostatic fluid.

   e. The first fraction emitted should be collected to ensure adequate sperm motility.

2. *Blood in the canine ejaculate may be associated with any of the following **except**:*

   a. prostatitis

   b. urethritis

   c. seminal vesiculitis

   d. orchitis

   e. ruptured blood vessel on the surface of the penis

3. *Semen is most often collected from dogs by:*

   a. electroejaculation

   b. rectal massage

   c. penile massage

   d. prostatic stimulation

   e. magnetic resonance impulsing

Correct answers are on pages 319-320.

4. *In transvaginal artificial insemination in the bitch, using fresh semen, semen should be deposited into the:*

   a. uterus
   b. vestibule
   c. cervical body
   d. cranial vagina
   e. oviduct

5. *An initial rise in plasma progesterone levels in a bitch indicates that:*

   a. ovulation has occurred and it is too late to breed the bitch
   b. ovulation is imminent and the bitch should be bred in the next few days
   c. the bitch is pregnant
   d. the bitch is due to whelp within 3 days
   e. the bitch has entered proestrus and should be bred immediately

6. *Erection persists in some male dogs after mating because hair adheres to the penis and the preputial orifice is inverted as the penis is withdrawn. Concerning this condition, which statement is most accurate?*

   a. This is an emergency condition and should receive prompt care to prevent permanent damage to the penis.
   b. This condition is usually self-correcting and resolves with rest.
   c. This condition is known as phimosis.
   d. Treatment should include tranquilization to increase blood pressure.
   e. Atropine is indicated to alleviate this condition, as erection is a sympathetic nervous system response and atropine is a sympatholytic drug.

7. *In managing breeding of dogs, several "rules of thumb" have proven valuable. Concerning dog breeding, which statement is **least** accurate?*

   a. Matings in which the male does not become "tied" to the female, by locking of the bulbis glandis in the vagina, are as fertile as those in which a "tie" does occur.

   b. Bitches should be bred on the first, third and fifth days of standing heat if vaginal smears and/or progesterone determinations are not available.
   c. Bitches should be introduced to the male's territory to maximize the chance of successful mating.
   d. Breeding on the 11th and 13th day or the 12th and 14th day after the bloody vulvar discharge is detected may not be adequate for all bitches to conceive.
   e. Bitches are most fertile between 3 and 5 years of age.

8. *Pseudopregnancy is a common clinical complaint in dogs. It is usually characterized by mammary development, lactation, nesting and possibly adoption of kittens or inanimate objects as surrogate puppies. It usually occurs within 60 days of the previous heat. Concerning pseudopregnancy in dogs, which statement is most accurate?*

   a. Pseudopregnancy is caused by abnormal hormone imbalance in the bitch.
   b. Repeated pseudopregnancy can lead to pyometra.
   c. Pseudopregnancy can occur after ovariohysterectomy performed 1-2 months after the previous heat.
   d. Pseudopregnancy must be treated with hormones.
   e. Bitches experiencing pseudopregnancy are permanently infertile.

9. *Various hormones have been used to control estrus in dogs and cats. Concerning drugs used in estrual animals, which statement is **least** accurate?*

   a. Megestrol acetate can be used to prevent or suppress heat in dogs.
   b. Mibolerone can be used to prevent but not suppress heat in dogs.
   c. Megestrol acetate can be used to suppress or postpone heat in cats.
   d. Mibolerone should not be used in cats because it can be nephrotoxic and hepatotoxic.
   e. Estrogens are safe and effective for inducing fertile heat in dogs.

10. *Hormones used to control estrus and prevent or terminate pregnancy in dogs can have potentially harmful side effects. Concerning such use of hormones, which statement is **least** accurate?*

    a. Mibolerone should not be given to a pregnant bitch because it may maculinize the female pups.
    b. Megestrol acetate should not be given to bitches in advanced estrus because pyometra may result.
    c. Overdoses of estrogen used to treat mismating can lead to anemia, reduced platelet numbers and hemorrhaging in bitches.
    d. Use of prostaglandins to treat pyometra or terminate pregnancy in bitches can have fatal results if the bitch is overdosed or if the bitch has a heart condition.
    e. Testosterone can be safely administered to prepubertal bitches to increase growth and muscle mass without affecting reproductive cycles and fertility.

11. *Dystocia (difficult or abnormal birth) can be related to maternal or fetal factors. Which condition is **least** likely to cause dystocia in a bitch?*

    a. dead puppy blocking the birth canal
    b. uterine inertia
    c. a single-puppy litter
    d. previous pelvic fracture
    e. a multiple-puppy litter

12. *In most bitches, the entire estrous cycle spans:*

    a. 4-7 months
    b. 21 days
    c. 7 days
    d. 28 days
    e. 63 days

13. *In dogs, gestation lasts approximately:*

    a. 21 days
    b. 30 days
    c. 63 days
    d. 90 days

    e. 115 days

14. *In a vaginal smear of a bitch in standing heat, what is the predominant epithelial cell type?*

    a. parabasal cell
    b. noncornified small intermediate cell
    c. cornified, large intermediate and superficial cell
    d. red blood cell
    e. white blood cell

15. *Which of the following is **not** an indication for cesarean section in a queen?*

    a. pregnancy lasting more than 67 days
    b. period of more than 4 hours since delivery of the previous kitten
    c. foul-smelling, hemorrhagic vulvar discharge
    d. constant straining to deliver a kitten
    e. nonodoriferous, brownish vulvar discharge after delivery of the second kitten

16. *Concerning reproduction in cats, which statement is **least** accurate?*

    a. Cats ovulate in response to vaginal stimulation.
    b. In the Northern Hemisphere, cats are polyestrous from late January to fall.
    c. In a nonpregnant cat, the corpus luteum produces progesterone for 10 days between heats.
    d. Cats that have been bred but that are not pregnant may develop pseudopregnancy and show signs of pregnancy.
    e. Cats that have been bred but that are not pregnant cease cycling for several months.

17. *In cats, classic signs of estrus include all of the following **except**:*

    a. vocalization, rear-leg treading
    b. mounting of the male by the female
    c. rubbing and rolling
    d. elevated hindquarters (lordosis), tail deflected
    e. attraction of male cats

Correct answers are on pages 319-320.

18. In cats, normal signs of copulation, but not necessarily conception, include all of the following **except**:

   a. the male's biting queen's neck while holding the queen between his front legs

   b. the queen's crying out and turning to strike at the tom as he dismounts

   c. the queen's rolling and licking at her vulva in a frenzied manner

   d. the queen's rejecting the tom for 20-60 minutes

   e. draining of white blood-flecked mucus from the queen's vulva

19. Concerning reproduction in cats, which statement is **least** accurate?

   a. The estrous cycle lasts about 14 days.

   b. Cats remain in standing heat (estrus) about 3-6 days if not bred.

   c. Corpora lutea formed after sterile matings last 60-90 days.

   d. Progesterone is produced for 20-44 days after matings with a vasectomized tom.

   e. Nonbred queens go through a period of "nonestrus," but not diestrus, between heats.

20. In queens, pregnancy lasts approximately:

   a. 21 days

   b. 65 days

   c. 90 days

   d. 120 days

   e. 150 days

21. Concerning cytologic examination of feline vaginal smears, which statement is most accurate?

   a. Smears should not be collected because this may alter the duration of heat.

   b. Cellular changes are similar to those in bitches.

   c. Papanicolaou, new methylene blue and Diff-Quik stains are not acceptable for staining vaginal smears.

   d. Queens in anestrus have a high percentage of anuclear, flat, cornified cells in vaginal smears.

   e. Spermatozoa cannot be seen in vaginal smears from cats bred 2 hours previously.

22. Signs of queening (parturition) in cats include all of the following **except**:

   a. fall in rectal temperature in the first stage of labor

   b. nesting behavior

   c. increased appetite

   d. frequent licking of the vulva

   e. straining

23. The contraceptive method of choice for an adult queen whose owner does **not** intend to breed her is:

   a. ovariohysterectomy

   b. progesterone injection

   c. estrogen injection

   d. androgen implants

   e. prostaglandin suppositories

24. Concerning anesthesia of a cat for cesarean section, which statement is **least** accurate?

   a. Impingement of the large, pregnant uterus on the diaphragm can reduce the functional residual capacity of the lungs, leading to decreased oxygen reserves.

   b. Oxygen uptake is increased during pregnancy and labor.

   c. Anesthetics decrease arterial blood pressure, and placing a cat in dorsal recumbency can cause hypotension.

   d. Fetal hypoxia can delay respiration in kittens after delivery.

   e. Even though fetal drug metabolism is limited, most anesthetics are safe for cesarean section because they do not cross the placenta.

25. Concerning vaccination of queens and bitches during pregnancy, which statement is most accurate?

a. Modified-live-virus vaccines should not be given to pregnant females.

b. Modified-live-virus rabies vaccine is safe in pregnant dogs but not in pregnant queens.

c. Modified-live-virus canine distemper vaccine is safe in pregnant dogs.

d. Modified-live-virus panleukopenia vaccine is safe in pregnant queens.

e. Modified-live-virus feline viral rhinotracheitis vaccine is acceptable for use in pregnant cats.

26. *In female dogs, the entire estrous cycle spans:*

a. 2-4 months
b. 4-7 months
c. 7-9 months
d. 8-12 months
e. 10-14 months

27. *In female cats, the entire estrous cycle spans:*

a. 18 days
b. 21 days
c. 24 days
d. 28 days
e. 32 days

28. *Though there may be considerable individual variation, the average gestation length in cats and dogs is:*

a. 58 days
b. 54 days
c. 63 days
d. 66 days
e. 69 days

29. *Signs of proestrus in the bitch include all of the following **except**:*

a. vulvar swelling
b. bloody vulvar discharge
c. attraction of males
d. courtship play
e. standing to be mounted

30. *The earliest time in gestation that radiographs can be used to diagnose pregnancy in dogs and cats is:*

a. 20 days
b. 25 days
c. 35 days
d. 45 days
e. 55 days

31. *Another term for false pregnancy is:*

a. pseudogestation
b. nymphomania
c. pseudocyesis
d. pseudoestrogenism
e. feminization

Answers

1. e
2. c
3. c
4. d
5. b
6. a
7. a
8. c
9. e
10. e
11. e
12. a
13. c
14. c
15. e
16. c

17. **b**

18. **e**

19. **c**

20. **b**

21. **b**

22. **c**

23. **a**

24. **e**

25. **a**

26. **b**

27. **b**

28. **c**

29. **e** Standing to be mounted is characteristic of estrus.

30. **d**

31. **c**

Notes

Section 16

Urology and Nephrology

K.C. Bovée

Recommended Reading

Bovée KC: *Canine Nephrology*. Harwal Publishing, Media, PA, 1984.

Breitschwerdt EB: *Nephrology and Urology*. Churchill Livingstone, New York, 1986.

Cunningham JG: *Textbook of Veterinary Physiology*. Saunders, Philadelphia, 1992.

Guyton AC: *Textbook of Medical Physiology*. 8th ed. Saunders, Philadelphia, 1991.

Swenson MJ: *Dukes' Physiology of Domestic Animals*. 10th ed. Comstock Publishing, Ithaca, NY, 1984.

> ### *Practice answer sheet is on page 363.*

Questions

1. *Which portion of the nephron has the most complex brush border membrane?*

   a. distal tubule
   b. collecting duct
   c. proximal tubule
   d. loop of Henle
   e. ascending limb of Henle

2. *There are several anatomic components of the juxtaglomerular apparatus of the kidney. Which is the portion contributed by the distal tubule?*

   a. vasa recta
   b. macula densa
   c. afferent arteriole
   d. efferent arteriole
   e. mesangial or polkissen cell

3. *The extracellular fluid volume in mammals represents approximately what percentage of total body weight?*

   a. 20%
   b. 30%
   c. 40%
   d. 10%
   e. 60%

Correct answers are on page 327.

321

4. *The major difference in electrolyte composition between plasma and intracellular fluid is that intracellular fluid contains a:*

   a. higher sodium concentration
   b. higher bicarbonate concentration
   c. lower phosphate concentration
   d. lower magnesium concentration
   e. higher potassium concentration

5. *In dogs, the normal value for plasma osmolarity, expressed as mOsm/kg of water, is:*

   a. 270
   b. 290
   c. 315
   d. 325
   e. 250

6. *Starling's hypothesis of fluid distribution between blood plasma and interstitial compartments states that the hydrostatic pressure on the venule side of the capillary is:*

   a. 20 mm Hg
   b. 10 mm Hg
   c. 40 mm Hg
   d. overshadowed by oncotic pressure
   e. influenced principally by lymphatic pressure in normal animals

7. *The renal medullary efferent arteriole contains smooth muscle and divides into:*

   a. a single vas rectum surrounding the proximal tubule
   b. multiple vasa recta that penetrate deep into the medulla
   c. a capillary network that absorbs large volumes of fluid from the distal tubule in the cortex
   d. multiple vasa recta that are controlled by the renin-angiotensin system
   e. peritubular capillaries distributed in the cortex and medulla

8. *Renal plasma flow is:*

   a. measured by clearance of creatinine corrected for the hematocrit
   b. measured by renal clearance of inulin
   c. essentially the same as total renal blood flow
   d. approximately 200 ml/min/kg body weight in dogs
   e. measured by renal clearance of para-aminohippurate

9. *The rate of blood flow to the renal medulla is important because it influences:*

   a. urine-concentrating capacity and urinary sodium excretion
   b. acid/base balance
   c. the osmolarity of final urine, which is approximately 100 mOsm/L
   d. 50% of blood flow to the kidney
   e. the multiple endocrine functions of the kidney

10. *Autoregulation of renal blood flow is:*

    a. controlled by myogenic tone of the efferent arteriole, dependent on the juxtaglomerular apparatus and angiotensinogen
    b. effective within the range of approximately 80-180 mm Hg renal arterial pressure
    c. effective between a renal arterial pressure of 60 to 120 mm Hg
    d. directly dependent on oxygen extraction by the kidney
    e. controlled by the same factors that control autoregulation of cerebral blood flow

11. *Which vasoactive agent is most likely to* ***decrease*** *total renal blood flow?*

    a. acetylcholine
    b. bradykinin
    c. dopamine
    d. norepinephrine
    e. angiotensinogen

12. *The profile of hydrostatic pressure along the renal circulation is characterized by:*

    a. the largest fall in pressure across the afferent arteriole
    b. a peritubular capillary pressure of 40 mm Hg
    c. the largest pressure fall across the glomerular capillary

d. an efferent arterial pressure similar to afferent pressure

e. an aortic pressure of approximately 50 mm Hg

13. *The selective permeability of the glomerular capillary wall to various macromolecules in dogs allows the highest clearance of:*

a. myoglobin
b. hemoglobin
c. albumin
d. inulin
e. globulin

14. *The dynamics of glomerular filtration are best characterized by:*

a. clearance of para-aminohippurate
b. clearance of creatinine and sodium
c. the role of mesangial cells
d. increasing net ultrafiltration pressure throughout the length of the glomerular capillary
e. increasing plasma oncotic pressure along the length of the glomerular capillary

15. *The mean glomerular hydrostatic pressure in dogs is:*

a. secondary to the glomerular filtration rate and the tone of the efferent arteriole
b. increased to 80 mm Hg when vasoconstriction of the afferent arteriole is maximal
c. equal to plasma oncotic pressure
d. the same as net ultrafiltration
e. approximately 60 mm Hg and remains unchanged throughout the glomerular capillary

16. *The mesangial cells of the renal glomerulus are:*

a. the major filter of the glomerular membrane
b. located within the basement membrane
c. a nutrient source to epithelial cells
d. located between the basement membrane of adjoining capillaries, with processes that extend between the basement membrane and endothelial cells

e. located between the basement membrane of adjoining capillaries, with processes that extend into the epithelial cells

17. *If the renal clearance of creatinine is 20 ml/minute for a given animal, one would then expect the clearance of:*

a. para-aminohippurate to be 100 ml/minute
b. para-aminohippurate to be 250 ml/minute
c. glucose to be the same as for creatinine
d. inulin to be 50 ml/minute
e. inulin to be approximately the same as for para-aminohippurate

18. *Resorption of sodium in the proximal tubule is normally:*

a. 65% of the filtered load of sodium
b. 90% of the filtered load of sodium
c. closely linked to the renal concentrating mechanism
d. influenced by aldosterone
e. 99.9% of the filtered load of sodium

19. *The net movement of sodium ions from the tubular lumen into proximal tubule cells is associated with all of the following solutes except:*

a. arginine
b. creatinine
c. glucose
d. chloride
e. bicarbonate

20. *Aldosterone influences tubular transport of sodium and potassium by:*

a. maintaining high sodium resorption in the proximal tubule
b. decreasing sodium resorption in the distal tubule
c. increasing potassium resorption in the proximal tubule
d. increasing sodium resorption in the distal tubule, representing approximately 5% of the filtered load
e. enhancing sodium resorption in the distal tubule, representing approximately 30% of the filtered load

Correct answers are on page 327.

21. The primary influence of parathyroid hormone on renal tubular electrolyte transport is to:

    a. enhance potassium resorption
    b. decrease calcium resorption
    c. decrease phosphate resorption
    d. enhance bicarbonate resorption and hydrogen ion secretion
    e. enhance sodium resorption of approximately 20% of the filtered load

22. Which site within the nephron is associated with active transport of chloride?

    a. cortical collecting duct
    b. distal tubule
    c. descending limb of Henle
    d. proximal straight tubule
    e. diluting segment of the ascending limb of Henle

23. The kidney's urine-concentrating mechanism is **reduced** with:

    a. isosmotic proximal tubular sodium resorption
    b. high medullary blood flow
    c. low medullary blood flow
    d. excessive parathyroid hormone
    e. metabolic acidosis

24. Prostaglandin E_1 acts primarily in the kidney to:

    a. enhance the renin-angiotensin system
    b. decrease renal plasma flow
    c. decrease urine flow
    d. increase sodium resorption
    e. increase urinary sodium excretion

25. The renal tubular mechanism in the proximal tubule and distal tubule that creates titratable acid is associated with:

    a. secretion of hydrogen ion associated with glutamine
    b. a natriuretic hormone
    c. potassium secretion
    d. calcium resorption
    e. phosphate resorption

26. The osmolarity of fluid within the lumen of the nephron normally varies throughout the length of the nephron, so that an osmolarity of:

    a. 200 mOsm/kg would be expected in the collecting duct
    b. 100 mOsm/kg would be expected in the proximal tubule
    c. 400 mOsm/kg would be expected throughout the length of the proximal tubule
    d. 600 mOsm/kg would be expected at the tip of the loop of Henle
    e. 300 mOsm/kg would be expected in Bowman's space

27. Which of the following is most likely to activate the renin-angiotensin system?

    a. extracellular fluid volume depletion
    b. increased renal arterial pressure
    c. decreased sympathetic tone
    d. extracellular fluid volume expansion
    e. a mean arterial pressure of 100 mm Hg

28. The tissue renin-angiotensin system is present in all of the following **except**:

    a. brain
    b. pituitary gland
    c. adrenal gland
    d. kidney
    e. anterior chamber of the eye

29. Which of the following is most likely to cause release of atrial natriuretic factor?

    a. reduced production of antidiuretic hormone
    b. extracellular fluid volume expansion
    c. extracellular fluid volume depletion
    d. renal ischemia
    e. diabetes insipidus

30. The most potent vasoconstrictor known is:

    a. angiotensin I
    b. angiotensin II
    c. endothelin
    d. angiotensin III
    e. prostaglandin E_2

31. Which of the following is **not** a cause of prerenal azotemia?

   a. shock
   b. acute hemorrhage
   c. dehydration
   d. acute tubular necrosis
   e. myocardial failure

32. Which of the following is most consistent with massive proteinuria, hypoalbuminemia, edema and hypercholesterolemia?

   a. nephrolithiasis
   b. urinary tract infection
   c. nephrotic syndrome
   d. acute renal failure
   e. chronic urinary tract obstruction

33. The normal glomerular filtration rate in domestic animals is approximately:

   a. 2 ml/min/kg body weight
   b. 4 ml/min/kg body weight
   c. 8 ml/min/kg body weight
   d. 12 ml/min/kg body weight
   e. 20 ml/min/kg body weight

34. Thirty days after 75% nephrectomy, one would expect creatinine clearance to be:

   a. 20% of normal
   b. 40% of normal
   c. 60% of normal
   d. 95% of normal
   e. 120% of normal

35. Which species normally has the highest urine specific gravity (1.065)?

   a. horses
   b. cattle
   c. pigs
   d. dogs
   e. cats

36. Measurement of protein levels in urine using 24-hour urine collection allows absolute quantitation of daily protein excretion. In an animal with a urinary protein/creatinine ratio of 2.0, the daily rate of protein excretion is likely to be:

   a. 10 mg/kg
   b. 60 mg/kg
   c. 1.0 mg/kg
   d. 500 mg/kg
   e. 1 g/kg

37. When performing a urinalysis with the standard dipstick reagent pads for heme pigments, a positive color test indicates:

   a. intact erythrocytes, free hemoglobin and free myoglobin
   b. free myoglobin and free hemoglobin only
   c. free hemoglobin only
   d. free hemoglobin and intact erythrocytes
   e. intact erythrocytes only

38. White blood cell casts in the urinary sediment are strongly suggestive of:

   a. glomerulonephritis
   b. amyloidosis
   c. lower urinary tract infection
   d. prostatitis
   e. pyelonephritis

39. A dog has a urine specific gravity of 1.005. The most likely cause of this finding is:

   a. chronic renal failure
   b. diabetes mellitus
   c. pyelonephritis
   d. renal glycosuria
   e. diabetes insipidus

40. The species with the highest incidence of congenital polycystic kidneys is:

   a. dogs
   b. sheep
   c. horses
   d. cats
   e. pigs

Correct answers are on page 327.

41. The type of urolith most frequently associated with bacterial urinary tract infection is:

    a. cystine
    b. ammonium acid urate
    c. calcium phosphate
    d. calcium oxalate
    e. magnesium ammonium phosphate

42. After 48 hours of complete lower urinary tract obstruction, one would expect renal blood flow to be approximately:

    a. 10% of normal
    b. 50% of normal
    c. 90% of normal
    d. normal
    e. essentially zero, resulting in acute tubular necrosis

43. After relief of acute urinary obstruction of 24 hours' duration, followed by 48 hours of endogenous postobstructive diuresis, which plasma electrolyte change is most likely?

    a. hypernatremia
    b. hyperkalemia
    c. hypokalemia
    d. hypophosphatemia
    e. hypocalcemia

44. Which class of antimicrobials is considered the most common nephrotoxin in domestic animals?

    a. sulfonamides
    b. tetracyclines
    c. penicillins
    d. aminoglycosides
    e. fluoroquinolones

45. Concerning glomerulonephritis in dogs, which statement is most accurate?

    a. It is effectively controlled with corticosteroids.
    b. It is effectively controlled with immunosuppressive agents.
    c. It is effectively controlled with anticoagulants and vasoactive amine inhibitors.
    d. It is effectively controlled with a high-protein diet.
    e. It cannot be effectively controlled by any of the above.

46. During progression of chronic renal failure, as the filtered load of sodium changes, one would expect the fractional resorption of sodium to:

    a. increase to 100%
    b. decrease to approximately 90%
    c. decrease to 20%
    d. remain normal until more than 60% of renal mass is lost
    e. decrease in parallel to glomerular filtration rate

47. In secondary hyperparathyroidism associated with chronic renal failure,:

    a. tubular resorption of phosphate is increased to 99% of the filtered load
    b. tubular resorption of phosphate falls from 90% to 40% as the glomerular filtration rate declines
    c. phosphate is secreted through the tubules
    d. resorption of tubular phosphate is inhibited by calcium resorption
    e. the first alteration in tubular movement of phosphate is signaled by hyperphosphatemia

48. The slight hyperglycemia seen during chronic renal failure in dogs is due to:

    a. altered tubular movement of glucose
    b. moderate acidosis
    c. severe acidosis
    d. peripheral insensitivity to the action of insulin
    e. hyperglucagonemia

49. The most important cause of the anemia in chronic renal failure is:

a. insidious blood loss through the gastrointestinal tract

b. reduced lifespan of red blood cells

c. folate deficiency because of increased excretion

d. inadequate production of erythropoietin

e. excessive parathyroid hormone

50. *Gastrointestinal malabsorption of several solutes has been investigated in animals with chronic renal failure. Osteodystrophy is related to malabsorption of:*

a. vitamin D

b. phosphate

c. calcium

d. protein

e. potassium

Answers

1. **c**

2. **b**

3. **a**

4. **e**

5. **b**

6. **b**

7. **b**

8. **e**

9. **a**

10. **b**

11. **d**

12. **a**

13. **d**

14. **e**

15. **e**

16. **d**

17. **a**

18. **a**

19. **b**

20. **d**

21. **c**

22. **e**

23. **b**

24. **e**

25. **e**

26. **e**

27. **a**

28. **e**

29. **b**

30. **c**

31. **d**

32. **c**

33. **b**

34. **c**

35. **e**

36. **b** There is no absolute calculation possible from the premise. One must know the normal values of the 2 measures and their relation to each other.

37. **a**

38. **e**

39. **e**

40. **d**

41. **e**

42. **b** This level of blood flow provides nutrient flow and prevents tubular necrosis.

43. **c**

44. **d**

45. **e**

46. **b** Fractional resorption of sodium rarely falls lower even when the glomerular filtration rate is 10% of normal, which allows a small population of nephrons to control sodium balance.

47. **b**

48. **d**

49. **d**

50. **c**

Notes

Section 1
Anesthesiology

Fill in a circled letter to indicate your answer choice.

1. ⓐ ⓑ ⓒ ⓓ ⓔ	17. ⓐ ⓑ ⓒ ⓓ ⓔ	33. ⓐ ⓑ ⓒ ⓓ ⓔ	49. ⓐ ⓑ ⓒ ⓓ ⓔ
2. ⓐ ⓑ ⓒ ⓓ ⓔ	18. ⓐ ⓑ ⓒ ⓓ ⓔ	34. ⓐ ⓑ ⓒ ⓓ ⓔ	50. ⓐ ⓑ ⓒ ⓓ ⓔ
3. ⓐ ⓑ ⓒ ⓓ ⓔ	19. ⓐ ⓑ ⓒ ⓓ ⓔ	35. ⓐ ⓑ ⓒ ⓓ ⓔ	51. ⓐ ⓑ ⓒ ⓓ ⓔ
4. ⓐ ⓑ ⓒ ⓓ ⓔ	20. ⓐ ⓑ ⓒ ⓓ ⓔ	36. ⓐ ⓑ ⓒ ⓓ ⓔ	52. ⓐ ⓑ ⓒ ⓓ ⓔ
5. ⓐ ⓑ ⓒ ⓓ ⓔ	21. ⓐ ⓑ ⓒ ⓓ ⓔ	37. ⓐ ⓑ ⓒ ⓓ ⓔ	53. ⓐ ⓑ ⓒ ⓓ ⓔ
6. ⓐ ⓑ ⓒ ⓓ ⓔ	22. ⓐ ⓑ ⓒ ⓓ ⓔ	38. ⓐ ⓑ ⓒ ⓓ ⓔ	54. ⓐ ⓑ ⓒ ⓓ ⓔ
7. ⓐ ⓑ ⓒ ⓓ ⓔ	23. ⓐ ⓑ ⓒ ⓓ ⓔ	39. ⓐ ⓑ ⓒ ⓓ ⓔ	55. ⓐ ⓑ ⓒ ⓓ ⓔ
8. ⓐ ⓑ ⓒ ⓓ ⓔ	24. ⓐ ⓑ ⓒ ⓓ ⓔ	40. ⓐ ⓑ ⓒ ⓓ ⓔ	56. ⓐ ⓑ ⓒ ⓓ ⓔ
9. ⓐ ⓑ ⓒ ⓓ ⓔ	25. ⓐ ⓑ ⓒ ⓓ ⓔ	41. ⓐ ⓑ ⓒ ⓓ ⓔ	57. ⓐ ⓑ ⓒ ⓓ ⓔ
10. ⓐ ⓑ ⓒ ⓓ ⓔ	26. ⓐ ⓑ ⓒ ⓓ ⓔ	42. ⓐ ⓑ ⓒ ⓓ ⓔ	58. ⓐ ⓑ ⓒ ⓓ ⓔ
11. ⓐ ⓑ ⓒ ⓓ ⓔ	27. ⓐ ⓑ ⓒ ⓓ ⓔ	43. ⓐ ⓑ ⓒ ⓓ ⓔ	59. ⓐ ⓑ ⓒ ⓓ ⓔ
12. ⓐ ⓑ ⓒ ⓓ ⓔ	28. ⓐ ⓑ ⓒ ⓓ ⓔ	44. ⓐ ⓑ ⓒ ⓓ ⓔ	
13. ⓐ ⓑ ⓒ ⓓ ⓔ	29. ⓐ ⓑ ⓒ ⓓ ⓔ	45. ⓐ ⓑ ⓒ ⓓ ⓔ	
14. ⓐ ⓑ ⓒ ⓓ ⓔ	30. ⓐ ⓑ ⓒ ⓓ ⓔ	46. ⓐ ⓑ ⓒ ⓓ ⓔ	
15. ⓐ ⓑ ⓒ ⓓ ⓔ	31. ⓐ ⓑ ⓒ ⓓ ⓔ	47. ⓐ ⓑ ⓒ ⓓ ⓔ	
16. ⓐ ⓑ ⓒ ⓓ ⓔ	32. ⓐ ⓑ ⓒ ⓓ ⓔ	48. ⓐ ⓑ ⓒ ⓓ ⓔ	

This page intentionally left blank.

Practice Answer Sheet

Section 2

Cardiology

Fill in a circled letter to indicate your answer choice.

1. (a) (b) (c) (d) (e)
2. (a) (b) (c) (d) (e)
3. (a) (b) (c) (d) (e)
4. (a) (b) (c) (d) (e)
5. (a) (b) (c) (d) (e)
6. (a) (b) (c) (d) (e)
7. (a) (b) (c) (d) (e)
8. (a) (b) (c) (d) (e)

9. (a) (b) (c) (d) (e)
10. (a) (b) (c) (d) (e)
11. (a) (b) (c) (d) (e)
12. (a) (b) (c) (d) (e)
13. (a) (b) (c) (d) (e)
14. (a) (b) (c) (d) (e)
15. (a) (b) (c) (d) (e)
16. (a) (b) (c) (d) (e)

17. (a) (b) (c) (d) (e)
18. (a) (b) (c) (d) (e)
19. (a) (b) (c) (d) (e)
20. (a) (b) (c) (d) (e)
21. (a) (b) (c) (d) (e)
22. (a) (b) (c) (d) (e)
23. (a) (b) (c) (d) (e)
24. (a) (b) (c) (d) (e)

25. (a) (b) (c) (d) (e)

This page intentionally left blank.

Section 3

Clinical Pathology

Fill in a circled letter to indicate your answer choice.

1. ⓐ ⓑ ⓒ ⓓ ⓔ	27. ⓐ ⓑ ⓒ ⓓ ⓔ	53. ⓐ ⓑ ⓒ ⓓ ⓔ	79. ⓐ ⓑ ⓒ ⓓ ⓔ
2. ⓐ ⓑ ⓒ ⓓ ⓔ	28. ⓐ ⓑ ⓒ ⓓ ⓔ	54. ⓐ ⓑ ⓒ ⓓ ⓔ	80. ⓐ ⓑ ⓒ ⓓ ⓔ
3. ⓐ ⓑ ⓒ ⓓ ⓔ	29. ⓐ ⓑ ⓒ ⓓ ⓔ	55. ⓐ ⓑ ⓒ ⓓ ⓔ	81. ⓐ ⓑ ⓒ ⓓ ⓔ
4. ⓐ ⓑ ⓒ ⓓ ⓔ	30. ⓐ ⓑ ⓒ ⓓ ⓔ	56. ⓐ ⓑ ⓒ ⓓ ⓔ	82. ⓐ ⓑ ⓒ ⓓ ⓔ
5. ⓐ ⓑ ⓒ ⓓ ⓔ	31. ⓐ ⓑ ⓒ ⓓ ⓔ	57. ⓐ ⓑ ⓒ ⓓ ⓔ	83. ⓐ ⓑ ⓒ ⓓ ⓔ
6. ⓐ ⓑ ⓒ ⓓ ⓔ	32. ⓐ ⓑ ⓒ ⓓ ⓔ	58. ⓐ ⓑ ⓒ ⓓ ⓔ	84. ⓐ ⓑ ⓒ ⓓ ⓔ
7. ⓐ ⓑ ⓒ ⓓ ⓔ	33. ⓐ ⓑ ⓒ ⓓ ⓔ	59. ⓐ ⓑ ⓒ ⓓ ⓔ	85. ⓐ ⓑ ⓒ ⓓ ⓔ
8. ⓐ ⓑ ⓒ ⓓ ⓔ	34. ⓐ ⓑ ⓒ ⓓ ⓔ	60. ⓐ ⓑ ⓒ ⓓ ⓔ	86. ⓐ ⓑ ⓒ ⓓ ⓔ
9. ⓐ ⓑ ⓒ ⓓ ⓔ	35. ⓐ ⓑ ⓒ ⓓ ⓔ	61. ⓐ ⓑ ⓒ ⓓ ⓔ	87. ⓐ ⓑ ⓒ ⓓ ⓔ
10. ⓐ ⓑ ⓒ ⓓ ⓔ	36. ⓐ ⓑ ⓒ ⓓ ⓔ	62. ⓐ ⓑ ⓒ ⓓ ⓔ	88. ⓐ ⓑ ⓒ ⓓ ⓔ
11. ⓐ ⓑ ⓒ ⓓ ⓔ	37. ⓐ ⓑ ⓒ ⓓ ⓔ	63. ⓐ ⓑ ⓒ ⓓ ⓔ	89. ⓐ ⓑ ⓒ ⓓ ⓔ
12. ⓐ ⓑ ⓒ ⓓ ⓔ	38. ⓐ ⓑ ⓒ ⓓ ⓔ	64. ⓐ ⓑ ⓒ ⓓ ⓔ	90. ⓐ ⓑ ⓒ ⓓ ⓔ
13. ⓐ ⓑ ⓒ ⓓ ⓔ	39. ⓐ ⓑ ⓒ ⓓ ⓔ	65. ⓐ ⓑ ⓒ ⓓ ⓔ	91. ⓐ ⓑ ⓒ ⓓ ⓔ
14. ⓐ ⓑ ⓒ ⓓ ⓔ	40. ⓐ ⓑ ⓒ ⓓ ⓔ	66. ⓐ ⓑ ⓒ ⓓ ⓔ	92. ⓐ ⓑ ⓒ ⓓ ⓔ
15. ⓐ ⓑ ⓒ ⓓ ⓔ	41. ⓐ ⓑ ⓒ ⓓ ⓔ	67. ⓐ ⓑ ⓒ ⓓ ⓔ	93. ⓐ ⓑ ⓒ ⓓ ⓔ
16. ⓐ ⓑ ⓒ ⓓ ⓔ	42. ⓐ ⓑ ⓒ ⓓ ⓔ	68. ⓐ ⓑ ⓒ ⓓ ⓔ	94. ⓐ ⓑ ⓒ ⓓ ⓔ
17. ⓐ ⓑ ⓒ ⓓ ⓔ	43. ⓐ ⓑ ⓒ ⓓ ⓔ	69. ⓐ ⓑ ⓒ ⓓ ⓔ	95. ⓐ ⓑ ⓒ ⓓ ⓔ
18. ⓐ ⓑ ⓒ ⓓ ⓔ	44. ⓐ ⓑ ⓒ ⓓ ⓔ	70. ⓐ ⓑ ⓒ ⓓ ⓔ	96. ⓐ ⓑ ⓒ ⓓ ⓔ
19. ⓐ ⓑ ⓒ ⓓ ⓔ	45. ⓐ ⓑ ⓒ ⓓ ⓔ	71. ⓐ ⓑ ⓒ ⓓ ⓔ	97. ⓐ ⓑ ⓒ ⓓ ⓔ
20. ⓐ ⓑ ⓒ ⓓ ⓔ	46. ⓐ ⓑ ⓒ ⓓ ⓔ	72. ⓐ ⓑ ⓒ ⓓ ⓔ	98. ⓐ ⓑ ⓒ ⓓ ⓔ
21. ⓐ ⓑ ⓒ ⓓ ⓔ	47. ⓐ ⓑ ⓒ ⓓ ⓔ	73. ⓐ ⓑ ⓒ ⓓ ⓔ	99. ⓐ ⓑ ⓒ ⓓ ⓔ
22. ⓐ ⓑ ⓒ ⓓ ⓔ	48. ⓐ ⓑ ⓒ ⓓ ⓔ	74. ⓐ ⓑ ⓒ ⓓ ⓔ	100. ⓐ ⓑ ⓒ ⓓ ⓔ
23. ⓐ ⓑ ⓒ ⓓ ⓔ	49. ⓐ ⓑ ⓒ ⓓ ⓔ	75. ⓐ ⓑ ⓒ ⓓ ⓔ	
24. ⓐ ⓑ ⓒ ⓓ ⓔ	50. ⓐ ⓑ ⓒ ⓓ ⓔ	76. ⓐ ⓑ ⓒ ⓓ ⓔ	
25. ⓐ ⓑ ⓒ ⓓ ⓔ	51. ⓐ ⓑ ⓒ ⓓ ⓔ	77. ⓐ ⓑ ⓒ ⓓ ⓔ	
26. ⓐ ⓑ ⓒ ⓓ ⓔ	52. ⓐ ⓑ ⓒ ⓓ ⓔ	78. ⓐ ⓑ ⓒ ⓓ ⓔ	

This page intentionally left blank.

Practice Answer Sheet
Section 4
Dentistry

Fill in a circled letter to indicate your answer choice.

1. ⓐ ⓑ ⓒ ⓓ ⓔ	25. ⓐ ⓑ ⓒ ⓓ ⓔ	49. ⓐ ⓑ ⓒ ⓓ ⓔ	73. ⓐ ⓑ ⓒ ⓓ ⓔ
2. ⓐ ⓑ ⓒ ⓓ ⓔ	26. ⓐ ⓑ ⓒ ⓓ ⓔ	50. ⓐ ⓑ ⓒ ⓓ ⓔ	74. ⓐ ⓑ ⓒ ⓓ ⓔ
3. ⓐ ⓑ ⓒ ⓓ ⓔ	27. ⓐ ⓑ ⓒ ⓓ ⓔ	51. ⓐ ⓑ ⓒ ⓓ ⓔ	75. ⓐ ⓑ ⓒ ⓓ ⓔ
4. ⓐ ⓑ ⓒ ⓓ ⓔ	28. ⓐ ⓑ ⓒ ⓓ ⓔ	52. ⓐ ⓑ ⓒ ⓓ ⓔ	76. ⓐ ⓑ ⓒ ⓓ ⓔ
5. ⓐ ⓑ ⓒ ⓓ ⓔ	29. ⓐ ⓑ ⓒ ⓓ ⓔ	53. ⓐ ⓑ ⓒ ⓓ ⓔ	77. ⓐ ⓑ ⓒ ⓓ ⓔ
6. ⓐ ⓑ ⓒ ⓓ ⓔ	30. ⓐ ⓑ ⓒ ⓓ ⓔ	54. ⓐ ⓑ ⓒ ⓓ ⓔ	78. ⓐ ⓑ ⓒ ⓓ ⓔ
7. ⓐ ⓑ ⓒ ⓓ ⓔ	31. ⓐ ⓑ ⓒ ⓓ ⓔ	55. ⓐ ⓑ ⓒ ⓓ ⓔ	79. ⓐ ⓑ ⓒ ⓓ ⓔ
8. ⓐ ⓑ ⓒ ⓓ ⓔ	32. ⓐ ⓑ ⓒ ⓓ ⓔ	56. ⓐ ⓑ ⓒ ⓓ ⓔ	80. ⓐ ⓑ ⓒ ⓓ ⓔ
9. ⓐ ⓑ ⓒ ⓓ ⓔ	33. ⓐ ⓑ ⓒ ⓓ ⓔ	57. ⓐ ⓑ ⓒ ⓓ ⓔ	81. ⓐ ⓑ ⓒ ⓓ ⓔ
10. ⓐ ⓑ ⓒ ⓓ ⓔ	34. ⓐ ⓑ ⓒ ⓓ ⓔ	58. ⓐ ⓑ ⓒ ⓓ ⓔ	82. ⓐ ⓑ ⓒ ⓓ ⓔ
11. ⓐ ⓑ ⓒ ⓓ ⓔ	35. ⓐ ⓑ ⓒ ⓓ ⓔ	59. ⓐ ⓑ ⓒ ⓓ ⓔ	83. ⓐ ⓑ ⓒ ⓓ ⓔ
12. ⓐ ⓑ ⓒ ⓓ ⓔ	36. ⓐ ⓑ ⓒ ⓓ ⓔ	60. ⓐ ⓑ ⓒ ⓓ ⓔ	84. ⓐ ⓑ ⓒ ⓓ ⓔ
13. ⓐ ⓑ ⓒ ⓓ ⓔ	37. ⓐ ⓑ ⓒ ⓓ ⓔ	61. ⓐ ⓑ ⓒ ⓓ ⓔ	85. ⓐ ⓑ ⓒ ⓓ ⓔ
14. ⓐ ⓑ ⓒ ⓓ ⓔ	38. ⓐ ⓑ ⓒ ⓓ ⓔ	62. ⓐ ⓑ ⓒ ⓓ ⓔ	86. ⓐ ⓑ ⓒ ⓓ ⓔ
15. ⓐ ⓑ ⓒ ⓓ ⓔ	39. ⓐ ⓑ ⓒ ⓓ ⓔ	63. ⓐ ⓑ ⓒ ⓓ ⓔ	87. ⓐ ⓑ ⓒ ⓓ ⓔ
16. ⓐ ⓑ ⓒ ⓓ ⓔ	40. ⓐ ⓑ ⓒ ⓓ ⓔ	64. ⓐ ⓑ ⓒ ⓓ ⓔ	88. ⓐ ⓑ ⓒ ⓓ ⓔ
17. ⓐ ⓑ ⓒ ⓓ ⓔ	41. ⓐ ⓑ ⓒ ⓓ ⓔ	65. ⓐ ⓑ ⓒ ⓓ ⓔ	89. ⓐ ⓑ ⓒ ⓓ ⓔ
18. ⓐ ⓑ ⓒ ⓓ ⓔ	42. ⓐ ⓑ ⓒ ⓓ ⓔ	66. ⓐ ⓑ ⓒ ⓓ ⓔ	90. ⓐ ⓑ ⓒ ⓓ ⓔ
19. ⓐ ⓑ ⓒ ⓓ ⓔ	43. ⓐ ⓑ ⓒ ⓓ ⓔ	67. ⓐ ⓑ ⓒ ⓓ ⓔ	91. ⓐ ⓑ ⓒ ⓓ ⓔ
20. ⓐ ⓑ ⓒ ⓓ ⓔ	44. ⓐ ⓑ ⓒ ⓓ ⓔ	68. ⓐ ⓑ ⓒ ⓓ ⓔ	92. ⓐ ⓑ ⓒ ⓓ ⓔ
21. ⓐ ⓑ ⓒ ⓓ ⓔ	45. ⓐ ⓑ ⓒ ⓓ ⓔ	69. ⓐ ⓑ ⓒ ⓓ ⓔ	93. ⓐ ⓑ ⓒ ⓓ ⓔ
22. ⓐ ⓑ ⓒ ⓓ ⓔ	46. ⓐ ⓑ ⓒ ⓓ ⓔ	70. ⓐ ⓑ ⓒ ⓓ ⓔ	94. ⓐ ⓑ ⓒ ⓓ ⓔ
23. ⓐ ⓑ ⓒ ⓓ ⓔ	47. ⓐ ⓑ ⓒ ⓓ ⓔ	71. ⓐ ⓑ ⓒ ⓓ ⓔ	95. ⓐ ⓑ ⓒ ⓓ ⓔ
24. ⓐ ⓑ ⓒ ⓓ ⓔ	48. ⓐ ⓑ ⓒ ⓓ ⓔ	72. ⓐ ⓑ ⓒ ⓓ ⓔ	96. ⓐ ⓑ ⓒ ⓓ ⓔ

This page intentionally left blank.

Dermatology

Fill in a circled letter to indicate your answer choice.

1. ⓐ ⓑ ⓒ ⓓ ⓔ	15. ⓐ ⓑ ⓒ ⓓ ⓔ	29. ⓐ ⓑ ⓒ ⓓ ⓔ	43. ⓐ ⓑ ⓒ ⓓ ⓔ
2. ⓐ ⓑ ⓒ ⓓ ⓔ	16. ⓐ ⓑ ⓒ ⓓ ⓔ	30. ⓐ ⓑ ⓒ ⓓ ⓔ	44. ⓐ ⓑ ⓒ ⓓ ⓔ
3. ⓐ ⓑ ⓒ ⓓ ⓔ	17. ⓐ ⓑ ⓒ ⓓ ⓔ	31. ⓐ ⓑ ⓒ ⓓ ⓔ	45. ⓐ ⓑ ⓒ ⓓ ⓔ
4. ⓐ ⓑ ⓒ ⓓ ⓔ	18. ⓐ ⓑ ⓒ ⓓ ⓔ	32. ⓐ ⓑ ⓒ ⓓ ⓔ	46. ⓐ ⓑ ⓒ ⓓ ⓔ
5. ⓐ ⓑ ⓒ ⓓ ⓔ	19. ⓐ ⓑ ⓒ ⓓ ⓔ	33. ⓐ ⓑ ⓒ ⓓ ⓔ	47. ⓐ ⓑ ⓒ ⓓ ⓔ
6. ⓐ ⓑ ⓒ ⓓ ⓔ	20. ⓐ ⓑ ⓒ ⓓ ⓔ	34. ⓐ ⓑ ⓒ ⓓ ⓔ	48. ⓐ ⓑ ⓒ ⓓ ⓔ
7. ⓐ ⓑ ⓒ ⓓ ⓔ	21. ⓐ ⓑ ⓒ ⓓ ⓔ	35. ⓐ ⓑ ⓒ ⓓ ⓔ	49. ⓐ ⓑ ⓒ ⓓ ⓔ
8. ⓐ ⓑ ⓒ ⓓ ⓔ	22. ⓐ ⓑ ⓒ ⓓ ⓔ	36. ⓐ ⓑ ⓒ ⓓ ⓔ	50. ⓐ ⓑ ⓒ ⓓ ⓔ
9. ⓐ ⓑ ⓒ ⓓ ⓔ	23. ⓐ ⓑ ⓒ ⓓ ⓔ	37. ⓐ ⓑ ⓒ ⓓ ⓔ	
10. ⓐ ⓑ ⓒ ⓓ ⓔ	24. ⓐ ⓑ ⓒ ⓓ ⓔ	38. ⓐ ⓑ ⓒ ⓓ ⓔ	
11. ⓐ ⓑ ⓒ ⓓ ⓔ	25. ⓐ ⓑ ⓒ ⓓ ⓔ	39. ⓐ ⓑ ⓒ ⓓ ⓔ	
12. ⓐ ⓑ ⓒ ⓓ ⓔ	26. ⓐ ⓑ ⓒ ⓓ ⓔ	40. ⓐ ⓑ ⓒ ⓓ ⓔ	
13. ⓐ ⓑ ⓒ ⓓ ⓔ	27. ⓐ ⓑ ⓒ ⓓ ⓔ	41. ⓐ ⓑ ⓒ ⓓ ⓔ	
14. ⓐ ⓑ ⓒ ⓓ ⓔ	28. ⓐ ⓑ ⓒ ⓓ ⓔ	42. ⓐ ⓑ ⓒ ⓓ ⓔ	

This page intentionally left blank.

Practice Answer Sheet
Section 6
Hematology

Fill in a circled letter to indicate your answer choice.

1. ⓐ ⓑ ⓒ ⓓ ⓔ	15. ⓐ ⓑ ⓒ ⓓ ⓔ	29. ⓐ ⓑ ⓒ ⓓ ⓔ	43. ⓐ ⓑ ⓒ ⓓ ⓔ
2. ⓐ ⓑ ⓒ ⓓ ⓔ	16. ⓐ ⓑ ⓒ ⓓ ⓔ	30. ⓐ ⓑ ⓒ ⓓ ⓔ	44. ⓐ ⓑ ⓒ ⓓ ⓔ
3. ⓐ ⓑ ⓒ ⓓ ⓔ	17. ⓐ ⓑ ⓒ ⓓ ⓔ	31. ⓐ ⓑ ⓒ ⓓ ⓔ	45. ⓐ ⓑ ⓒ ⓓ ⓔ
4. ⓐ ⓑ ⓒ ⓓ ⓔ	18. ⓐ ⓑ ⓒ ⓓ ⓔ	32. ⓐ ⓑ ⓒ ⓓ ⓔ	46. ⓐ ⓑ ⓒ ⓓ ⓔ
5. ⓐ ⓑ ⓒ ⓓ ⓔ	19. ⓐ ⓑ ⓒ ⓓ ⓔ	33. ⓐ ⓑ ⓒ ⓓ ⓔ	47. ⓐ ⓑ ⓒ ⓓ ⓔ
6. ⓐ ⓑ ⓒ ⓓ ⓔ	20. ⓐ ⓑ ⓒ ⓓ ⓔ	34. ⓐ ⓑ ⓒ ⓓ ⓔ	48. ⓐ ⓑ ⓒ ⓓ ⓔ
7. ⓐ ⓑ ⓒ ⓓ ⓔ	21. ⓐ ⓑ ⓒ ⓓ ⓔ	35. ⓐ ⓑ ⓒ ⓓ ⓔ	49. ⓐ ⓑ ⓒ ⓓ ⓔ
8. ⓐ ⓑ ⓒ ⓓ ⓔ	22. ⓐ ⓑ ⓒ ⓓ ⓔ	36. ⓐ ⓑ ⓒ ⓓ ⓔ	50. ⓐ ⓑ ⓒ ⓓ ⓔ
9. ⓐ ⓑ ⓒ ⓓ ⓔ	23. ⓐ ⓑ ⓒ ⓓ ⓔ	37. ⓐ ⓑ ⓒ ⓓ ⓔ	
10. ⓐ ⓑ ⓒ ⓓ ⓔ	24. ⓐ ⓑ ⓒ ⓓ ⓔ	38. ⓐ ⓑ ⓒ ⓓ ⓔ	
11. ⓐ ⓑ ⓒ ⓓ ⓔ	25. ⓐ ⓑ ⓒ ⓓ ⓔ	39. ⓐ ⓑ ⓒ ⓓ ⓔ	
12. ⓐ ⓑ ⓒ ⓓ ⓔ	26. ⓐ ⓑ ⓒ ⓓ ⓔ	40. ⓐ ⓑ ⓒ ⓓ ⓔ	
13. ⓐ ⓑ ⓒ ⓓ ⓔ	27. ⓐ ⓑ ⓒ ⓓ ⓔ	41. ⓐ ⓑ ⓒ ⓓ ⓔ	
14. ⓐ ⓑ ⓒ ⓓ ⓔ	28. ⓐ ⓑ ⓒ ⓓ ⓔ	42. ⓐ ⓑ ⓒ ⓓ ⓔ	

This page intentionally left blank.

Section 7
Medical Diseases
Fill in a circled letter to indicate your answer choice.

#						#						#						#					
1.	ⓐ	ⓑ	ⓒ	ⓓ	ⓔ	47.	ⓐ	ⓑ	ⓒ	ⓓ	ⓔ	93.	ⓐ	ⓑ	ⓒ	ⓓ	ⓔ	139.	ⓐ	ⓑ	ⓒ	ⓓ	ⓔ
2.	ⓐ	ⓑ	ⓒ	ⓓ	ⓔ	48.	ⓐ	ⓑ	ⓒ	ⓓ	ⓔ	94.	ⓐ	ⓑ	ⓒ	ⓓ	ⓔ	140.	ⓐ	ⓑ	ⓒ	ⓓ	ⓔ
3.	ⓐ	ⓑ	ⓒ	ⓓ	ⓔ	49.	ⓐ	ⓑ	ⓒ	ⓓ	ⓔ	95.	ⓐ	ⓑ	ⓒ	ⓓ	ⓔ	141.	ⓐ	ⓑ	ⓒ	ⓓ	ⓔ
4.	ⓐ	ⓑ	ⓒ	ⓓ	ⓔ	50.	ⓐ	ⓑ	ⓒ	ⓓ	ⓔ	96.	ⓐ	ⓑ	ⓒ	ⓓ	ⓔ	142.	ⓐ	ⓑ	ⓒ	ⓓ	ⓔ
5.	ⓐ	ⓑ	ⓒ	ⓓ	ⓔ	51.	ⓐ	ⓑ	ⓒ	ⓓ	ⓔ	97.	ⓐ	ⓑ	ⓒ	ⓓ	ⓔ	143.	ⓐ	ⓑ	ⓒ	ⓓ	ⓔ
6.	ⓐ	ⓑ	ⓒ	ⓓ	ⓔ	52.	ⓐ	ⓑ	ⓒ	ⓓ	ⓔ	98.	ⓐ	ⓑ	ⓒ	ⓓ	ⓔ	144.	ⓐ	ⓑ	ⓒ	ⓓ	ⓔ
7.	ⓐ	ⓑ	ⓒ	ⓓ	ⓔ	53.	ⓐ	ⓑ	ⓒ	ⓓ	ⓔ	99.	ⓐ	ⓑ	ⓒ	ⓓ	ⓔ	145.	ⓐ	ⓑ	ⓒ	ⓓ	ⓔ
8.	ⓐ	ⓑ	ⓒ	ⓓ	ⓔ	54.	ⓐ	ⓑ	ⓒ	ⓓ	ⓔ	100.	ⓐ	ⓑ	ⓒ	ⓓ	ⓔ	146.	ⓐ	ⓑ	ⓒ	ⓓ	ⓔ
9.	ⓐ	ⓑ	ⓒ	ⓓ	ⓔ	55.	ⓐ	ⓑ	ⓒ	ⓓ	ⓔ	101.	ⓐ	ⓑ	ⓒ	ⓓ	ⓔ	147.	ⓐ	ⓑ	ⓒ	ⓓ	ⓔ
10.	ⓐ	ⓑ	ⓒ	ⓓ	ⓔ	56.	ⓐ	ⓑ	ⓒ	ⓓ	ⓔ	102.	ⓐ	ⓑ	ⓒ	ⓓ	ⓔ	148.	ⓐ	ⓑ	ⓒ	ⓓ	ⓔ
11.	ⓐ	ⓑ	ⓒ	ⓓ	ⓔ	57.	ⓐ	ⓑ	ⓒ	ⓓ	ⓔ	103.	ⓐ	ⓑ	ⓒ	ⓓ	ⓔ	149.	ⓐ	ⓑ	ⓒ	ⓓ	ⓔ
12.	ⓐ	ⓑ	ⓒ	ⓓ	ⓔ	58.	ⓐ	ⓑ	ⓒ	ⓓ	ⓔ	104.	ⓐ	ⓑ	ⓒ	ⓓ	ⓔ	150.	ⓐ	ⓑ	ⓒ	ⓓ	ⓔ
13.	ⓐ	ⓑ	ⓒ	ⓓ	ⓔ	59.	ⓐ	ⓑ	ⓒ	ⓓ	ⓔ	105.	ⓐ	ⓑ	ⓒ	ⓓ	ⓔ	151.	ⓐ	ⓑ	ⓒ	ⓓ	ⓔ
14.	ⓐ	ⓑ	ⓒ	ⓓ	ⓔ	60.	ⓐ	ⓑ	ⓒ	ⓓ	ⓔ	106.	ⓐ	ⓑ	ⓒ	ⓓ	ⓔ	152.	ⓐ	ⓑ	ⓒ	ⓓ	ⓔ
15.	ⓐ	ⓑ	ⓒ	ⓓ	ⓔ	61.	ⓐ	ⓑ	ⓒ	ⓓ	ⓔ	107.	ⓐ	ⓑ	ⓒ	ⓓ	ⓔ	153.	ⓐ	ⓑ	ⓒ	ⓓ	ⓔ
16.	ⓐ	ⓑ	ⓒ	ⓓ	ⓔ	62.	ⓐ	ⓑ	ⓒ	ⓓ	ⓔ	108.	ⓐ	ⓑ	ⓒ	ⓓ	ⓔ	154.	ⓐ	ⓑ	ⓒ	ⓓ	ⓔ
17.	ⓐ	ⓑ	ⓒ	ⓓ	ⓔ	63.	ⓐ	ⓑ	ⓒ	ⓓ	ⓔ	109.	ⓐ	ⓑ	ⓒ	ⓓ	ⓔ	155.	ⓐ	ⓑ	ⓒ	ⓓ	ⓔ
18.	ⓐ	ⓑ	ⓒ	ⓓ	ⓔ	64.	ⓐ	ⓑ	ⓒ	ⓓ	ⓔ	110.	ⓐ	ⓑ	ⓒ	ⓓ	ⓔ	156.	ⓐ	ⓑ	ⓒ	ⓓ	ⓔ
19.	ⓐ	ⓑ	ⓒ	ⓓ	ⓔ	65.	ⓐ	ⓑ	ⓒ	ⓓ	ⓔ	111.	ⓐ	ⓑ	ⓒ	ⓓ	ⓔ	157.	ⓐ	ⓑ	ⓒ	ⓓ	ⓔ
20.	ⓐ	ⓑ	ⓒ	ⓓ	ⓔ	66.	ⓐ	ⓑ	ⓒ	ⓓ	ⓔ	112.	ⓐ	ⓑ	ⓒ	ⓓ	ⓔ	158.	ⓐ	ⓑ	ⓒ	ⓓ	ⓔ
21.	ⓐ	ⓑ	ⓒ	ⓓ	ⓔ	67.	ⓐ	ⓑ	ⓒ	ⓓ	ⓔ	113.	ⓐ	ⓑ	ⓒ	ⓓ	ⓔ	159.	ⓐ	ⓑ	ⓒ	ⓓ	ⓔ
22.	ⓐ	ⓑ	ⓒ	ⓓ	ⓔ	68.	ⓐ	ⓑ	ⓒ	ⓓ	ⓔ	114.	ⓐ	ⓑ	ⓒ	ⓓ	ⓔ	160.	ⓐ	ⓑ	ⓒ	ⓓ	ⓔ
23.	ⓐ	ⓑ	ⓒ	ⓓ	ⓔ	69.	ⓐ	ⓑ	ⓒ	ⓓ	ⓔ	115.	ⓐ	ⓑ	ⓒ	ⓓ	ⓔ	161.	ⓐ	ⓑ	ⓒ	ⓓ	ⓔ
24.	ⓐ	ⓑ	ⓒ	ⓓ	ⓔ	70.	ⓐ	ⓑ	ⓒ	ⓓ	ⓔ	116.	ⓐ	ⓑ	ⓒ	ⓓ	ⓔ	162.	ⓐ	ⓑ	ⓒ	ⓓ	ⓔ
25.	ⓐ	ⓑ	ⓒ	ⓓ	ⓔ	71.	ⓐ	ⓑ	ⓒ	ⓓ	ⓔ	117.	ⓐ	ⓑ	ⓒ	ⓓ	ⓔ	163.	ⓐ	ⓑ	ⓒ	ⓓ	ⓔ
26.	ⓐ	ⓑ	ⓒ	ⓓ	ⓔ	72.	ⓐ	ⓑ	ⓒ	ⓓ	ⓔ	118.	ⓐ	ⓑ	ⓒ	ⓓ	ⓔ	164.	ⓐ	ⓑ	ⓒ	ⓓ	ⓔ
27.	ⓐ	ⓑ	ⓒ	ⓓ	ⓔ	73.	ⓐ	ⓑ	ⓒ	ⓓ	ⓔ	119.	ⓐ	ⓑ	ⓒ	ⓓ	ⓔ	165.	ⓐ	ⓑ	ⓒ	ⓓ	ⓔ
28.	ⓐ	ⓑ	ⓒ	ⓓ	ⓔ	74.	ⓐ	ⓑ	ⓒ	ⓓ	ⓔ	120.	ⓐ	ⓑ	ⓒ	ⓓ	ⓔ	166.	ⓐ	ⓑ	ⓒ	ⓓ	ⓔ
29.	ⓐ	ⓑ	ⓒ	ⓓ	ⓔ	75.	ⓐ	ⓑ	ⓒ	ⓓ	ⓔ	121.	ⓐ	ⓑ	ⓒ	ⓓ	ⓔ	167.	ⓐ	ⓑ	ⓒ	ⓓ	ⓔ
30.	ⓐ	ⓑ	ⓒ	ⓓ	ⓔ	76.	ⓐ	ⓑ	ⓒ	ⓓ	ⓔ	122.	ⓐ	ⓑ	ⓒ	ⓓ	ⓔ	168.	ⓐ	ⓑ	ⓒ	ⓓ	ⓔ
31.	ⓐ	ⓑ	ⓒ	ⓓ	ⓔ	77.	ⓐ	ⓑ	ⓒ	ⓓ	ⓔ	123.	ⓐ	ⓑ	ⓒ	ⓓ	ⓔ	169.	ⓐ	ⓑ	ⓒ	ⓓ	ⓔ
32.	ⓐ	ⓑ	ⓒ	ⓓ	ⓔ	78.	ⓐ	ⓑ	ⓒ	ⓓ	ⓔ	124.	ⓐ	ⓑ	ⓒ	ⓓ	ⓔ	170.	ⓐ	ⓑ	ⓒ	ⓓ	
33.	ⓐ	ⓑ	ⓒ	ⓓ	ⓔ	79.	ⓐ	ⓑ	ⓒ	ⓓ	ⓔ	125.	ⓐ	ⓑ	ⓒ	ⓓ	ⓔ	171.	ⓐ	ⓑ	ⓒ	ⓓ	
34.	ⓐ	ⓑ	ⓒ	ⓓ	ⓔ	80.	ⓐ	ⓑ	ⓒ	ⓓ	ⓔ	126.	ⓐ	ⓑ	ⓒ	ⓓ	ⓔ	172.	ⓐ	ⓑ	ⓒ	ⓓ	
35.	ⓐ	ⓑ	ⓒ	ⓓ	ⓔ	81.	ⓐ	ⓑ	ⓒ	ⓓ	ⓔ	127.	ⓐ	ⓑ	ⓒ	ⓓ	ⓔ	173.	ⓐ	ⓑ	ⓒ	ⓓ	
36.	ⓐ	ⓑ	ⓒ	ⓓ	ⓔ	82.	ⓐ	ⓑ	ⓒ	ⓓ	ⓔ	128.	ⓐ	ⓑ	ⓒ	ⓓ	ⓔ	174.	ⓐ	ⓑ	ⓒ	ⓓ	ⓔ
37.	ⓐ	ⓑ	ⓒ	ⓓ	ⓔ	83.	ⓐ	ⓑ	ⓒ	ⓓ	ⓔ	129.	ⓐ	ⓑ	ⓒ	ⓓ	ⓔ	175.	ⓐ	ⓑ	ⓒ	ⓓ	ⓔ
38.	ⓐ	ⓑ	ⓒ	ⓓ	ⓔ	84.	ⓐ	ⓑ	ⓒ	ⓓ	ⓔ	130.	ⓐ	ⓑ	ⓒ	ⓓ	ⓔ	176.	ⓐ	ⓑ	ⓒ	ⓓ	ⓔ
39.	ⓐ	ⓑ	ⓒ	ⓓ	ⓔ	85.	ⓐ	ⓑ	ⓒ	ⓓ	ⓔ	131.	ⓐ	ⓑ	ⓒ	ⓓ	ⓔ	177.	ⓐ	ⓑ	ⓒ	ⓓ	ⓔ
40.	ⓐ	ⓑ	ⓒ	ⓓ	ⓔ	86.	ⓐ	ⓑ	ⓒ	ⓓ	ⓔ	132.	ⓐ	ⓑ	ⓒ	ⓓ	ⓔ	178.	ⓐ	ⓑ	ⓒ	ⓓ	ⓔ
41.	ⓐ	ⓑ	ⓒ	ⓓ	ⓔ	87.	ⓐ	ⓑ	ⓒ	ⓓ		133.	ⓐ	ⓑ	ⓒ	ⓓ	ⓔ	179.	ⓐ	ⓑ	ⓒ	ⓓ	ⓔ
42.	ⓐ	ⓑ	ⓒ	ⓓ	ⓔ	88.	ⓐ	ⓑ	ⓒ	ⓓ		134.	ⓐ	ⓑ	ⓒ	ⓓ	ⓔ	180.	ⓐ	ⓑ	ⓒ	ⓓ	ⓔ
43.	ⓐ	ⓑ	ⓒ	ⓓ	ⓔ	89.	ⓐ	ⓑ	ⓒ	ⓓ		135.	ⓐ	ⓑ	ⓒ	ⓓ	ⓔ	181.	ⓐ	ⓑ	ⓒ	ⓓ	ⓔ
44.	ⓐ	ⓑ	ⓒ	ⓓ	ⓔ	90.	ⓐ	ⓑ	ⓒ	ⓓ		136.	ⓐ	ⓑ	ⓒ	ⓓ	ⓔ	182.	ⓐ	ⓑ	ⓒ	ⓓ	ⓔ
45.	ⓐ	ⓑ	ⓒ	ⓓ	ⓔ	91.	ⓐ	ⓑ	ⓒ	ⓓ	ⓔ	137.	ⓐ	ⓑ	ⓒ	ⓓ	ⓔ	183.	ⓐ	ⓑ	ⓒ	ⓓ	ⓔ
46.	ⓐ	ⓑ	ⓒ	ⓓ	ⓔ	92.	ⓐ	ⓑ	ⓒ	ⓓ	ⓔ	138.	ⓐ	ⓑ	ⓒ	ⓓ	ⓔ	184.	ⓐ	ⓑ	ⓒ	ⓓ	ⓔ

Continued

342

Medical Diseases, continued

185. ⓐ ⓑ ⓒ ⓓ ⓔ	231. ⓐ ⓑ ⓒ ⓓ ⓔ	277. ⓐ ⓑ ⓒ ⓓ ⓔ	323. ⓐ ⓑ ⓒ ⓓ ⓔ
186. ⓐ ⓑ ⓒ ⓓ ⓔ	232. ⓐ ⓑ ⓒ ⓓ ⓔ	278. ⓐ ⓑ ⓒ ⓓ ⓔ	324. ⓐ ⓑ ⓒ ⓓ ⓔ
187. ⓐ ⓑ ⓒ ⓓ ⓔ	233. ⓐ ⓑ ⓒ ⓓ ⓔ	279. ⓐ ⓑ ⓒ ⓓ ⓔ	325. ⓐ ⓑ ⓒ ⓓ ⓔ
188. ⓐ ⓑ ⓒ ⓓ ⓔ	234. ⓐ ⓑ ⓒ ⓓ ⓔ	280. ⓐ ⓑ ⓒ ⓓ ⓔ	326. ⓐ ⓑ ⓒ ⓓ ⓔ
189. ⓐ ⓑ ⓒ ⓓ ⓔ	235. ⓐ ⓑ ⓒ ⓓ ⓔ	281. ⓐ ⓑ ⓒ ⓓ ⓔ	327. ⓐ ⓑ ⓒ ⓓ ⓔ
190. ⓐ ⓑ ⓒ ⓓ ⓔ	236. ⓐ ⓑ ⓒ ⓓ ⓔ	282. ⓐ ⓑ ⓒ ⓓ ⓔ	328. ⓐ ⓑ ⓒ ⓓ ⓔ
191. ⓐ ⓑ ⓒ ⓓ ⓔ	237. ⓐ ⓑ ⓒ ⓓ ⓔ	283. ⓐ ⓑ ⓒ ⓓ ⓔ	329. ⓐ ⓑ ⓒ ⓓ ⓔ
192. ⓐ ⓑ ⓒ ⓓ ⓔ	238. ⓐ ⓑ ⓒ ⓓ ⓔ	284. ⓐ ⓑ ⓒ ⓓ ⓔ	330. ⓐ ⓑ ⓒ ⓓ ⓔ
193. ⓐ ⓑ ⓒ ⓓ ⓔ	239. ⓐ ⓑ ⓒ ⓓ ⓔ	285. ⓐ ⓑ ⓒ ⓓ ⓔ	331. ⓐ ⓑ ⓒ ⓓ ⓔ
194. ⓐ ⓑ ⓒ ⓓ ⓔ	240. ⓐ ⓑ ⓒ ⓓ ⓔ	286. ⓐ ⓑ ⓒ ⓓ ⓔ	332. ⓐ ⓑ ⓒ ⓓ ⓔ
195. ⓐ ⓑ ⓒ ⓓ	241. ⓐ ⓑ ⓒ ⓓ ⓔ	287. ⓐ ⓑ ⓒ ⓓ ⓔ	333. ⓐ ⓑ ⓒ ⓓ ⓔ
196. ⓐ ⓑ ⓒ ⓓ	242. ⓐ ⓑ ⓒ ⓓ ⓔ	288. ⓐ ⓑ ⓒ ⓓ ⓔ	334. ⓐ ⓑ ⓒ ⓓ ⓔ
197. ⓐ ⓑ ⓒ ⓓ	243. ⓐ ⓑ ⓒ ⓓ ⓔ	289. ⓐ ⓑ ⓒ ⓓ ⓔ	335. ⓐ ⓑ ⓒ ⓓ ⓔ
198. ⓐ ⓑ ⓒ ⓓ	244. ⓐ ⓑ ⓒ ⓓ ⓔ	290. ⓐ ⓑ ⓒ ⓓ ⓔ	336. ⓐ ⓑ ⓒ ⓓ ⓔ
199. ⓐ ⓑ ⓒ ⓓ ⓔ	245. ⓐ ⓑ ⓒ ⓓ ⓔ	291. ⓐ ⓑ ⓒ ⓓ ⓔ	337. ⓐ ⓑ ⓒ ⓓ ⓔ
200. ⓐ ⓑ ⓒ ⓓ ⓔ	246. ⓐ ⓑ ⓒ ⓓ ⓔ	292. ⓐ ⓑ ⓒ ⓓ ⓔ	338. ⓐ ⓑ ⓒ ⓓ ⓔ
201. ⓐ ⓑ ⓒ ⓓ ⓔ	247. ⓐ ⓑ ⓒ ⓓ ⓔ	293. ⓐ ⓑ ⓒ ⓓ ⓔ	339. ⓐ ⓑ ⓒ ⓓ ⓔ
202. ⓐ ⓑ ⓒ ⓓ ⓔ	248. ⓐ ⓑ ⓒ ⓓ ⓔ	294. ⓐ ⓑ ⓒ ⓓ ⓔ	340. ⓐ ⓑ ⓒ ⓓ ⓔ
203. ⓐ ⓑ ⓒ ⓓ ⓔ	249. ⓐ ⓑ ⓒ ⓓ ⓔ	295. ⓐ ⓑ ⓒ ⓓ ⓔ	341. ⓐ ⓑ ⓒ ⓓ ⓔ
204. ⓐ ⓑ ⓒ ⓓ ⓔ	250. ⓐ ⓑ ⓒ ⓓ ⓔ	296. ⓐ ⓑ ⓒ ⓓ ⓔ	342. ⓐ ⓑ ⓒ ⓓ ⓔ
205. ⓐ ⓑ ⓒ ⓓ ⓔ	251. ⓐ ⓑ ⓒ ⓓ ⓔ	297. ⓐ ⓑ ⓒ ⓓ ⓔ	343. ⓐ ⓑ ⓒ ⓓ ⓔ
206. ⓐ ⓑ ⓒ ⓓ ⓔ	252. ⓐ ⓑ ⓒ ⓓ ⓔ	298. ⓐ ⓑ ⓒ ⓓ ⓔ	344. ⓐ ⓑ ⓒ ⓓ ⓔ
207. ⓐ ⓑ ⓒ ⓓ ⓔ	253. ⓐ ⓑ ⓒ ⓓ ⓔ	299. ⓐ ⓑ ⓒ ⓓ ⓔ	345. ⓐ ⓑ ⓒ ⓓ ⓔ
208. ⓐ ⓑ ⓒ ⓓ ⓔ	254. ⓐ ⓑ ⓒ ⓓ ⓔ	300. ⓐ ⓑ ⓒ ⓓ ⓔ	346. ⓐ ⓑ ⓒ ⓓ ⓔ
209. ⓐ ⓑ ⓒ ⓓ ⓔ	255. ⓐ ⓑ ⓒ ⓓ ⓔ	301. ⓐ ⓑ ⓒ ⓓ ⓔ	347. ⓐ ⓑ ⓒ ⓓ ⓔ
210. ⓐ ⓑ ⓒ ⓓ ⓔ	256. ⓐ ⓑ ⓒ ⓓ ⓔ	302. ⓐ ⓑ ⓒ ⓓ ⓔ	348. ⓐ ⓑ ⓒ ⓓ ⓔ
211. ⓐ ⓑ ⓒ ⓓ ⓔ	257. ⓐ ⓑ ⓒ ⓓ ⓔ	303. ⓐ ⓑ ⓒ ⓓ ⓔ	349. ⓐ ⓑ ⓒ ⓓ ⓔ
212. ⓐ ⓑ ⓒ ⓓ ⓔ	258. ⓐ ⓑ ⓒ ⓓ ⓔ	304. ⓐ ⓑ ⓒ ⓓ ⓔ	350. ⓐ ⓑ ⓒ ⓓ ⓔ
213. ⓐ ⓑ ⓒ ⓓ ⓔ	259. ⓐ ⓑ ⓒ ⓓ ⓔ	305. ⓐ ⓑ ⓒ ⓓ ⓔ	351. ⓐ ⓑ ⓒ ⓓ ⓔ
214. ⓐ ⓑ ⓒ ⓓ ⓔ	260. ⓐ ⓑ ⓒ ⓓ ⓔ	306. ⓐ ⓑ ⓒ ⓓ ⓔ	352. ⓐ ⓑ ⓒ ⓓ ⓔ
215. ⓐ ⓑ ⓒ ⓓ ⓔ	261. ⓐ ⓑ ⓒ ⓓ ⓔ	307. ⓐ ⓑ ⓒ ⓓ ⓔ	353. ⓐ ⓑ ⓒ ⓓ ⓔ
216. ⓐ ⓑ ⓒ ⓓ ⓔ	262. ⓐ ⓑ ⓒ ⓓ ⓔ	308. ⓐ ⓑ ⓒ ⓓ ⓔ	354. ⓐ ⓑ ⓒ ⓓ ⓔ
217. ⓐ ⓑ ⓒ ⓓ ⓔ	263. ⓐ ⓑ ⓒ ⓓ ⓔ	309. ⓐ ⓑ ⓒ ⓓ ⓔ	355. ⓐ ⓑ ⓒ ⓓ ⓔ
218. ⓐ ⓑ ⓒ ⓓ ⓔ	264. ⓐ ⓑ ⓒ ⓓ ⓔ	310. ⓐ ⓑ ⓒ ⓓ ⓔ	356. ⓐ ⓑ ⓒ ⓓ ⓔ
219. ⓐ ⓑ ⓒ ⓓ ⓔ	265. ⓐ ⓑ ⓒ ⓓ ⓔ	311. ⓐ ⓑ ⓒ ⓓ ⓔ	357. ⓐ ⓑ ⓒ ⓓ ⓔ
220. ⓐ ⓑ ⓒ ⓓ ⓔ	266. ⓐ ⓑ ⓒ ⓓ ⓔ	312. ⓐ ⓑ ⓒ ⓓ ⓔ	358. ⓐ ⓑ ⓒ ⓓ ⓔ
221. ⓐ ⓑ ⓒ ⓓ ⓔ	267. ⓐ ⓑ ⓒ ⓓ ⓔ	313. ⓐ ⓑ ⓒ ⓓ ⓔ	359. ⓐ ⓑ ⓒ ⓓ ⓔ
222. ⓐ ⓑ ⓒ ⓓ ⓔ	268. ⓐ ⓑ ⓒ ⓓ ⓔ	314. ⓐ ⓑ ⓒ ⓓ ⓔ	360. ⓐ ⓑ ⓒ ⓓ ⓔ
223. ⓐ ⓑ ⓒ ⓓ ⓔ	269. ⓐ ⓑ ⓒ ⓓ ⓔ	315. ⓐ ⓑ ⓒ ⓓ ⓔ	361. ⓐ ⓑ ⓒ ⓓ ⓔ
224. ⓐ ⓑ ⓒ ⓓ ⓔ	270. ⓐ ⓑ ⓒ ⓓ ⓔ	316. ⓐ ⓑ ⓒ ⓓ ⓔ	362. ⓐ ⓑ ⓒ ⓓ ⓔ
225. ⓐ ⓑ ⓒ ⓓ ⓔ	271. ⓐ ⓑ ⓒ ⓓ ⓔ	317. ⓐ ⓑ ⓒ ⓓ ⓔ	363. ⓐ ⓑ ⓒ ⓓ ⓔ
226. ⓐ ⓑ ⓒ ⓓ ⓔ	272. ⓐ ⓑ ⓒ ⓓ ⓔ	318. ⓐ ⓑ ⓒ ⓓ ⓔ	364. ⓐ ⓑ ⓒ ⓓ ⓔ
227. ⓐ ⓑ ⓒ ⓓ ⓔ	273. ⓐ ⓑ ⓒ ⓓ ⓔ	319. ⓐ ⓑ ⓒ ⓓ ⓔ	365. ⓐ ⓑ ⓒ ⓓ ⓔ
228. ⓐ ⓑ ⓒ ⓓ ⓔ	274. ⓐ ⓑ ⓒ ⓓ ⓔ	320. ⓐ ⓑ ⓒ ⓓ ⓔ	366. ⓐ ⓑ ⓒ ⓓ ⓔ
229. ⓐ ⓑ ⓒ ⓓ ⓔ	275. ⓐ ⓑ ⓒ ⓓ ⓔ	321. ⓐ ⓑ ⓒ ⓓ ⓔ	367. ⓐ ⓑ ⓒ ⓓ ⓔ
230. ⓐ ⓑ ⓒ ⓓ ⓔ	276. ⓐ ⓑ ⓒ ⓓ ⓔ	322. ⓐ ⓑ ⓒ ⓓ ⓔ	368. ⓐ ⓑ ⓒ ⓓ ⓔ

369. (a) (b) (c) (d) (e)	415. (a) (b) (c) (d) (e)	461. (a) (b) (c) (d) (e)	507. (a) (b) (c) (d) (e)
370. (a) (b) (c) (d) (e)	416. (a) (b) (c) (d) (e)	462. (a) (b) (c) (d) (e)	508. (a) (b) (c) (d) (e)
371. (a) (b) (c) (d) (e)	417. (a) (b) (c) (d) (e)	463. (a) (b) (c) (d) (e)	509. (a) (b) (c) (d) (e)
372. (a) (b) (c) (d) (e)	418. (a) (b) (c) (d) (e)	464. (a) (b) (c) (d) (e)	510. (a) (b) (c) (d) (e)
373. (a) (b) (c) (d) (e)	419. (a) (b) (c) (d) (e)	465. (a) (b) (c) (d) (e)	511. (a) (b) (c) (d) (e)
374. (a) (b) (c) (d) (e)	420. (a) (b) (c) (d) (e)	466. (a) (b) (c) (d) (e)	512. (a) (b) (c) (d) (e)
375. (a) (b) (c) (d) (e)	421. (a) (b) (c) (d) (e)	467. (a) (b) (c) (d) (e)	513. (a) (b) (c) (d) (e)
376. (a) (b) (c) (d) (e)	422. (a) (b) (c) (d) (e)	468. (a) (b) (c) (d) (e)	514. (a) (b) (c) (d) (e)
377. (a) (b) (c) (d) (e)	423. (a) (b) (c) (d) (e)	469. (a) (b) (c) (d) (e)	515. (a) (b) (c) (d) (e)
378. (a) (b) (c) (d) (e)	424. (a) (b) (c) (d) (e)	470. (a) (b) (c) (d) (e)	516. (a) (b) (c) (d) (e)
379. (a) (b) (c) (d) (e)	425. (a) (b) (c) (d) (e)	471. (a) (b) (c) (d) (e)	517. (a) (b) (c) (d) (e)
380. (a) (b) (c) (d) (e)	426. (a) (b) (c) (d) (e)	472. (a) (b) (c) (d) (e)	518. (a) (b) (c) (d) (e)
381. (a) (b) (c) (d) (e)	427. (a) (b) (c) (d) (e)	473. (a) (b) (c) (d) (e)	519. (a) (b) (c) (d) (e)
382. (a) (b) (c) (d) (e)	428. (a) (b) (c) (d) (e)	474. (a) (b) (c) (d) (e)	520. (a) (b) (c) (d) (e)
383. (a) (b) (c) (d) (e)	429. (a) (b) (c) (d) (e)	475. (a) (b) (c) (d) (e)	521. (a) (b) (c) (d) (e)
384. (a) (b) (c) (d) (e)	430. (a) (b) (c) (d) (e)	476. (a) (b) (c) (d) (e)	522. (a) (b) (c) (d) (e)
385. (a) (b) (c) (d) (e)	431. (a) (b) (c) (d) (e)	477. (a) (b) (c) (d) (e)	523. (a) (b) (c) (d) (e)
386. (a) (b) (c) (d) (e)	432. (a) (b) (c) (d) (e)	478. (a) (b) (c) (d) (e)	524. (a) (b) (c) (d) (e)
387. (a) (b) (c) (d) (e)	433. (a) (b) (c) (d) (e)	479. (a) (b) (c) (d) (e)	525. (a) (b) (c) (d) (e)
388. (a) (b) (c) (d) (e)	434. (a) (b) (c) (d) (e)	480. (a) (b) (c) (d) (e)	526. (a) (b) (c) (d) (e)
389. (a) (b) (c) (d) (e)	435. (a) (b) (c) (d) (e)	481. (a) (b) (c) (d) (e)	527. (a) (b) (c) (d) (e)
390. (a) (b) (c) (d) (e)	436. (a) (b) (c) (d) (e)	482. (a) (b) (c) (d) (e)	528. (a) (b) (c) (d) (e)
391. (a) (b) (c) (d) (e)	437. (a) (b) (c) (d) (e)	483. (a) (b) (c) (d) (e)	529. (a) (b) (c) (d) (e)
392. (a) (b) (c) (d) (e)	438. (a) (b) (c) (d) (e)	484. (a) (b) (c) (d) (e)	530. (a) (b) (c) (d) (e)
393. (a) (b) (c) (d) (e)	439. (a) (b) (c) (d) (e)	485. (a) (b) (c) (d) (e)	531. (a) (b) (c) (d) (e)
394. (a) (b) (c) (d) (e)	440. (a) (b) (c) (d) (e)	486. (a) (b) (c) (d) (e)	532. (a) (b) (c) (d) (e)
395. (a) (b) (c) (d) (e)	441. (a) (b) (c) (d) (e)	487. (a) (b) (c) (d) (e)	533. (a) (b) (c) (d) (e)
396. (a) (b) (c) (d) (e)	442. (a) (b) (c) (d) (e)	488. (a) (b) (c) (d) (e)	534. (a) (b) (c) (d) (e)
397. (a) (b) (c) (d) (e)	443. (a) (b) (c) (d) (e)	489. (a) (b) (c) (d) (e)	535. (a) (b) (c) (d) (e)
398. (a) (b) (c) (d) (e)	444. (a) (b) (c) (d) (e)	490. (a) (b) (c) (d) (e)	536. (a) (b) (c) (d) (e)
399. (a) (b) (c) (d) (e)	445. (a) (b) (c) (d) (e)	491. (a) (b) (c) (d) (e)	537. (a) (b) (c) (d) (e)
400. (a) (b) (c) (d) (e)	446. (a) (b) (c) (d) (e)	492. (a) (b) (c) (d) (e)	538. (a) (b) (c) (d) (e)
401. (a) (b) (c) (d) (e)	447. (a) (b) (c) (d) (e)	493. (a) (b) (c) (d) (e)	539. (a) (b) (c) (d) (e)
402. (a) (b) (c) (d) (e)	448. (a) (b) (c) (d) (e)	494. (a) (b) (c) (d) (e)	540. (a) (b) (c) (d) (e)
403. (a) (b) (c) (d) (e)	449. (a) (b) (c) (d) (e)	495. (a) (b) (c) (d) (e)	541. (a) (b) (c) (d) (e)
404. (a) (b) (c) (d) (e)	450. (a) (b) (c) (d) (e)	496. (a) (b) (c) (d) (e)	542. (a) (b) (c) (d) (e)
405. (a) (b) (c) (d) (e)	451. (a) (b) (c) (d) (e)	497. (a) (b) (c) (d) (e)	543. (a) (b) (c) (d) (e)
406. (a) (b) (c) (d) (e)	452. (a) (b) (c) (d) (e)	498. (a) (b) (c) (d) (e)	544. (a) (b) (c) (d) (e)
407. (a) (b) (c) (d) (e)	453. (a) (b) (c) (d) (e)	499. (a) (b) (c) (d) (e)	545. (a) (b) (c) (d) (e)
408. (a) (b) (c) (d) (e)	454. (a) (b) (c) (d) (e)	500. (a) (b) (c) (d) (e)	546. (a) (b) (c) (d) (e)
409. (a) (b) (c) (d) (e)	455. (a) (b) (c) (d) (e)	501. (a) (b) (c) (d) (e)	547. (a) (b) (c) (d) (e)
410. (a) (b) (c) (d) (e)	456. (a) (b) (c) (d) (e)	502. (a) (b) (c) (d) (e)	548. (a) (b) (c) (d) (e)
411. (a) (b) (c) (d) (e)	457. (a) (b) (c) (d) (e)	503. (a) (b) (c) (d) (e)	549. (a) (b) (c) (d) (e)
412. (a) (b) (c) (d) (e)	458. (a) (b) (c) (d) (e)	504. (a) (b) (c) (d) (e)	550. (a) (b) (c) (d) (e)
413. (a) (b) (c) (d) (e)	459. (a) (b) (c) (d) (e)	505. (a) (b) (c) (d) (e)	551. (a) (b) (c) (d) (e)
414. (a) (b) (c) (d) (e)	460. (a) (b) (c) (d) (e)	506. (a) (b) (c) (d) (e)	552. (a) (b) (c) (d) (e)

Continued

Medical Diseases, continued

553. ⓐ ⓑ ⓒ ⓓ ⓔ	603. ⓐ ⓑ ⓒ ⓓ ⓔ	653. ⓐ ⓑ ⓒ ⓓ ⓔ	703. ⓐ ⓑ ⓒ ⓓ ⓔ
554. ⓐ ⓑ ⓒ ⓓ ⓔ	604. ⓐ ⓑ ⓒ ⓓ ⓔ	654. ⓐ ⓑ ⓒ ⓓ ⓔ	704. ⓐ ⓑ ⓒ ⓓ ⓔ
555. ⓐ ⓑ ⓒ ⓓ ⓔ	605. ⓐ ⓑ ⓒ ⓓ ⓔ	655. ⓐ ⓑ ⓒ ⓓ ⓔ	705. ⓐ ⓑ ⓒ ⓓ ⓔ
556. ⓐ ⓑ ⓒ ⓓ ⓔ	606. ⓐ ⓑ ⓒ ⓓ ⓔ	656. ⓐ ⓑ ⓒ ⓓ ⓔ	706. ⓐ ⓑ ⓒ ⓓ ⓔ
557. ⓐ ⓑ ⓒ ⓓ ⓔ	607. ⓐ ⓑ ⓒ ⓓ ⓔ	657. ⓐ ⓑ ⓒ ⓓ ⓔ	707. ⓐ ⓑ ⓒ ⓓ ⓔ
558. ⓐ ⓑ ⓒ ⓓ ⓔ	608. ⓐ ⓑ ⓒ ⓓ ⓔ	658. ⓐ ⓑ ⓒ ⓓ ⓔ	708. ⓐ ⓑ ⓒ ⓓ ⓔ
559. ⓐ ⓑ ⓒ ⓓ ⓔ	609. ⓐ ⓑ ⓒ ⓓ ⓔ	659. ⓐ ⓑ ⓒ ⓓ ⓔ	709. ⓐ ⓑ ⓒ ⓓ ⓔ
560. ⓐ ⓑ ⓒ ⓓ ⓔ	610. ⓐ ⓑ ⓒ ⓓ ⓔ	660. ⓐ ⓑ ⓒ ⓓ ⓔ	710. ⓐ ⓑ ⓒ ⓓ ⓔ
561. ⓐ ⓑ ⓒ ⓓ ⓔ	611. ⓐ ⓑ ⓒ ⓓ ⓔ	661. ⓐ ⓑ ⓒ ⓓ ⓔ	711. ⓐ ⓑ ⓒ ⓓ ⓔ
562. ⓐ ⓑ ⓒ ⓓ ⓔ	612. ⓐ ⓑ ⓒ ⓓ ⓔ	662. ⓐ ⓑ ⓒ ⓓ ⓔ	712. ⓐ ⓑ ⓒ ⓓ ⓔ
563. ⓐ ⓑ ⓒ ⓓ ⓔ	613. ⓐ ⓑ ⓒ ⓓ ⓔ	663. ⓐ ⓑ ⓒ ⓓ ⓔ	713. ⓐ ⓑ ⓒ ⓓ ⓔ
564. ⓐ ⓑ ⓒ ⓓ ⓔ	614. ⓐ ⓑ ⓒ ⓓ ⓔ	664. ⓐ ⓑ ⓒ ⓓ ⓔ	714. ⓐ ⓑ ⓒ ⓓ ⓔ
565. ⓐ ⓑ ⓒ ⓓ ⓔ	615. ⓐ ⓑ ⓒ ⓓ ⓔ	665. ⓐ ⓑ ⓒ ⓓ ⓔ	715. ⓐ ⓑ ⓒ ⓓ ⓔ
566. ⓐ ⓑ ⓒ ⓓ ⓔ	616. ⓐ ⓑ ⓒ ⓓ ⓔ	666. ⓐ ⓑ ⓒ ⓓ ⓔ	716. ⓐ ⓑ ⓒ ⓓ ⓔ
567. ⓐ ⓑ ⓒ ⓓ ⓔ	617. ⓐ ⓑ ⓒ ⓓ ⓔ	667. ⓐ ⓑ ⓒ ⓓ ⓔ	717. ⓐ ⓑ ⓒ ⓓ ⓔ
568. ⓐ ⓑ ⓒ ⓓ ⓔ	618. ⓐ ⓑ ⓒ ⓓ ⓔ	668. ⓐ ⓑ ⓒ ⓓ ⓔ	718. ⓐ ⓑ ⓒ ⓓ ⓔ
569. ⓐ ⓑ ⓒ ⓓ ⓔ	619. ⓐ ⓑ ⓒ ⓓ ⓔ	669. ⓐ ⓑ ⓒ ⓓ ⓔ	719. ⓐ ⓑ ⓒ ⓓ ⓔ
570. ⓐ ⓑ ⓒ ⓓ ⓔ	620. ⓐ ⓑ ⓒ ⓓ ⓔ	670. ⓐ ⓑ ⓒ ⓓ ⓔ	720. ⓐ ⓑ ⓒ ⓓ ⓔ
571. ⓐ ⓑ ⓒ ⓓ ⓔ	621. ⓐ ⓑ ⓒ ⓓ ⓔ	671. ⓐ ⓑ ⓒ ⓓ ⓔ	721. ⓐ ⓑ ⓒ ⓓ ⓔ
572. ⓐ ⓑ ⓒ ⓓ ⓔ	622. ⓐ ⓑ ⓒ ⓓ ⓔ	672. ⓐ ⓑ ⓒ ⓓ ⓔ	722. ⓐ ⓑ ⓒ ⓓ ⓔ
573. ⓐ ⓑ ⓒ ⓓ ⓔ	623. ⓐ ⓑ ⓒ ⓓ ⓔ	673. ⓐ ⓑ ⓒ ⓓ ⓔ	723. ⓐ ⓑ ⓒ ⓓ ⓔ
574. ⓐ ⓑ ⓒ ⓓ ⓔ	624. ⓐ ⓑ ⓒ ⓓ ⓔ	674. ⓐ ⓑ ⓒ ⓓ ⓔ	724. ⓐ ⓑ ⓒ ⓓ ⓔ
575. ⓐ ⓑ ⓒ ⓓ ⓔ	625. ⓐ ⓑ ⓒ ⓓ ⓔ	675. ⓐ ⓑ ⓒ ⓓ ⓔ	725. ⓐ ⓑ ⓒ ⓓ ⓔ
576. ⓐ ⓑ ⓒ ⓓ ⓔ	626. ⓐ ⓑ ⓒ ⓓ ⓔ	676. ⓐ ⓑ ⓒ ⓓ ⓔ	726. ⓐ ⓑ ⓒ ⓓ ⓔ
577. ⓐ ⓑ ⓒ ⓓ ⓔ	627. ⓐ ⓑ ⓒ ⓓ ⓔ	677. ⓐ ⓑ ⓒ ⓓ ⓔ	727. ⓐ ⓑ ⓒ ⓓ ⓔ
578. ⓐ ⓑ ⓒ ⓓ ⓔ	628. ⓐ ⓑ ⓒ ⓓ ⓔ	678. ⓐ ⓑ ⓒ ⓓ ⓔ	728. ⓐ ⓑ ⓒ ⓓ ⓔ
579. ⓐ ⓑ ⓒ ⓓ ⓔ	629. ⓐ ⓑ ⓒ ⓓ ⓔ	679. ⓐ ⓑ ⓒ ⓓ ⓔ	729. ⓐ ⓑ ⓒ ⓓ ⓔ
580. ⓐ ⓑ ⓒ ⓓ ⓔ	630. ⓐ ⓑ ⓒ ⓓ ⓔ	680. ⓐ ⓑ ⓒ ⓓ ⓔ	730. ⓐ ⓑ ⓒ ⓓ ⓔ
581. ⓐ ⓑ ⓒ ⓓ ⓔ	631. ⓐ ⓑ ⓒ ⓓ ⓔ	681. ⓐ ⓑ ⓒ ⓓ ⓔ	731. ⓐ ⓑ ⓒ ⓓ ⓔ
582. ⓐ ⓑ ⓒ ⓓ ⓔ	632. ⓐ ⓑ ⓒ ⓓ ⓔ	682. ⓐ ⓑ ⓒ ⓓ ⓔ	732. ⓐ ⓑ ⓒ ⓓ ⓔ
583. ⓐ ⓑ ⓒ ⓓ ⓔ	633. ⓐ ⓑ ⓒ ⓓ ⓔ	683. ⓐ ⓑ ⓒ ⓓ ⓔ	733. ⓐ ⓑ ⓒ ⓓ ⓔ
584. ⓐ ⓑ ⓒ ⓓ ⓔ	634. ⓐ ⓑ ⓒ ⓓ ⓔ	684. ⓐ ⓑ ⓒ ⓓ ⓔ	734. ⓐ ⓑ ⓒ ⓓ ⓔ
585. ⓐ ⓑ ⓒ ⓓ ⓔ	635. ⓐ ⓑ ⓒ ⓓ ⓔ	685. ⓐ ⓑ ⓒ ⓓ ⓔ	735. ⓐ ⓑ ⓒ ⓓ ⓔ
586. ⓐ ⓑ ⓒ ⓓ ⓔ	636. ⓐ ⓑ ⓒ ⓓ ⓔ	686. ⓐ ⓑ ⓒ ⓓ ⓔ	736. ⓐ ⓑ ⓒ ⓓ ⓔ
587. ⓐ ⓑ ⓒ ⓓ ⓔ	637. ⓐ ⓑ ⓒ ⓓ ⓔ	687. ⓐ ⓑ ⓒ ⓓ ⓔ	737. ⓐ ⓑ ⓒ ⓓ ⓔ
588. ⓐ ⓑ ⓒ ⓓ ⓔ	638. ⓐ ⓑ ⓒ ⓓ ⓔ	688. ⓐ ⓑ ⓒ ⓓ ⓔ	738. ⓐ ⓑ ⓒ ⓓ ⓔ
589. ⓐ ⓑ ⓒ ⓓ ⓔ	639. ⓐ ⓑ ⓒ ⓓ ⓔ	689. ⓐ ⓑ ⓒ ⓓ ⓔ	739. ⓐ ⓑ ⓒ ⓓ ⓔ
590. ⓐ ⓑ ⓒ ⓓ ⓔ	640. ⓐ ⓑ ⓒ ⓓ ⓔ	690. ⓐ ⓑ ⓒ ⓓ ⓔ	740. ⓐ ⓑ ⓒ ⓓ ⓔ
591. ⓐ ⓑ ⓒ ⓓ ⓔ	641. ⓐ ⓑ ⓒ ⓓ ⓔ	691. ⓐ ⓑ ⓒ ⓓ ⓔ	741. ⓐ ⓑ ⓒ ⓓ ⓔ
592. ⓐ ⓑ ⓒ ⓓ ⓔ	642. ⓐ ⓑ ⓒ ⓓ ⓔ	692. ⓐ ⓑ ⓒ ⓓ ⓔ	742. ⓐ ⓑ ⓒ ⓓ ⓔ
593. ⓐ ⓑ ⓒ ⓓ ⓔ	643. ⓐ ⓑ ⓒ ⓓ ⓔ	693. ⓐ ⓑ ⓒ ⓓ ⓔ	743. ⓐ ⓑ ⓒ ⓓ ⓔ
594. ⓐ ⓑ ⓒ ⓓ ⓔ	644. ⓐ ⓑ ⓒ ⓓ ⓔ	694. ⓐ ⓑ ⓒ ⓓ ⓔ	744. ⓐ ⓑ ⓒ ⓓ ⓔ
595. ⓐ ⓑ ⓒ ⓓ ⓔ	645. ⓐ ⓑ ⓒ ⓓ ⓔ	695. ⓐ ⓑ ⓒ ⓓ ⓔ	745. ⓐ ⓑ ⓒ ⓓ ⓔ
596. ⓐ ⓑ ⓒ ⓓ ⓔ	646. ⓐ ⓑ ⓒ ⓓ ⓔ	696. ⓐ ⓑ ⓒ ⓓ ⓔ ⓕ	746. ⓐ ⓑ ⓒ ⓓ ⓔ
597. ⓐ ⓑ ⓒ ⓓ ⓔ	647. ⓐ ⓑ ⓒ ⓓ ⓔ	697. ⓐ ⓑ ⓒ ⓓ ⓔ ⓕ	747. ⓐ ⓑ ⓒ ⓓ ⓔ
598. ⓐ ⓑ ⓒ ⓓ ⓔ	648. ⓐ ⓑ ⓒ ⓓ ⓔ	698. ⓐ ⓑ ⓒ ⓓ ⓔ ⓕ	748. ⓐ ⓑ ⓒ ⓓ ⓔ
599. ⓐ ⓑ ⓒ ⓓ ⓔ	649. ⓐ ⓑ ⓒ ⓓ ⓔ	699. ⓐ ⓑ ⓒ ⓓ ⓔ ⓕ	
600. ⓐ ⓑ ⓒ ⓓ ⓔ	650. ⓐ ⓑ ⓒ ⓓ ⓔ	700. ⓐ ⓑ ⓒ ⓓ ⓔ ⓕ	
601. ⓐ ⓑ ⓒ ⓓ ⓔ	651. ⓐ ⓑ ⓒ ⓓ ⓔ	701. ⓐ ⓑ ⓒ ⓓ ⓔ ⓕ	
602. ⓐ ⓑ ⓒ ⓓ ⓔ	652. ⓐ ⓑ ⓒ ⓓ ⓔ	702. ⓐ ⓑ ⓒ ⓓ ⓔ	

Section 8
Neurology

Fill in a circled letter to indicate your answer choice.

1. ⓐ ⓑ ⓒ ⓓ ⓔ	15. ⓐ ⓑ ⓒ ⓓ ⓔ	29. ⓐ ⓑ ⓒ ⓓ ⓔ	43. ⓐ ⓑ ⓒ ⓓ ⓔ
2. ⓐ ⓑ ⓒ ⓓ ⓔ	16. ⓐ ⓑ ⓒ ⓓ ⓔ	30. ⓐ ⓑ ⓒ ⓓ ⓔ	44. ⓐ ⓑ ⓒ ⓓ ⓔ
3. ⓐ ⓑ ⓒ ⓓ ⓔ	17. ⓐ ⓑ ⓒ ⓓ ⓔ	31. ⓐ ⓑ ⓒ ⓓ ⓔ	45. ⓐ ⓑ ⓒ ⓓ ⓔ
4. ⓐ ⓑ ⓒ ⓓ ⓔ	18. ⓐ ⓑ ⓒ ⓓ ⓔ	32. ⓐ ⓑ ⓒ ⓓ ⓔ	46. ⓐ ⓑ ⓒ ⓓ ⓔ
5. ⓐ ⓑ ⓒ ⓓ ⓔ	19. ⓐ ⓑ ⓒ ⓓ ⓔ	33. ⓐ ⓑ ⓒ ⓓ ⓔ	47. ⓐ ⓑ ⓒ ⓓ ⓔ
6. ⓐ ⓑ ⓒ ⓓ ⓔ	20. ⓐ ⓑ ⓒ ⓓ ⓔ	34. ⓐ ⓑ ⓒ ⓓ ⓔ	48. ⓐ ⓑ ⓒ ⓓ ⓔ
7. ⓐ ⓑ ⓒ ⓓ ⓔ	21. ⓐ ⓑ ⓒ ⓓ ⓔ	35. ⓐ ⓑ ⓒ ⓓ ⓔ	49. ⓐ ⓑ ⓒ ⓓ ⓔ
8. ⓐ ⓑ ⓒ ⓓ ⓔ	22. ⓐ ⓑ ⓒ ⓓ ⓔ	36. ⓐ ⓑ ⓒ ⓓ ⓔ	50. ⓐ ⓑ ⓒ ⓓ ⓔ
9. ⓐ ⓑ ⓒ ⓓ ⓔ	23. ⓐ ⓑ ⓒ ⓓ ⓔ	37. ⓐ ⓑ ⓒ ⓓ ⓔ	51. ⓐ ⓑ ⓒ ⓓ ⓔ
10. ⓐ ⓑ ⓒ ⓓ ⓔ	24. ⓐ ⓑ ⓒ ⓓ ⓔ	38. ⓐ ⓑ ⓒ ⓓ ⓔ	52. ⓐ ⓑ ⓒ ⓓ ⓔ
11. ⓐ ⓑ ⓒ ⓓ ⓔ	25. ⓐ ⓑ ⓒ ⓓ ⓔ	39. ⓐ ⓑ ⓒ ⓓ ⓔ	53. ⓐ ⓑ ⓒ ⓓ ⓔ
12. ⓐ ⓑ ⓒ ⓓ ⓔ	26. ⓐ ⓑ ⓒ ⓓ ⓔ	40. ⓐ ⓑ ⓒ ⓓ ⓔ	54. ⓐ ⓑ ⓒ ⓓ ⓔ
13. ⓐ ⓑ ⓒ ⓓ ⓔ	27. ⓐ ⓑ ⓒ ⓓ ⓔ	41. ⓐ ⓑ ⓒ ⓓ ⓔ	
14. ⓐ ⓑ ⓒ ⓓ ⓔ	28. ⓐ ⓑ ⓒ ⓓ ⓔ	42. ⓐ ⓑ ⓒ ⓓ ⓔ	

This page intentionally left blank.

Oncology

Fill in a circled letter to indicate your answer choice.

1. ⓐ ⓑ ⓒ ⓓ ⓔ	21. ⓐ ⓑ ⓒ ⓓ ⓔ	41. ⓐ ⓑ ⓒ ⓓ ⓔ	61. ⓐ ⓑ ⓒ ⓓ ⓔ
2. ⓐ ⓑ ⓒ ⓓ ⓔ	22. ⓐ ⓑ ⓒ ⓓ ⓔ	42. ⓐ ⓑ ⓒ ⓓ ⓔ	62. ⓐ ⓑ ⓒ ⓓ ⓔ
3. ⓐ ⓑ ⓒ ⓓ ⓔ	23. ⓐ ⓑ ⓒ ⓓ ⓔ	43. ⓐ ⓑ ⓒ ⓓ ⓔ	63. ⓐ ⓑ ⓒ ⓓ ⓔ
4. ⓐ ⓑ ⓒ ⓓ ⓔ	24. ⓐ ⓑ ⓒ ⓓ ⓔ	44. ⓐ ⓑ ⓒ ⓓ ⓔ	64. ⓐ ⓑ ⓒ ⓓ ⓔ
5. ⓐ ⓑ ⓒ ⓓ ⓔ	25. ⓐ ⓑ ⓒ ⓓ ⓔ	45. ⓐ ⓑ ⓒ ⓓ ⓔ	65. ⓐ ⓑ ⓒ ⓓ ⓔ
6. ⓐ ⓑ ⓒ ⓓ ⓔ	26. ⓐ ⓑ ⓒ ⓓ ⓔ	46. ⓐ ⓑ ⓒ ⓓ ⓔ	66. ⓐ ⓑ ⓒ ⓓ ⓔ
7. ⓐ ⓑ ⓒ ⓓ ⓔ	27. ⓐ ⓑ ⓒ ⓓ ⓔ	47. ⓐ ⓑ ⓒ ⓓ ⓔ	67. ⓐ ⓑ ⓒ ⓓ ⓔ
8. ⓐ ⓑ ⓒ ⓓ ⓔ	28. ⓐ ⓑ ⓒ ⓓ ⓔ	48. ⓐ ⓑ ⓒ ⓓ ⓔ	68. ⓐ ⓑ ⓒ ⓓ ⓔ
9. ⓐ ⓑ ⓒ ⓓ ⓔ	29. ⓐ ⓑ ⓒ ⓓ ⓔ	49. ⓐ ⓑ ⓒ ⓓ ⓔ	69. ⓐ ⓑ ⓒ ⓓ ⓔ
10. ⓐ ⓑ ⓒ ⓓ ⓔ	30. ⓐ ⓑ ⓒ ⓓ ⓔ	50. ⓐ ⓑ ⓒ ⓓ ⓔ	70. ⓐ ⓑ ⓒ ⓓ ⓔ
11. ⓐ ⓑ ⓒ ⓓ ⓔ	31. ⓐ ⓑ ⓒ ⓓ ⓔ	51. ⓐ ⓑ ⓒ ⓓ ⓔ	71. ⓐ ⓑ ⓒ ⓓ ⓔ
12. ⓐ ⓑ ⓒ ⓓ ⓔ	32. ⓐ ⓑ ⓒ ⓓ ⓔ	52. ⓐ ⓑ ⓒ ⓓ ⓔ	72. ⓐ ⓑ ⓒ ⓓ ⓔ
13. ⓐ ⓑ ⓒ ⓓ ⓔ	33. ⓐ ⓑ ⓒ ⓓ ⓔ	53. ⓐ ⓑ ⓒ ⓓ ⓔ	73. ⓐ ⓑ ⓒ ⓓ ⓔ
14. ⓐ ⓑ ⓒ ⓓ ⓔ	34. ⓐ ⓑ ⓒ ⓓ ⓔ	54. ⓐ ⓑ ⓒ ⓓ ⓔ	74. ⓐ ⓑ ⓒ ⓓ ⓔ
15. ⓐ ⓑ ⓒ ⓓ ⓔ	35. ⓐ ⓑ ⓒ ⓓ ⓔ	55. ⓐ ⓑ ⓒ ⓓ ⓔ	75. ⓐ ⓑ ⓒ ⓓ ⓔ
16. ⓐ ⓑ ⓒ ⓓ ⓔ	36. ⓐ ⓑ ⓒ ⓓ ⓔ	56. ⓐ ⓑ ⓒ ⓓ ⓔ	
17. ⓐ ⓑ ⓒ ⓓ ⓔ	37. ⓐ ⓑ ⓒ ⓓ ⓔ	57. ⓐ ⓑ ⓒ ⓓ ⓔ	
18. ⓐ ⓑ ⓒ ⓓ ⓔ	38. ⓐ ⓑ ⓒ ⓓ ⓔ	58. ⓐ ⓑ ⓒ ⓓ ⓔ	
19. ⓐ ⓑ ⓒ ⓓ ⓔ	39. ⓐ ⓑ ⓒ ⓓ ⓔ	59. ⓐ ⓑ ⓒ ⓓ ⓔ	
20. ⓐ ⓑ ⓒ ⓓ ⓔ	40. ⓐ ⓑ ⓒ ⓓ ⓔ	60. ⓐ ⓑ ⓒ ⓓ ⓔ	

This page intentionally left blank.

Section 10

Ophthalmology

Fill in a circled letter to indicate your answer choice.

1. ⓐ ⓑ ⓒ ⓓ ⓔ	15. ⓐ ⓑ ⓒ ⓓ ⓔ	29. ⓐ ⓑ ⓒ ⓓ ⓔ	43. ⓐ ⓑ ⓒ ⓓ ⓔ
2. ⓐ ⓑ ⓒ ⓓ ⓔ	16. ⓐ ⓑ ⓒ ⓓ ⓔ	30. ⓐ ⓑ ⓒ ⓓ ⓔ	44. ⓐ ⓑ ⓒ ⓓ ⓔ
3. ⓐ ⓑ ⓒ ⓓ ⓔ	17. ⓐ ⓑ ⓒ ⓓ ⓔ	31. ⓐ ⓑ ⓒ ⓓ ⓔ	45. ⓐ ⓑ ⓒ ⓓ ⓔ
4. ⓐ ⓑ ⓒ ⓓ ⓔ	18. ⓐ ⓑ ⓒ ⓓ ⓔ	32. ⓐ ⓑ ⓒ ⓓ ⓔ	46. ⓐ ⓑ ⓒ ⓓ ⓔ
5. ⓐ ⓑ ⓒ ⓓ ⓔ	19. ⓐ ⓑ ⓒ ⓓ ⓔ	33. ⓐ ⓑ ⓒ ⓓ ⓔ	47. ⓐ ⓑ ⓒ ⓓ ⓔ
6. ⓐ ⓑ ⓒ ⓓ ⓔ	20. ⓐ ⓑ ⓒ ⓓ ⓔ	34. ⓐ ⓑ ⓒ ⓓ ⓔ	48. ⓐ ⓑ ⓒ ⓓ ⓔ
7. ⓐ ⓑ ⓒ ⓓ ⓔ	21. ⓐ ⓑ ⓒ ⓓ ⓔ	35. ⓐ ⓑ ⓒ ⓓ ⓔ	49. ⓐ ⓑ ⓒ ⓓ ⓔ
8. ⓐ ⓑ ⓒ ⓓ ⓔ	22. ⓐ ⓑ ⓒ ⓓ ⓔ	36. ⓐ ⓑ ⓒ ⓓ ⓔ	50. ⓐ ⓑ ⓒ ⓓ ⓔ
9. ⓐ ⓑ ⓒ ⓓ ⓔ	23. ⓐ ⓑ ⓒ ⓓ ⓔ	37. ⓐ ⓑ ⓒ ⓓ ⓔ	
10. ⓐ ⓑ ⓒ ⓓ ⓔ	24. ⓐ ⓑ ⓒ ⓓ ⓔ	38. ⓐ ⓑ ⓒ ⓓ ⓔ	
11. ⓐ ⓑ ⓒ ⓓ ⓔ	25. ⓐ ⓑ ⓒ ⓓ ⓔ	39. ⓐ ⓑ ⓒ ⓓ ⓔ	
12. ⓐ ⓑ ⓒ ⓓ ⓔ	26. ⓐ ⓑ ⓒ ⓓ ⓔ	40. ⓐ ⓑ ⓒ ⓓ ⓔ	
13. ⓐ ⓑ ⓒ ⓓ ⓔ	27. ⓐ ⓑ ⓒ ⓓ ⓔ	41. ⓐ ⓑ ⓒ ⓓ ⓔ	
14. ⓐ ⓑ ⓒ ⓓ ⓔ	28. ⓐ ⓑ ⓒ ⓓ ⓔ	42. ⓐ ⓑ ⓒ ⓓ ⓔ	

This page intentionally left blank.

Section 11

Pharmacology and Pharmacy Procedures

Fill in a circled letter to indicate your answer choice.

1. ⓐ ⓑ ⓒ ⓓ ⓔ	19. ⓐ ⓑ ⓒ ⓓ ⓔ	37. ⓐ ⓑ ⓒ ⓓ ⓔ	55. ⓐ ⓑ ⓒ ⓓ ⓔ
2. ⓐ ⓑ ⓒ ⓓ ⓔ	20. ⓐ ⓑ ⓒ ⓓ ⓔ	38. ⓐ ⓑ ⓒ ⓓ ⓔ	56. ⓐ ⓑ ⓒ ⓓ ⓔ
3. ⓐ ⓑ ⓒ ⓓ ⓔ	21. ⓐ ⓑ ⓒ ⓓ ⓔ	39. ⓐ ⓑ ⓒ ⓓ ⓔ	57. ⓐ ⓑ ⓒ ⓓ ⓔ
4. ⓐ ⓑ ⓒ ⓓ ⓔ	22. ⓐ ⓑ ⓒ ⓓ ⓔ	40. ⓐ ⓑ ⓒ ⓓ ⓔ	58. ⓐ ⓑ ⓒ ⓓ ⓔ
5. ⓐ ⓑ ⓒ ⓓ ⓔ	23. ⓐ ⓑ ⓒ ⓓ ⓔ	41. ⓐ ⓑ ⓒ ⓓ ⓔ	59. ⓐ ⓑ ⓒ ⓓ ⓔ
6. ⓐ ⓑ ⓒ ⓓ ⓔ	24. ⓐ ⓑ ⓒ ⓓ ⓔ	42. ⓐ ⓑ ⓒ ⓓ ⓔ	60. ⓐ ⓑ ⓒ ⓓ ⓔ
7. ⓐ ⓑ ⓒ ⓓ ⓔ	25. ⓐ ⓑ ⓒ ⓓ ⓔ	43. ⓐ ⓑ ⓒ ⓓ ⓔ	61. ⓐ ⓑ ⓒ ⓓ ⓔ
8. ⓐ ⓑ ⓒ ⓓ ⓔ	26. ⓐ ⓑ ⓒ ⓓ ⓔ	44. ⓐ ⓑ ⓒ ⓓ ⓔ	62. ⓐ ⓑ ⓒ ⓓ ⓔ
9. ⓐ ⓑ ⓒ ⓓ ⓔ	27. ⓐ ⓑ ⓒ ⓓ ⓔ	45. ⓐ ⓑ ⓒ ⓓ ⓔ	63. ⓐ ⓑ ⓒ ⓓ ⓔ
10. ⓐ ⓑ ⓒ ⓓ ⓔ	28. ⓐ ⓑ ⓒ ⓓ ⓔ	46. ⓐ ⓑ ⓒ ⓓ ⓔ	64. ⓐ ⓑ ⓒ ⓓ ⓔ
11. ⓐ ⓑ ⓒ ⓓ ⓔ	29. ⓐ ⓑ ⓒ ⓓ ⓔ	47. ⓐ ⓑ ⓒ ⓓ ⓔ	65. ⓐ ⓑ ⓒ ⓓ ⓔ
12. ⓐ ⓑ ⓒ ⓓ ⓔ	30. ⓐ ⓑ ⓒ ⓓ ⓔ	48. ⓐ ⓑ ⓒ ⓓ ⓔ	66. ⓐ ⓑ ⓒ ⓓ ⓔ
13. ⓐ ⓑ ⓒ ⓓ ⓔ	31. ⓐ ⓑ ⓒ ⓓ ⓔ	49. ⓐ ⓑ ⓒ ⓓ ⓔ	67. ⓐ ⓑ ⓒ ⓓ ⓔ
14. ⓐ ⓑ ⓒ ⓓ ⓔ	32. ⓐ ⓑ ⓒ ⓓ ⓔ	50. ⓐ ⓑ ⓒ ⓓ ⓔ	
15. ⓐ ⓑ ⓒ ⓓ ⓔ	33. ⓐ ⓑ ⓒ ⓓ ⓔ	51. ⓐ ⓑ ⓒ ⓓ ⓔ	
16. ⓐ ⓑ ⓒ ⓓ ⓔ	34. ⓐ ⓑ ⓒ ⓓ ⓔ	52. ⓐ ⓑ ⓒ ⓓ ⓔ	
17. ⓐ ⓑ ⓒ ⓓ ⓔ	35. ⓐ ⓑ ⓒ ⓓ ⓔ	53. ⓐ ⓑ ⓒ ⓓ ⓔ	
18. ⓐ ⓑ ⓒ ⓓ ⓔ	36. ⓐ ⓑ ⓒ ⓓ ⓔ	54. ⓐ ⓑ ⓒ ⓓ ⓔ	

352

This page intentionally left blank.

Section 12
Preventive Medicine

Fill in a circled letter to indicate your answer choice.

1. ⓐ ⓑ ⓒ ⓓ ⓔ	23. ⓐ ⓑ ⓒ ⓓ ⓔ	45. ⓐ ⓑ ⓒ ⓓ ⓔ	67. ⓐ ⓑ ⓒ ⓓ ⓔ
2. ⓐ ⓑ ⓒ ⓓ ⓔ	24. ⓐ ⓑ ⓒ ⓓ ⓔ	46. ⓐ ⓑ ⓒ ⓓ ⓔ	68. ⓐ ⓑ ⓒ ⓓ ⓔ
3. ⓐ ⓑ ⓒ ⓓ ⓔ	25. ⓐ ⓑ ⓒ ⓓ ⓔ	47. ⓐ ⓑ ⓒ ⓓ ⓔ	69. ⓐ ⓑ ⓒ ⓓ ⓔ
4. ⓐ ⓑ ⓒ ⓓ ⓔ	26. ⓐ ⓑ ⓒ ⓓ ⓔ	48. ⓐ ⓑ ⓒ ⓓ ⓔ	70. ⓐ ⓑ ⓒ ⓓ ⓔ
5. ⓐ ⓑ ⓒ ⓓ ⓔ	27. ⓐ ⓑ ⓒ ⓓ ⓔ	49. ⓐ ⓑ ⓒ ⓓ ⓔ	71. ⓐ ⓑ ⓒ ⓓ ⓔ
6. ⓐ ⓑ ⓒ ⓓ ⓔ	28. ⓐ ⓑ ⓒ ⓓ ⓔ	50. ⓐ ⓑ ⓒ ⓓ ⓔ	72. ⓐ ⓑ ⓒ ⓓ ⓔ
7. ⓐ ⓑ ⓒ ⓓ ⓔ	29. ⓐ ⓑ ⓒ ⓓ ⓔ	51. ⓐ ⓑ ⓒ ⓓ ⓔ	73. ⓐ ⓑ ⓒ ⓓ ⓔ
8. ⓐ ⓑ ⓒ ⓓ ⓔ	30. ⓐ ⓑ ⓒ ⓓ ⓔ	52. ⓐ ⓑ ⓒ ⓓ ⓔ	74. ⓐ ⓑ ⓒ ⓓ ⓔ
9. ⓐ ⓑ ⓒ ⓓ ⓔ	31. ⓐ ⓑ ⓒ ⓓ ⓔ	53. ⓐ ⓑ ⓒ ⓓ ⓔ	75. ⓐ ⓑ ⓒ ⓓ ⓔ
10. ⓐ ⓑ ⓒ ⓓ ⓔ	32. ⓐ ⓑ ⓒ ⓓ ⓔ	54. ⓐ ⓑ ⓒ ⓓ ⓔ	76. ⓐ ⓑ ⓒ ⓓ ⓔ
11. ⓐ ⓑ ⓒ ⓓ ⓔ	33. ⓐ ⓑ ⓒ ⓓ ⓔ	55. ⓐ ⓑ ⓒ ⓓ ⓔ	77. ⓐ ⓑ ⓒ ⓓ ⓔ
12. ⓐ ⓑ ⓒ ⓓ ⓔ	34. ⓐ ⓑ ⓒ ⓓ ⓔ	56. ⓐ ⓑ ⓒ ⓓ ⓔ	78. ⓐ ⓑ ⓒ ⓓ ⓔ
13. ⓐ ⓑ ⓒ ⓓ ⓔ	35. ⓐ ⓑ ⓒ ⓓ ⓔ	57. ⓐ ⓑ ⓒ ⓓ ⓔ	79. ⓐ ⓑ ⓒ ⓓ ⓔ
14. ⓐ ⓑ ⓒ ⓓ ⓔ	36. ⓐ ⓑ ⓒ ⓓ ⓔ	58. ⓐ ⓑ ⓒ ⓓ ⓔ	80. ⓐ ⓑ ⓒ ⓓ ⓔ
15. ⓐ ⓑ ⓒ ⓓ ⓔ	37. ⓐ ⓑ ⓒ ⓓ ⓔ	59. ⓐ ⓑ ⓒ ⓓ ⓔ	81. ⓐ ⓑ ⓒ ⓓ ⓔ
16. ⓐ ⓑ ⓒ ⓓ ⓔ	38. ⓐ ⓑ ⓒ ⓓ ⓔ	60. ⓐ ⓑ ⓒ ⓓ ⓔ	82. ⓐ ⓑ ⓒ ⓓ ⓔ
17. ⓐ ⓑ ⓒ ⓓ ⓔ	39. ⓐ ⓑ ⓒ ⓓ ⓔ	61. ⓐ ⓑ ⓒ ⓓ ⓔ	83. ⓐ ⓑ ⓒ ⓓ ⓔ
18. ⓐ ⓑ ⓒ ⓓ ⓔ	40. ⓐ ⓑ ⓒ ⓓ ⓔ	62. ⓐ ⓑ ⓒ ⓓ ⓔ	84. ⓐ ⓑ ⓒ ⓓ ⓔ
19. ⓐ ⓑ ⓒ ⓓ ⓔ	41. ⓐ ⓑ ⓒ ⓓ ⓔ	63. ⓐ ⓑ ⓒ ⓓ ⓔ	85. ⓐ ⓑ ⓒ ⓓ ⓔ
20. ⓐ ⓑ ⓒ ⓓ ⓔ	42. ⓐ ⓑ ⓒ ⓓ ⓔ	64. ⓐ ⓑ ⓒ ⓓ ⓔ	86. ⓐ ⓑ ⓒ ⓓ ⓔ
21. ⓐ ⓑ ⓒ ⓓ ⓔ	43. ⓐ ⓑ ⓒ ⓓ ⓔ	65. ⓐ ⓑ ⓒ ⓓ ⓔ	87. ⓐ ⓑ ⓒ ⓓ ⓔ
22. ⓐ ⓑ ⓒ ⓓ ⓔ	44. ⓐ ⓑ ⓒ ⓓ ⓔ	66. ⓐ ⓑ ⓒ ⓓ ⓔ	

This page intentionally left blank.

Principles of Surgery

Fill in a circled letter to indicate your answer choice.

1. a b c d e	27. a b c d e	53. a b c d e	79. a b c d e
2. a b c d e	28. a b c d e	54. a b c d e	80. a b c d e
3. a b c d e	29. a b c d e	55. a b c d e	81. a b c d e
4. a b c d e	30. a b c d e	56. a b c d e	82. a b c d e
5. a b c d e	31. a b c d e	57. a b c d e	83. a b c d e
6. a b c d e	32. a b c d e	58. a b c d e	84. a b c d e
7. a b c d e	33. a b c d e	59. a b c d e	85. a b c d e
8. a b c d e	34. a b c d e	60. a b c d e	86. a b c d e
9. a b c d e	35. a b c d e	61. a b c d e	87. a b c d e
10. a b c d e	36. a b c d e	62. a b c d e	88. a b c d e
11. a b c d e	37. a b c d e	63. a b c d e	89. a b c d e
12. a b c d e	38. a b c d e	64. a b c d e	90. a b c d e
13. a b c d e	39. a b c d e	65. a b c d e	91. a b c d e
14. a b c d e	40. a b c d e	66. a b c d e	92. a b c d e
15. a b c d e	41. a b c d e	67. a b c d e	93. a b c d e
16. a b c d e	42. a b c d e	68. a b c d e	94. a b c d e
17. a b c d e	43. a b c d e	69. a b c d e	95. a b c d e
18. a b c d e	44. a b c d e	70. a b c d e	96. a b c d e
19. a b c d e	45. a b c d e	71. a b c d e	97. a b c d e
20. a b c d e	46. a b c d e	72. a b c d e	98. a b c d e
21. a b c d e	47. a b c d e	73. a b c d e	
22. a b c d e	48. a b c d e	74. a b c d e	
23. a b c d e	49. a b c d e	75. a b c d e	
24. a b c d e	50. a b c d e	76. a b c d e	
25. a b c d e	51. a b c d e	77. a b c d e	
26. a b c d e	52. a b c d e	78. a b c d e	

This page intentionally left blank.

Section 14
Surgical Diseases

Fill in a circled letter to indicate your answer choice.

1. ⓐ ⓑ ⓒ ⓓ ⓔ	47. ⓐ ⓑ ⓒ ⓓ ⓔ	93. ⓐ ⓑ ⓒ ⓓ ⓔ	139. ⓐ ⓑ ⓒ ⓓ ⓔ
2. ⓐ ⓑ ⓒ ⓓ ⓔ	48. ⓐ ⓑ ⓒ ⓓ ⓔ	94. ⓐ ⓑ ⓒ ⓓ ⓔ	140. ⓐ ⓑ ⓒ ⓓ ⓔ
3. ⓐ ⓑ ⓒ ⓓ ⓔ	49. ⓐ ⓑ ⓒ ⓓ ⓔ	95. ⓐ ⓑ ⓒ ⓓ ⓔ	141. ⓐ ⓑ ⓒ ⓓ ⓔ
4. ⓐ ⓑ ⓒ ⓓ ⓔ	50. ⓐ ⓑ ⓒ ⓓ ⓔ	96. ⓐ ⓑ ⓒ ⓓ ⓔ	142. ⓐ ⓑ ⓒ ⓓ ⓔ
5. ⓐ ⓑ ⓒ ⓓ ⓔ	51. ⓐ ⓑ ⓒ ⓓ ⓔ	97. ⓐ ⓑ ⓒ ⓓ ⓔ	143. ⓐ ⓑ ⓒ ⓓ ⓔ
6. ⓐ ⓑ ⓒ ⓓ ⓔ	52. ⓐ ⓑ ⓒ ⓓ ⓔ	98. ⓐ ⓑ ⓒ ⓓ ⓔ	144. ⓐ ⓑ ⓒ ⓓ ⓔ
7. ⓐ ⓑ ⓒ ⓓ ⓔ	53. ⓐ ⓑ ⓒ ⓓ	99. ⓐ ⓑ ⓒ ⓓ ⓔ	145. ⓐ ⓑ ⓒ ⓓ ⓔ
8. ⓐ ⓑ ⓒ ⓓ ⓔ	54. ⓐ ⓑ ⓒ ⓓ	100. ⓐ ⓑ ⓒ ⓓ ⓔ	146. ⓐ ⓑ ⓒ ⓓ ⓔ
9. ⓐ ⓑ ⓒ ⓓ ⓔ	55. ⓐ ⓑ ⓒ ⓓ	101. ⓐ ⓑ ⓒ ⓓ ⓔ	147. ⓐ ⓑ ⓒ ⓓ ⓔ
10. ⓐ ⓑ ⓒ ⓓ ⓔ	56. ⓐ ⓑ ⓒ ⓓ	102. ⓐ ⓑ ⓒ ⓓ ⓔ	148. ⓐ ⓑ ⓒ ⓓ ⓔ
11. ⓐ ⓑ ⓒ ⓓ ⓔ	57. ⓐ ⓑ ⓒ ⓓ ⓔ	103. ⓐ ⓑ ⓒ ⓓ ⓔ	149. ⓐ ⓑ ⓒ ⓓ ⓔ
12. ⓐ ⓑ ⓒ ⓓ ⓔ	58. ⓐ ⓑ ⓒ ⓓ ⓔ	104. ⓐ ⓑ ⓒ ⓓ ⓔ	150. ⓐ ⓑ ⓒ ⓓ ⓔ
13. ⓐ ⓑ ⓒ ⓓ ⓔ	59. ⓐ ⓑ ⓒ ⓓ ⓔ	105. ⓐ ⓑ ⓒ ⓓ ⓔ	151. ⓐ ⓑ ⓒ ⓓ ⓔ
14. ⓐ ⓑ ⓒ ⓓ ⓔ	60. ⓐ ⓑ ⓒ ⓓ ⓔ	106. ⓐ ⓑ ⓒ ⓓ ⓔ	152. ⓐ ⓑ ⓒ ⓓ ⓔ
15. ⓐ ⓑ ⓒ ⓓ ⓔ	61. ⓐ ⓑ ⓒ ⓓ ⓔ	107. ⓐ ⓑ ⓒ ⓓ ⓔ	153. ⓐ ⓑ ⓒ ⓓ ⓔ
16. ⓐ ⓑ ⓒ ⓓ ⓔ	62. ⓐ ⓑ ⓒ ⓓ ⓔ	108. ⓐ ⓑ ⓒ ⓓ ⓔ	154. ⓐ ⓑ ⓒ ⓓ ⓔ
17. ⓐ ⓑ ⓒ ⓓ ⓔ	63. ⓐ ⓑ ⓒ ⓓ ⓔ	109. ⓐ ⓑ ⓒ ⓓ ⓔ	155. ⓐ ⓑ ⓒ ⓓ ⓔ
18. ⓐ ⓑ ⓒ ⓓ ⓔ	64. ⓐ ⓑ ⓒ ⓓ ⓔ	110. ⓐ ⓑ ⓒ ⓓ ⓔ	156. ⓐ ⓑ ⓒ ⓓ ⓔ
19. ⓐ ⓑ ⓒ ⓓ ⓔ	65. ⓐ ⓑ ⓒ ⓓ ⓔ	111. ⓐ ⓑ ⓒ ⓓ ⓔ	157. ⓐ ⓑ ⓒ ⓓ ⓔ
20. ⓐ ⓑ ⓒ ⓓ ⓔ	66. ⓐ ⓑ ⓒ ⓓ ⓔ	112. ⓐ ⓑ ⓒ ⓓ ⓔ	158. ⓐ ⓑ ⓒ ⓓ ⓔ
21. ⓐ ⓑ ⓒ ⓓ ⓔ	67. ⓐ ⓑ ⓒ ⓓ ⓔ	113. ⓐ ⓑ ⓒ ⓓ ⓔ	159. ⓐ ⓑ ⓒ ⓓ ⓔ
22. ⓐ ⓑ ⓒ ⓓ ⓔ	68. ⓐ ⓑ ⓒ ⓓ ⓔ	114. ⓐ ⓑ ⓒ ⓓ ⓔ	160. ⓐ ⓑ ⓒ ⓓ ⓔ
23. ⓐ ⓑ ⓒ ⓓ ⓔ	69. ⓐ ⓑ ⓒ ⓓ ⓔ	115. ⓐ ⓑ ⓒ ⓓ ⓔ	161. ⓐ ⓑ ⓒ ⓓ ⓔ
24. ⓐ ⓑ ⓒ ⓓ ⓔ	70. ⓐ ⓑ ⓒ ⓓ ⓔ	116. ⓐ ⓑ ⓒ ⓓ ⓔ	162. ⓐ ⓑ ⓒ ⓓ ⓔ
25. ⓐ ⓑ ⓒ ⓓ ⓔ	71. ⓐ ⓑ ⓒ ⓓ ⓔ	117. ⓐ ⓑ ⓒ ⓓ ⓔ	163. ⓐ ⓑ ⓒ ⓓ ⓔ
26. ⓐ ⓑ ⓒ ⓓ ⓔ	72. ⓐ ⓑ ⓒ ⓓ ⓔ	118. ⓐ ⓑ ⓒ ⓓ ⓔ	164. ⓐ ⓑ ⓒ ⓓ ⓔ
27. ⓐ ⓑ ⓒ ⓓ ⓔ	73. ⓐ ⓑ ⓒ ⓓ ⓔ	119. ⓐ ⓑ ⓒ ⓓ ⓔ	165. ⓐ ⓑ ⓒ ⓓ ⓔ
28. ⓐ ⓑ ⓒ ⓓ ⓔ	74. ⓐ ⓑ ⓒ ⓓ ⓔ	120. ⓐ ⓑ ⓒ ⓓ ⓔ	166. ⓐ ⓑ ⓒ ⓓ ⓔ
29. ⓐ ⓑ ⓒ ⓓ ⓔ	75. ⓐ ⓑ ⓒ ⓓ ⓔ	121. ⓐ ⓑ ⓒ ⓓ ⓔ	167. ⓐ ⓑ ⓒ ⓓ ⓔ
30. ⓐ ⓑ ⓒ ⓓ ⓔ	76. ⓐ ⓑ ⓒ ⓓ ⓔ	122. ⓐ ⓑ ⓒ ⓓ ⓔ	168. ⓐ ⓑ ⓒ ⓓ ⓔ
31. ⓐ ⓑ ⓒ ⓓ ⓔ	77. ⓐ ⓑ ⓒ ⓓ ⓔ	123. ⓐ ⓑ ⓒ ⓓ ⓔ	169. ⓐ ⓑ ⓒ ⓓ ⓔ
32. ⓐ ⓑ ⓒ ⓓ ⓔ	78. ⓐ ⓑ ⓒ ⓓ ⓔ	124. ⓐ ⓑ ⓒ ⓓ ⓔ	170. ⓐ ⓑ ⓒ ⓓ ⓔ
33. ⓐ ⓑ ⓒ ⓓ ⓔ	79. ⓐ ⓑ ⓒ ⓓ ⓔ	125. ⓐ ⓑ ⓒ ⓓ ⓔ	171. ⓐ ⓑ ⓒ ⓓ ⓔ
34. ⓐ ⓑ ⓒ ⓓ ⓔ	80. ⓐ ⓑ ⓒ ⓓ ⓔ	126. ⓐ ⓑ ⓒ ⓓ ⓔ	172. ⓐ ⓑ ⓒ ⓓ ⓔ
35. ⓐ ⓑ ⓒ ⓓ ⓔ	81. ⓐ ⓑ ⓒ ⓓ ⓔ	127. ⓐ ⓑ ⓒ ⓓ ⓔ	173. ⓐ ⓑ ⓒ ⓓ ⓔ
36. ⓐ ⓑ ⓒ ⓓ ⓔ	82. ⓐ ⓑ ⓒ ⓓ ⓔ	128. ⓐ ⓑ ⓒ ⓓ ⓔ	174. ⓐ ⓑ ⓒ ⓓ ⓔ
37. ⓐ ⓑ ⓒ ⓓ ⓔ	83. ⓐ ⓑ ⓒ ⓓ ⓔ	129. ⓐ ⓑ ⓒ ⓓ ⓔ	175. ⓐ ⓑ ⓒ ⓓ ⓔ
38. ⓐ ⓑ ⓒ ⓓ ⓔ	84. ⓐ ⓑ ⓒ ⓓ ⓔ	130. ⓐ ⓑ ⓒ ⓓ ⓔ	176. ⓐ ⓑ ⓒ ⓓ ⓔ
39. ⓐ ⓑ ⓒ ⓓ ⓔ	85. ⓐ ⓑ ⓒ ⓓ ⓔ	131. ⓐ ⓑ ⓒ ⓓ ⓔ	177. ⓐ ⓑ ⓒ ⓓ ⓔ
40. ⓐ ⓑ ⓒ ⓓ ⓔ	86. ⓐ ⓑ ⓒ ⓓ ⓔ	132. ⓐ ⓑ ⓒ ⓓ ⓔ	178. ⓐ ⓑ ⓒ ⓓ ⓔ
41. ⓐ ⓑ ⓒ ⓓ ⓔ	87. ⓐ ⓑ ⓒ ⓓ ⓔ	133. ⓐ ⓑ ⓒ ⓓ ⓔ	179. ⓐ ⓑ ⓒ ⓓ ⓔ
42. ⓐ ⓑ ⓒ ⓓ ⓔ	88. ⓐ ⓑ ⓒ ⓓ ⓔ	134. ⓐ ⓑ ⓒ ⓓ ⓔ	180. ⓐ ⓑ ⓒ ⓓ ⓔ
43. ⓐ ⓑ ⓒ ⓓ ⓔ	89. ⓐ ⓑ ⓒ ⓓ ⓔ	135. ⓐ ⓑ ⓒ ⓓ ⓔ	181. ⓐ ⓑ ⓒ ⓓ ⓔ
44. ⓐ ⓑ ⓒ ⓓ ⓔ	90. ⓐ ⓑ ⓒ ⓓ ⓔ	136. ⓐ ⓑ ⓒ ⓓ ⓔ	182. ⓐ ⓑ ⓒ ⓓ ⓔ
45. ⓐ ⓑ ⓒ ⓓ ⓔ	91. ⓐ ⓑ ⓒ ⓓ ⓔ	137. ⓐ ⓑ ⓒ ⓓ ⓔ	183. ⓐ ⓑ ⓒ ⓓ ⓔ
46. ⓐ ⓑ ⓒ ⓓ ⓔ	92. ⓐ ⓑ ⓒ ⓓ ⓔ	138. ⓐ ⓑ ⓒ ⓓ ⓔ	184. ⓐ ⓑ ⓒ ⓓ ⓔ

Continued

185. (a) (b) (c) (d) (e)	231. (a) (b) (c) (d) (e)	277. (a) (b) (c) (d) (e)	323. (a) (b) (c) (d) (e)
186. (a) (b) (c) (d) (e)	232. (a) (b) (c) (d) (e)	278. (a) (b) (c) (d) (e)	324. (a) (b) (c) (d) (e)
187. (a) (b) (c) (d) (e)	233. (a) (b) (c) (d) (e)	279. (a) (b) (c) (d) (e)	325. (a) (b) (c) (d) (e)
188. (a) (b) (c) (d) (e)	234. (a) (b) (c) (d) (e)	280. (a) (b) (c) (d) (e)	326. (a) (b) (c) (d) (e)
189. (a) (b) (c) (d) (e)	235. (a) (b) (c) (d) (e)	281. (a) (b) (c) (d) (e)	327. (a) (b) (c) (d) (e)
190. (a) (b) (c) (d) (e)	236. (a) (b) (c) (d) (e)	282. (a) (b) (c) (d) (e)	328. (a) (b) (c) (d) (e)
191. (a) (b) (c) (d) (e)	237. (a) (b) (c) (d) (e)	283. (a) (b) (c) (d) (e)	329. (a) (b) (c) (d) (e)
192. (a) (b) (c) (d) (e)	238. (a) (b) (c) (d) (e)	284. (a) (b) (c) (d) (e)	330. (a) (b) (c) (d) (e)
193. (a) (b) (c) (d) (e)	239. (a) (b) (c) (d) (e)	285. (a) (b) (c) (d) (e)	331. (a) (b) (c) (d) (e)
194. (a) (b) (c) (d) (e)	240. (a) (b) (c) (d) (e)	286. (a) (b) (c) (d) (e)	332. (a) (b) (c) (d) (e)
195. (a) (b) (c) (d) (e)	241. (a) (b) (c) (d) (e)	287. (a) (b) (c) (d) (e)	333. (a) (b) (c) (d) (e)
196. (a) (b) (c) (d) (e)	242. (a) (b) (c) (d) (e)	288. (a) (b) (c) (d) (e)	334. (a) (b) (c) (d) (e)
197. (a) (b) (c) (d) (e)	243. (a) (b) (c) (d) (e)	289. (a) (b) (c) (d) (e)	335. (a) (b) (c) (d) (e)
198. (a) (b) (c) (d) (e)	244. (a) (b) (c) (d) (e)	290. (a) (b) (c) (d) (e)	336. (a) (b) (c) (d) (e)
199. (a) (b) (c) (d) (e)	245. (a) (b) (c) (d) (e)	291. (a) (b) (c) (d) (e)	337. (a) (b) (c) (d) (e)
200. (a) (b) (c) (d) (e)	246. (a) (b) (c) (d) (e)	292. (a) (b) (c) (d) (e)	338. (a) (b) (c) (d) (e)
201. (a) (b) (c) (d) (e)	247. (a) (b) (c) (d) (e)	293. (a) (b) (c) (d) (e)	339. (a) (b) (c) (d) (e)
202. (a) (b) (c) (d) (e)	248. (a) (b) (c) (d) (e)	294. (a) (b) (c) (d) (e)	340. (a) (b) (c) (d) (e)
203. (a) (b) (c) (d) (e)	249. (a) (b) (c) (d) (e)	295. (a) (b) (c) (d) (e)	341. (a) (b) (c) (d) (e)
204. (a) (b) (c) (d) (e)	250. (a) (b) (c) (d) (e)	296. (a) (b) (c) (d) (e)	342. (a) (b) (c) (d) (e)
205. (a) (b) (c) (d) (e)	251. (a) (b) (c) (d) (e)	297. (a) (b) (c) (d) (e)	343. (a) (b) (c) (d) (e)
206. (a) (b) (c) (d) (e)	252. (a) (b) (c) (d) (e)	298. (a) (b) (c) (d) (e)	344. (a) (b) (c) (d) (e)
207. (a) (b) (c) (d) (e)	253. (a) (b) (c) (d) (e)	299. (a) (b) (c) (d) (e)	345. (a) (b) (c) (d) (e)
208. (a) (b) (c) (d) (e)	254. (a) (b) (c) (d) (e)	300. (a) (b) (c) (d) (e)	346. (a) (b) (c) (d) (e)
209. (a) (b) (c) (d) (e)	255. (a) (b) (c) (d) (e)	301. (a) (b) (c) (d) (e)	347. (a) (b) (c) (d) (e)
210. (a) (b) (c) (d) (e)	256. (a) (b) (c) (d) (e)	302. (a) (b) (c) (d) (e)	348. (a) (b) (c) (d) (e)
211. (a) (b) (c) (d) (e)	257. (a) (b) (c) (d) (e)	303. (a) (b) (c) (d) (e)	349. (a) (b) (c) (d) (e)
212. (a) (b) (c) (d) (e)	258. (a) (b) (c) (d) (e)	304. (a) (b) (c) (d) (e)	350. (a) (b) (c) (d) (e)
213. (a) (b) (c) (d) (e)	259. (a) (b) (c) (d) (e)	305. (a) (b) (c) (d) (e)	351. (a) (b) (c) (d) (e)
214. (a) (b) (c) (d) (e)	260. (a) (b) (c) (d) (e)	306. (a) (b) (c) (d) (e)	352. (a) (b) (c) (d) (e)
215. (a) (b) (c) (d) (e)	261. (a) (b) (c) (d) (e)	307. (a) (b) (c) (d) (e)	353. (a) (b) (c) (d) (e)
216. (a) (b) (c) (d) (e)	262. (a) (b) (c) (d) (e)	308. (a) (b) (c) (d) (e)	354. (a) (b) (c) (d) (e)
217. (a) (b) (c) (d) (e)	263. (a) (b) (c) (d) (e)	309. (a) (b) (c) (d) (e)	355. (a) (b) (c) (d) (e)
218. (a) (b) (c) (d) (e)	264. (a) (b) (c) (d) (e)	310. (a) (b) (c) (d) (e)	356. (a) (b) (c) (d) (e)
219. (a) (b) (c) (d) (e)	265. (a) (b) (c) (d) (e)	311. (a) (b) (c) (d) (e)	357. (a) (b) (c) (d) (e)
220. (a) (b) (c) (d) (e)	266. (a) (b) (c) (d) (e)	312. (a) (b) (c) (d) (e)	358. (a) (b) (c) (d) (e)
221. (a) (b) (c) (d) (e)	267. (a) (b) (c) (d) (e)	313. (a) (b) (c) (d) (e)	359. (a) (b) (c) (d) (e)
222. (a) (b) (c) (d) (e)	268. (a) (b) (c) (d) (e)	314. (a) (b) (c) (d) (e)	360. (a) (b) (c) (d) (e)
223. (a) (b) (c) (d) (e)	269. (a) (b) (c) (d) (e)	315. (a) (b) (c) (d) (e)	361. (a) (b) (c) (d) (e)
224. (a) (b) (c) (d) (e)	270. (a) (b) (c) (d) (e)	316. (a) (b) (c) (d) (e)	362. (a) (b) (c) (d) (e)
225. (a) (b) (c) (d) (e)	271. (a) (b) (c) (d) (e)	317. (a) (b) (c) (d) (e)	363. (a) (b) (c) (d) (e)
226. (a) (b) (c) (d) (e)	272. (a) (b) (c) (d) (e)	318. (a) (b) (c) (d) (e)	364. (a) (b) (c) (d) (e)
227. (a) (b) (c) (d) (e)	273. (a) (b) (c) (d) (e)	319. (a) (b) (c) (d) (e)	365. (a) (b) (c) (d) (e)
228. (a) (b) (c) (d) (e)	274. (a) (b) (c) (d) (e)	320. (a) (b) (c) (d) (e)	366. (a) (b) (c) (d) (e)
229. (a) (b) (c) (d) (e)	275. (a) (b) (c) (d) (e)	321. (a) (b) (c) (d) (e)	367. (a) (b) (c) (d) (e)
230. (a) (b) (c) (d) (e)	276. (a) (b) (c) (d) (e)	322. (a) (b) (c) (d) (e)	368. (a) (b) (c) (d) (e)

Theriogenology

Fill in a circled letter to indicate your answer choice.

1. ⓐ ⓑ ⓒ ⓓ ⓔ	9. ⓐ ⓑ ⓒ ⓓ ⓔ	17. ⓐ ⓑ ⓒ ⓓ ⓔ	25. ⓐ ⓑ ⓒ ⓓ ⓔ
2. ⓐ ⓑ ⓒ ⓓ ⓔ	10. ⓐ ⓑ ⓒ ⓓ ⓔ	18. ⓐ ⓑ ⓒ ⓓ ⓔ	26. ⓐ ⓑ ⓒ ⓓ ⓔ
3. ⓐ ⓑ ⓒ ⓓ ⓔ	11. ⓐ ⓑ ⓒ ⓓ ⓔ	19. ⓐ ⓑ ⓒ ⓓ ⓔ	27. ⓐ ⓑ ⓒ ⓓ ⓔ
4. ⓐ ⓑ ⓒ ⓓ ⓔ	12. ⓐ ⓑ ⓒ ⓓ ⓔ	20. ⓐ ⓑ ⓒ ⓓ ⓔ	28. ⓐ ⓑ ⓒ ⓓ ⓔ
5. ⓐ ⓑ ⓒ ⓓ ⓔ	13. ⓐ ⓑ ⓒ ⓓ ⓔ	21. ⓐ ⓑ ⓒ ⓓ ⓔ	29. ⓐ ⓑ ⓒ ⓓ ⓔ
6. ⓐ ⓑ ⓒ ⓓ ⓔ	14. ⓐ ⓑ ⓒ ⓓ ⓔ	22. ⓐ ⓑ ⓒ ⓓ ⓔ	30. ⓐ ⓑ ⓒ ⓓ ⓔ
7. ⓐ ⓑ ⓒ ⓓ ⓔ	15. ⓐ ⓑ ⓒ ⓓ ⓔ	23. ⓐ ⓑ ⓒ ⓓ ⓔ	31. ⓐ ⓑ ⓒ ⓓ ⓔ
8. ⓐ ⓑ ⓒ ⓓ ⓔ	16. ⓐ ⓑ ⓒ ⓓ ⓔ	24. ⓐ ⓑ ⓒ ⓓ ⓔ	

369. ⓐ ⓑ ⓒ ⓓ ⓔ	375. ⓐ ⓑ ⓒ ⓓ ⓔ	381. ⓐ ⓑ ⓒ ⓓ ⓔ	387. ⓐ ⓑ ⓒ ⓓ ⓔ
370. ⓐ ⓑ ⓒ ⓓ ⓔ	376. ⓐ ⓑ ⓒ ⓓ ⓔ	382. ⓐ ⓑ ⓒ ⓓ ⓔ	388. ⓐ ⓑ ⓒ ⓓ ⓔ
371. ⓐ ⓑ ⓒ ⓓ ⓔ	377. ⓐ ⓑ ⓒ ⓓ ⓔ	383. ⓐ ⓑ ⓒ ⓓ ⓔ	
372. ⓐ ⓑ ⓒ ⓓ ⓔ	378. ⓐ ⓑ ⓒ ⓓ ⓔ	384. ⓐ ⓑ ⓒ ⓓ ⓔ	
373. ⓐ ⓑ ⓒ ⓓ ⓔ	379. ⓐ ⓑ ⓒ ⓓ ⓔ	385. ⓐ ⓑ ⓒ ⓓ ⓔ	
374. ⓐ ⓑ ⓒ ⓓ ⓔ	380. ⓐ ⓑ ⓒ ⓓ ⓔ	386. ⓐ ⓑ ⓒ ⓓ ⓔ	

Section 15

Theriogenology

Fill in a circled letter to indicate your answer choice.

1. ⓐ ⓑ ⓒ ⓓ ⓔ	9. ⓐ ⓑ ⓒ ⓓ ⓔ	17. ⓐ ⓑ ⓒ ⓓ ⓔ	25. ⓐ ⓑ ⓒ ⓓ ⓔ
2. ⓐ ⓑ ⓒ ⓓ ⓔ	10. ⓐ ⓑ ⓒ ⓓ ⓔ	18. ⓐ ⓑ ⓒ ⓓ ⓔ	26. ⓐ ⓑ ⓒ ⓓ ⓔ
3. ⓐ ⓑ ⓒ ⓓ ⓔ	11. ⓐ ⓑ ⓒ ⓓ ⓔ	19. ⓐ ⓑ ⓒ ⓓ ⓔ	27. ⓐ ⓑ ⓒ ⓓ ⓔ
4. ⓐ ⓑ ⓒ ⓓ ⓔ	12. ⓐ ⓑ ⓒ ⓓ ⓔ	20. ⓐ ⓑ ⓒ ⓓ ⓔ	28. ⓐ ⓑ ⓒ ⓓ ⓔ
5. ⓐ ⓑ ⓒ ⓓ ⓔ	13. ⓐ ⓑ ⓒ ⓓ ⓔ	21. ⓐ ⓑ ⓒ ⓓ ⓔ	29. ⓐ ⓑ ⓒ ⓓ ⓔ
6. ⓐ ⓑ ⓒ ⓓ ⓔ	14. ⓐ ⓑ ⓒ ⓓ ⓔ	22. ⓐ ⓑ ⓒ ⓓ ⓔ	30. ⓐ ⓑ ⓒ ⓓ ⓔ
7. ⓐ ⓑ ⓒ ⓓ ⓔ	15. ⓐ ⓑ ⓒ ⓓ ⓔ	23. ⓐ ⓑ ⓒ ⓓ ⓔ	31. ⓐ ⓑ ⓒ ⓓ ⓔ
8. ⓐ ⓑ ⓒ ⓓ ⓔ	16. ⓐ ⓑ ⓒ ⓓ ⓔ	24. ⓐ ⓑ ⓒ ⓓ ⓔ	

This page intentionally left blank.

Section 16

Urology and Nephrology

Fill in a circled letter to indicate your answer choice.

1. (a) (b) (c) (d) (e)	15. (a) (b) (c) (d) (e)	29. (a) (b) (c) (d) (e)	43. (a) (b) (c) (d) (e)
2. (a) (b) (c) (d) (e)	16. (a) (b) (c) (d) (e)	30. (a) (b) (c) (d) (e)	44. (a) (b) (c) (d) (e)
3. (a) (b) (c) (d) (e)	17. (a) (b) (c) (d) (e)	31. (a) (b) (c) (d) (e)	45. (a) (b) (c) (d) (e)
4. (a) (b) (c) (d) (e)	18. (a) (b) (c) (d) (e)	32. (a) (b) (c) (d) (e)	46. (a) (b) (c) (d) (e)
5. (a) (b) (c) (d) (e)	19. (a) (b) (c) (d) (e)	33. (a) (b) (c) (d) (e)	47. (a) (b) (c) (d) (e)
6. (a) (b) (c) (d) (e)	20. (a) (b) (c) (d) (e)	34. (a) (b) (c) (d) (e)	48. (a) (b) (c) (d) (e)
7. (a) (b) (c) (d) (e)	21. (a) (b) (c) (d) (e)	35. (a) (b) (c) (d) (e)	49. (a) (b) (c) (d) (e)
8. (a) (b) (c) (d) (e)	22. (a) (b) (c) (d) (e)	36. (a) (b) (c) (d) (e)	50. (a) (b) (c) (d) (e)
9. (a) (b) (c) (d) (e)	23. (a) (b) (c) (d) (e)	37. (a) (b) (c) (d) (e)	
10. (a) (b) (c) (d) (e)	24. (a) (b) (c) (d) (e)	38. (a) (b) (c) (d) (e)	
11. (a) (b) (c) (d) (e)	25. (a) (b) (c) (d) (e)	39. (a) (b) (c) (d) (e)	
12. (a) (b) (c) (d) (e)	26. (a) (b) (c) (d) (e)	40. (a) (b) (c) (d) (e)	
13. (a) (b) (c) (d) (e)	27. (a) (b) (c) (d) (e)	41. (a) (b) (c) (d) (e)	
14. (a) (b) (c) (d) (e)	28. (a) (b) (c) (d) (e)	42. (a) (b) (c) (d) (e)	

We Welcome Your Comments

We value your opinion and encourage you to send us your comments, flattering or critical. Please let us know if you detect any errors or ambiguous statements, or if there is any way in which we can make *Review Questions & Answers For Veterinary Boards* more useful to you.

Paul W. Pratt, VMD
Editor and Publisher

Return to:
American Veterinary Publications
5782 Thornwood Drive
Goleta, CA 93117

Detach, fold and seal with tape.
No postage needed in the United States.

FOLD HERE

BUSINESS REPLY MAIL
FIRST CLASS MAIL PERMIT NO. 770 SANTA BARBARA, CA

POSTAGE WILL BE PAID BY ADDRESSEE

American Veterinary Publications
5782 Thornwood Drive
Goleta, CA 93117-9942

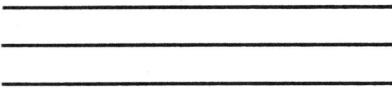

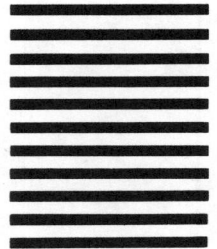

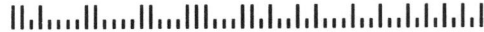

FOLD HERE

You may use this as a return
envelope. Detach at right and fold
as indicated. If a check is enclosed,
please tape the sides.

Review Questions & Answers For Veterinary Boards

Your key to success in

- State licensure examinations
- National Board Examination in Veterinary Medicine
- ECFVG certification examination
- ABVP examination

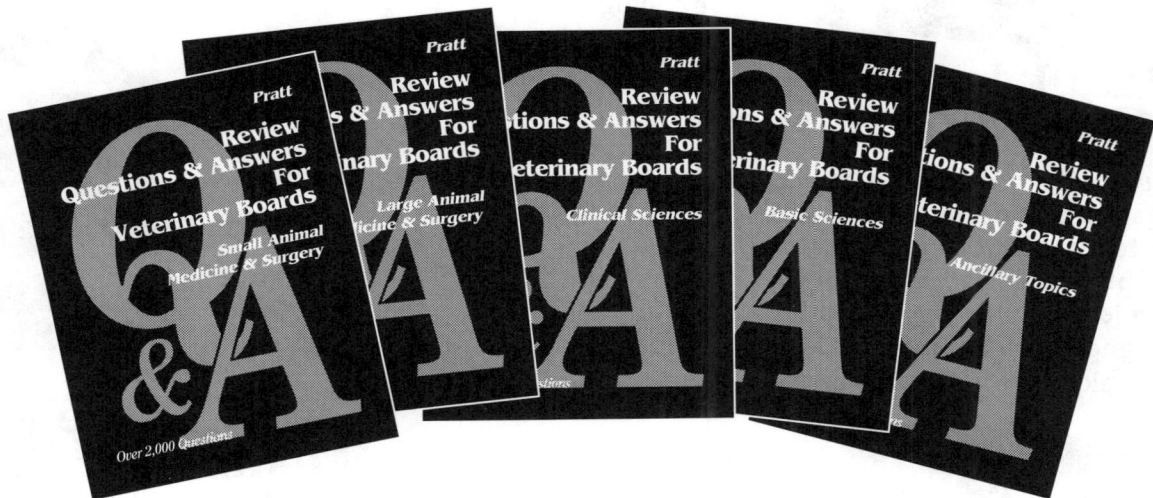

Recommended for

- *Veterinary students* preparing for final examinations
- *New graduates* preparing for licensure examinations
- *Practicing veterinarians* relocating to another state, or preparing for the American Board of Veterinary Practitioners examination
- *Non-practicing veterinarians* seeking licensure
- *Foreign graduates* preparing for ECFVG certification

√ *Over 9,400 multiple-choice questions, with accompanying answers.*

√ *Written by 112 veterinary educators, content-area specialists and experienced clinicians.*

√ *5 volumes cover nearly every aspect of veterinary medicine.*

Basic Sciences

Over 1,800 questions on Biochemistry, Embryology, Gross Anatomy, Microbiology, Microscopic Anatomy, Neuroanatomy, Parasitology, Pathology, Physiology, Terminology.

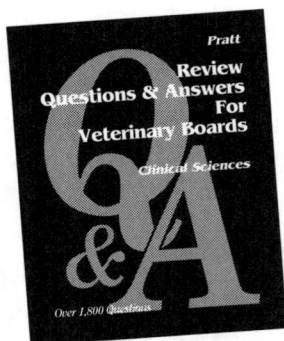

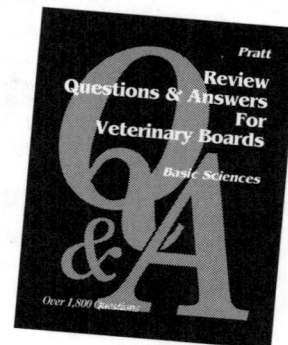

Clinical Sciences

Over 1,800 questions on Anesthesiology, Clinical Pathology, Cytology, Diagnostic Imaging, Hematology, Immunology, Nutrition, Pharmacology, Principles of Surgery, Theriogenology, Toxicology.

Small Animal Medicine & Surgery

Over 2,000 questions on medical and surgical diseases of dogs and cats. Disciplines include Anesthesiology, Cardiology, Clinical Pathology, Cytology, Dentistry, Dermatology, Hematology, Neurology, Oncology, Ophthalmology, Pharmacology, Preventive Medicine, Theriogenology, Urology/Nephrology. Questions on history taking, physical examination, diagnostic techniques, medical care, preoperative preparations, operative techniques, postoperative care, emergency care.

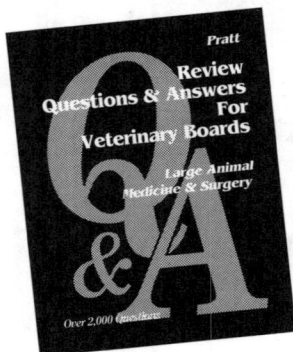

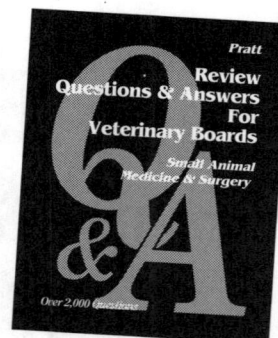

Large Animal Medicine & Surgery

Over 2,000 questions on medical and surgical diseases of horses, cattle, pigs, sheep and goats. Questions on history taking, physical examination, diagnostic techniques, medical care, preoperative preparations, operative techniques, postoperative care, emergency care.

Ancillary Topics

Over 1,800 questions on Behavior, Cage/Aviary Bird Medicine, Epidemiology, Ethics, Jurisprudence and Animal Welfare, Laboratory Animal Medicine, Necropsy, Physical Restraint, Poultry Medicine, Practice Management, Public Health and Regulatory Medicine, Zoo and Exotic Animal Medicine, Marine Mammal Medicine, Aquarium Fish.

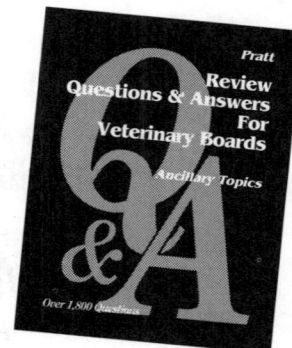

Order Form

Please send the following volumes of *Review Questions & Answers For Veterinary Boards:*

☐ ***Basic Sciences***
☐ ***Clinical Sciences***
☐ ***Small Animal Medicine & Surgery***
☐ ***Large Animal Medicine & Surgery***
☐ ***Ancillary Topics***

Any 1 volume:	$38 ($33 plus $5 shipping)
Any 2 volumes:	$69 ($64 plus $5 shipping)
Any 3 volumes:	$99 ($93 plus $6 shipping)
Any 4 volumes:	$127 ($120 plus $7 shipping)
All 5 volumes:	$152 ($145 plus $7 shipping)

(Non-U.S. orders, add $2 per volume.)

Payment or credit card information must be enclosed.
Sorry, we cannot bill you.

☐ Please charge my _____ VISA _____ MasterCard

Card # _____ Expiration _____

Signature _____

☐ Payment enclosed *(U.S. funds only) (California residents please add 7.25% sales tax)*

Name _____

Street _____

   ☐ Business   ☐ Residence

City/State/Zip _____

Telephone (_____) _____

For fastest service, call ***(805) 967-5988*** ***8 AM – 4 PM*** ***M-F, Pacific Time***	***Return to:*** ***American Veterinary Publications*** ***5782 Thornwood Dr.*** ***Goleta, CA 93117***

Detach order form, enclose payment, fold and seal with tape.
No postage needed if mailed in the United States.

FOLD HERE

NO POSTAGE
NECESSARY
IF MAILED
IN THE
UNITED STATES

BUSINESS REPLY MAIL
FIRST CLASS MAIL PERMIT NO. 770 SANTA BARBARA, CA

POSTAGE WILL BE PAID BY ADDRESSEE

American Veterinary Publications
5782 Thornwood Drive
Goleta, CA 93117-9942

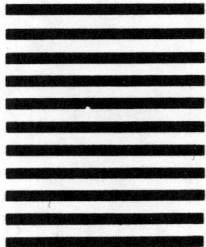

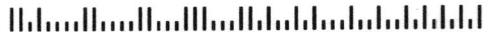

FOLD HERE

You may use this as a return
envelope. Detach at right and fold
as indicated. If a check is enclosed,
please tape the sides.